Systematic Musculoskeletal Examinations

Systematic Musculoskeletal Examinations

Developed at the UNIVERSITY OF IOWA

George V. Lawry, MD, FACP, FACR

Department of Internal Medicine
Division of Rheumatology
University of California, Irvine
Orange, California

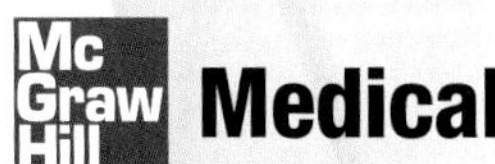

New York Chicago San Francisco Lisbon London Madrid Mexico City
Milan New Delhi Paris San Juan Seoul Singapore Sydney Toronto

The McGraw·Hill Companies

Systematic Musculoskeletal Examinations

1 2 3 4 5 6 7 8 9 10 CTP/CTP 15 14 13 12 11

ISBN 978- 0-07-174521-5
MHID 0-07-174521-1

This book was set in Berkeley Book by Cenveo Publisher Services.
The editors were Jim Shanahan and Karen G. Edmonson.
The production supervisor was Sherri Souffrance.
Project management was provided by Vastavikta Sharma, Cenveo Publisher Services.
The designer was Mary McKeon.
China Translation & Printing Ltd. was printer and binder.

This book is printed on acid-free paper.

Cataloging-in-Publication Data is on file with the Library of Congress.

To my wife, Judy, whose unending support made this labor of love possible.
Thank you for always being my biggest supporter.

Contents

Preface . . . . *ix*
Acknowledgments . . . . *xi*

Chapter 1 Introduction 1

Chapter 2 The Screening Musculoskeletal Examination 5

Chapter 3 The General Musculoskeletal Examination 25

Chapter 4 The Regional Musculoskeletal Examination of the Shoulder 87

Chapter 5 The Regional Musculoskeletal Examination of the Knee 131

Chapter 6 The Regional Musculoskeletal Examination of the Neck 183

Chapter 7 The Regional Musculoskeletal Examination of the Low Back 225

Suggested References 279

Index *281*

Preface

During my third year of Internal Medicine Residency, I encountered a patient with severe, long-standing psoriatic arthritis. After examining him (as best I could) and recording all his deformities (having only a vague idea of how to effectively describe them), I presented him to my attending. After patiently listening to me stumble through my findings, he asked "Geordie, was there any synovitis, any joint swelling?" I was dumbfounded. I had no idea. My Rheumatology fellowship followed shortly thereafter and for the first time I received excellent, systematic instruction in musculoskeletal physical examination techniques that I would build on for the rest of my life.

If you are reading this, you have a book in front of you. As such, it runs the risk of becoming "just another physical examination book." Physical examination techniques are not intellectual concepts but skills to be developed. As such, they require education of our eyes and hands, not just our brain. As with any activity involving our eyes and hands, increasing skill development only occurs with practice.

Systematic Musculoskeletal Examinations © is intended to bring a fresh approach to musculoskeletal examination instruction through the combined use of printed text (what you have before you), web-delivered self study programs (to parallel written material) with video instruction, graphics, animations and hotlinks to illustrative examples of key abnormalities plus additional web-delivered skill-building workshops (for supervised or independent hands-on practice).

My intention is that Systematic Musculoskeletal Examinations © meet three key requirements:

1) To develop a set of user-friendly, efficient, practical, and reproducibly effective basic examinations which can be readily integrated into the time demands of a busy outpatient practice.
2) To make effective use of on-demand, multimedia instruction to amplify and clarify static images on a printed page.
3) To provide learners a useful frame work for further skill development in musculoskeletal examination techniques for the rest of their careers.

It is my hope that this curriculum brings satisfaction and joy to you personally and greatly benefits patients with musculoskeletal problems who present for your assessment and management.

Geordie Lawry
July 2011

Acknowledgments

My earliest recollection of a "vocational calling" was my desire to become a train engine. My second, at the age of 5 or 6 (strongly influenced by my pediatrician, Dr. Harold Faber) was to become a doctor. I am forever grateful I pursued my second choice.

As a 4th year student on my sub-internship in Rheumatology, I met Dr. Mary Betty Stevens, a wonderful physician and teacher at Johns Hopkins. Dr. Stevens stunned all of us at the bedside by demonstrating the power of careful observation as the first step in physical diagnosis. There, during "Hand Rounds" at the Good Samaritan Hospital, my love and respect for Rheumatology and the musculoskeletal physical examination was born. That love and respect has continued to grow ever since.

In the summer of 1993 (just in time for the flood), I left private practice in California to join the Rheumatology faculty of the University of Iowa with a passion to help others discover the joy and power of the musculoskeletal physical examination. There I met some very special people who joined me to lend their considerable talents toward that end. This work is a product of our collaboration.

I am indebted to the members of the Division of Rheumatology, Department of Orthopaedics and Physical Therapy at the University of Iowa for suggestions regarding content and clarity, especially Drs. David Tearse, Brian Wolf, and Ernest Found and physical therapists Dennis Bewyer and Mike Shafer. Special thanks to students Ryan Carver, Hank Diggelman, Paul VanHeukelom, Amy Bois, and Emily Hall for their tireless (and thankfully lighthearted) submission of their bodies for filming, to the crew at Seashore Hall for our sessions in the studio, and especially to Brian Gilbert for the hours and hours we spent together in a small dark room editing. I am grateful for the invaluable assistance of Shawn Roach and Rich Tack, through whom many wonderful graphics and animations sprang to life.

Lastly, none of the pieces of this project could possibly have come together without the computer skills (and humor) of Phil Bailey and particularly the technological wizardry (and humor) of Greyson Purcell.

I am so grateful to all of you, not only for our shared destination, but especially for the joy of our journey together. I will never forget my 16 years at the University of Iowa!

George V. (Geordie) Lawry MD
Chief, Rheumatology Division
University of California, Irvine
July 2011

1

Introduction

I. WHY *SYSTEMATIC MUSCULOSKELETAL EXAMINATIONS*?

Musculoskeletal complaints and rheumatic diseases account for at least 15% to 20% of all visits to a physician. Because these problems are most often evaluated and treated by generalist physicians (internists, family physicians, and pediatricians) and physical therapists, it is essential for primary care providers to acquire an organized approach to the musculoskeletal examination.

Systematic Musculoskeletal Examinations is a three-part vertically integrated curriculum designed to teach essential and foundational skills of musculoskeletal physical assessment, particularly useful for students, residents in training, physical therapists, nurse practitioners, physician assistants, and practicing physicians.

I. **Screening musculoskeletal examination (SMSE):** a rapid assessment of structure and function
II. **General musculoskeletal examination (GMSE):** a comprehensive assessment of joint inflammation and arthritis
III. **Regional musculoskeletal examinations (RMSE):** focused assessments of structure and function combined with special testing of shoulder, knee, neck, and low back

The patient's history is the essential first step in all musculoskeletal diagnosis and directs the focus of an appropriate examination. The musculoskeletal physical examination is used to confirm or refute diagnostic hypotheses generated by a thoughtful history. Since the diagnosis of nearly all musculoskeletal problems depends on the demonstration of objective physical findings, the musculoskeletal examination has enormous importance. The patient's chief complaint and the clinical context will direct your initial choice of the screening, general, or regional musculoskeletal examinations.

II. SKILL BUILDING: MORE THAN "HEAD" KNOWLEDGE

The *screening musculoskeletal examination* (SMSE) is designed to provide an introduction to the physical assessment of musculoskeletal structures: joints, ligaments, tendons, muscles, and bones. It is intended to facilitate recognition of normal joint appearance and alignment, the spectrum of normal joint range of motion (ROM), and basic abnormalities of musculoskeletal structure and function. As a screening

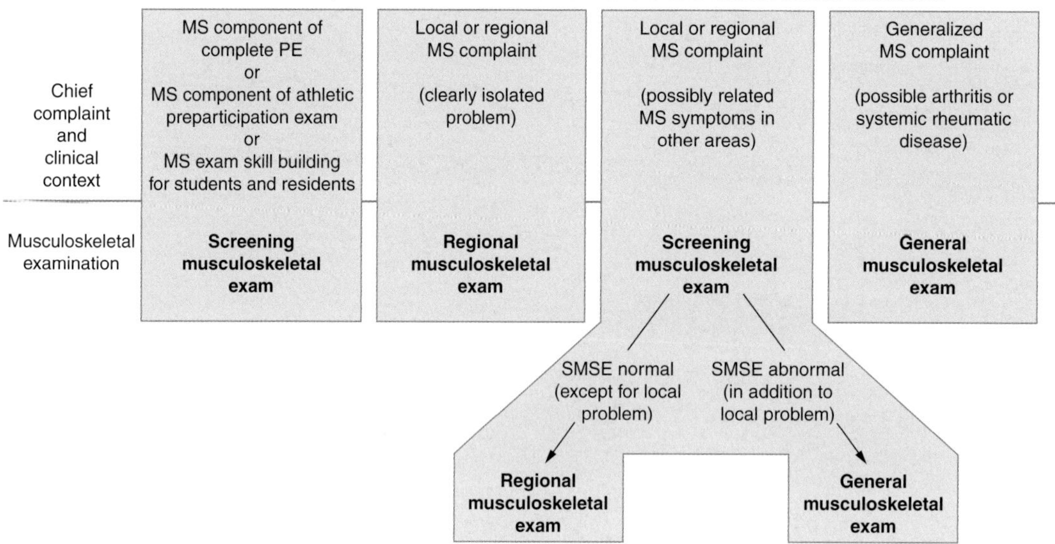

examination, it is brief yet systematic, is easily preformed, and increases examiner confidence that no important musculoskeletal findings have been overlooked. The SMSE is clinically useful as the musculoskeletal component of a complete physical examination (complete checkup) or athletic preparticipation physical examination. With practice, the SMSE can be performed in ~3 to 4 minutes.

The *general musculoskeletal examination* (GMSE) is designed to build directly on the sequence and techniques taught in the SMSE. It is intended to provide a comprehensive assessment of joint inflammation through the use of palpation and permits the recognition of joint swelling, essential to the physical diagnosis of arthritis. The skills involved require practice and careful attention to detail, but the proper techniques of joint palpation can be mastered on normal individuals. The GMSE is clinically useful as the initial examination in individuals with generalized musculoskeletal complaints (possible arthritis or connective tissue disease) and in individuals with apparently local or regional musculoskeletal complaints found to have additional abnormalities on the SMSE. With practice, the GMSE can be preformed in ~6 to 8 minutes.

The *regional musculoskeletal examinations* (RMSE) of the shoulder, knee, neck, and low back are designed to build on the sequences and techniques of the SMSE and GMSE. They are intended to provide comprehensive assessments of structure and function combined with special testing to permit evaluation of common, important musculoskeletal problems in the shoulder, knee, neck, and low back. The skills involved require practice and careful attention to technique; however, they can be learned and mastered on normal individuals. The RMSEs are clinically useful as the initial examination in individuals whose history clearly suggests a local or regional musculoskeletal problem of the shoulder, knee, neck, or low back. With practice, a systematic, efficient RMSE can be performed in ~3 to 4 minutes.

Since each of the three component examinations has specific diagnostic utility, this program encourages learners to develop the skills necessary to recognize which examination is most appropriate to a given chief complaint and clinical context.

III. VERTICALLY INTEGRATED LEARNING: MULTIPLE FEEDINGS OVER TIME

Presenting these examinations as a part of a carefully constructed, sequential curriculum offers learners exposure to core skills critical to clinical practice. Teaching builds systematically and sequentially at each successive level of training to maximize retention and utilization.

This three-part curriculum involves the following components:

Printed text for the SMSE, GMSE, and RMSE designed for individual learners and instructors for easy access and reference (this book).

Web-based tutorials for the SMSE, GMSE, and RMSE with content parallel to the text designed to provide individual learners an introduction, objectives, essential concepts, overview, and detailed presentation of component parts (utilizing narration, full-motion streaming video, graphics, etc) for each of the examinations. These tutorials are intended for self-study and preparation for hands-on, small group instructional workshops.

Web-based skill building workshops for the SMSE, GMSE, and RMSE intended for instruction of groups of learners. These workshops are designed to be pretimed, self-running, projectable programs for delivering hands-on instruction to groups of learners under faculty supervision. These workshops are intended to permit uniform and effective instruction while minimizing faculty time requirements for preparation and delivery.

Web-based instructor's manual for the SMSE, GMSE, and RMSE designed to provide a clear, easy-to-use resource for planning the timing and delivery of tutorial and workshop instruction.

Practical integration into existing curricula might include

Students (medical, osteopathic)

- **SMSE:** delivered during the first or second year as part of instruction in basic PE skills
- **GMSE:** delivered during the third year as part of internal medicine or family medicine core outpatient rotations
- **RMSE:** delivered during the third or fourth year as part of orthopedic or rheumatology core or elective rotations

Students (PA, ARNP, physical therapists, others)

- **SMSE, GMSE, and RMSE:** delivered during appropriate parts of 2- to 4-year curricula, prior to and during clinical contact with patients

Residents (internal medicine, family practice, pediatrics, and emergency medicine)

- SMSE and GMSE: delivered during the first 6 months of PGY 1 year
- RMSE: delivered during the first 6 to 12 months of PGY 1 year (review for trainees who received this instruction as students)

Rheumatology fellows

- SMSE and GMSE: delivered during orientation block RMSE: delivered during orientation or first 3 months of F1 year

Primary providers in practice (MD, DO, PA, ARNP, PT)

SMSE, GMSE, and RMSE: delivered in hands-on continuing medical education (CME) workshops (new instruction for many providers and review for others)

Using selected students, residents, and fellows as facilitators to work with faculty enhances vertically integrated education, reinforces the importance of physical examination skill development, and reduces direct faculty time requirements.

IV. ACCURATE DIAGNOSIS: STARTING POINT OF EFFECTIVE PATIENT CARE

Teaching practical and foundational musculoskeletal examination skills may have an impact on the interest in musculoskeletal problems among trainees, may increase confidence levels of practicing primary physicians, and, most importantly, greatly enhance the quality of care for all patients with musculoskeletal problems. The material presented here was designed to be learner-friendly, systematic, and, most of all practical, efficient, and clinically relevant.

Proficiency with all three components of this curriculum (screening, general, and regional examinations) may greatly increase physical diagnostic skills in evaluating patients with musculoskeletal problems. Indeed, it is nearly impossible to diagnose most musculoskeletal problems and rheumatic diseases in the absence of objective physical signs. Increasing powers of observation and techniques of palpation and manipulation will greatly enhance skills of pattern recognition in patients with musculoskeletal problems, directing differential diagnosis, focusing the choice of additional testing, and reducing reliance on costly (and frequently unnecessary) diagnostic laboratory and imaging studies.

V. DISCOVERY AND REDISCOVERY: THE FUN OF PHYSICAL EXAMINATION

Furthermore, improving physical diagnostic skills may significantly increase the pleasure and satisfaction in the practice of clinical medicine while caring for patients with musculoskeletal problems. It's time to rediscover the joy of this essential part of medicine!

2

The Screening Musculoskeletal Examination

INTRODUCTION

The *screening musculoskeletal examination* (SMSE) is designed to provide an introduction to the physical assessment of musculoskeletal structures and will enable you to recognize normal joint appearance and alignment, the spectrum of normal joint range of motion and will help you recognize basic abnormalities of musculoskeletal structure and function. As a screening examination, it is brief yet systematic, is easily performed, and increases examiner confidence that no important musculoskeletal findings have been overlooked. With practice, the SMSE can be performed in ~ 3 to 4 minutes. Furthermore, the screening examination provides the foundation for learning a more complete examination, the GMSE, at a later point in your training.

CLINICAL UTILITY

The SMSE is clinically useful as the musculoskeletal component of an *athletic preparticipation physical examination, as part of a complete physical examination, or as the initial examination in an individual with a local or regional musculoskeletal complaint with possible musculoskeletal symptoms in other sites.*

OBJECTIVES

This instructional program will emphasize *five categories of abnormality* and will define the important role of *symmetry* in assessing the musculoskeletal system. It will outline the principles of *active and passive range of motion* and illustrate the *neutral position* and the principal *direction of motion* for most peripheral joints and the axial spine. Most importantly, it will prepare you to perform a fully integrated SMSE.

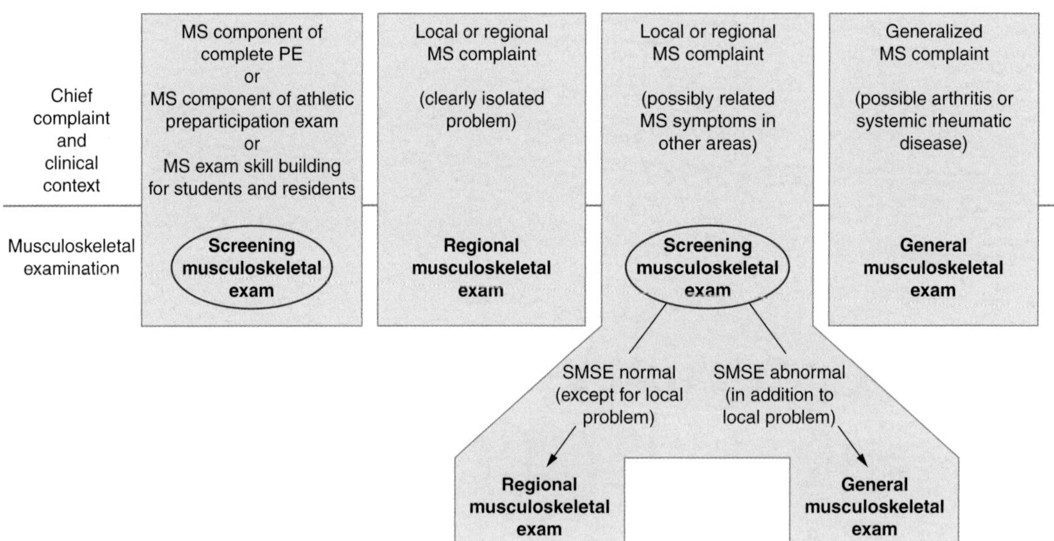

ESSENTIAL CONCEPTS

Categories of Abnormality The five basic categories of abnormality you will assess with the screening examination include

1. Deformity
2. Visible swelling
3. Muscle atrophy
4. Abnormalities of range of motion
5. Abnormalities of gait

Symmetry A central axial spine, paired peripheral joints, and symmetrical musculature provide the basis for essential side-to-side comparison during the musculoskeletal examination. Recognizing asymmetry is extremely important and may provide your first clue in diagnosing an abnormality.

Active and Passive Range of Motion Both active and passive range of motion are used to assess joint function. Active range of motion is patient-initiated movement of the joint. Active range of motion tests integrated function and requires intact innervation, muscle and tendon function, as well as joint mobility (Fig. 2–1A).

Passive range of motion is examiner-initiated movement of the joint, and tests only joint mobility. The combined use of passive as well as active range of motion minimizes the need for patient instruction and thus maximizes the speed and efficiency of the examination (Fig. 2–1B).

Whenever joint movement is anticipated to be painful, it is best to first observe active range of motion (patient-initiated movement) to appreciate the degree of pain and dysfunction before gently attempting passive range of motion (examiner-initiated manipulation).

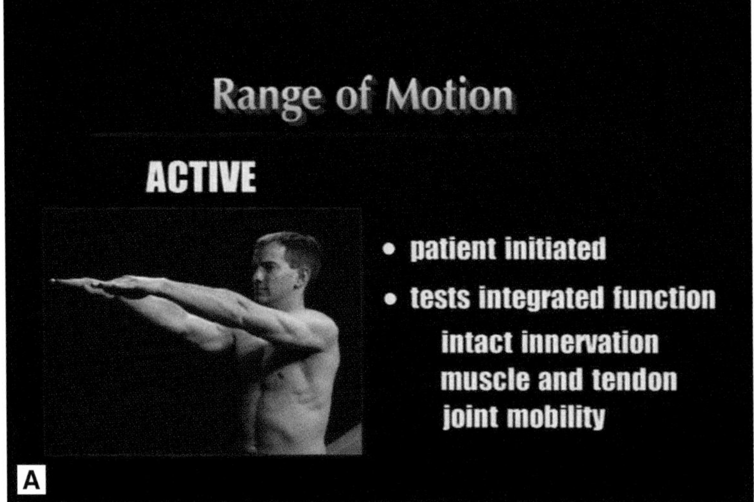

Fig. 2–1

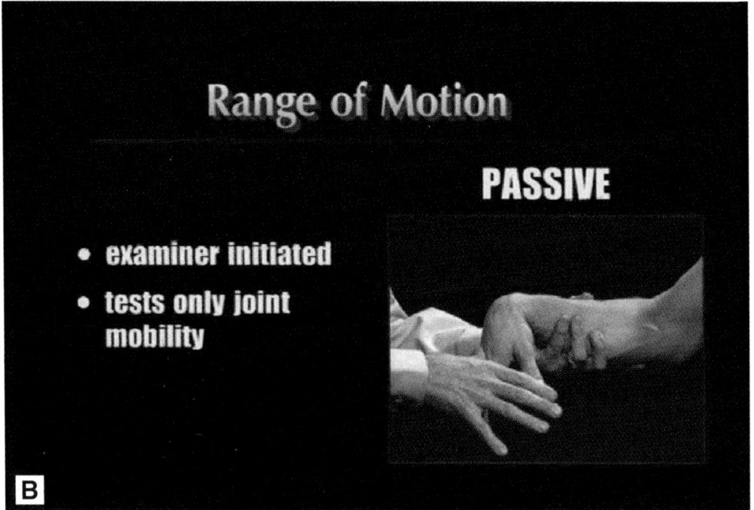

Fig. 2–1

Neutral Position, Plane, and Direction of Motion The neutral position for each joint is the anatomical position, defined as standing erect with face, palms, and feet directed forward and arms at the side (Fig. 2–2). Flexion, extension, abduction, and adduction are defined by the plane and direction of movement away from or toward this neutral position (Fig. 2–3).

With this background, you are now ready to learn the integrated SMSE.

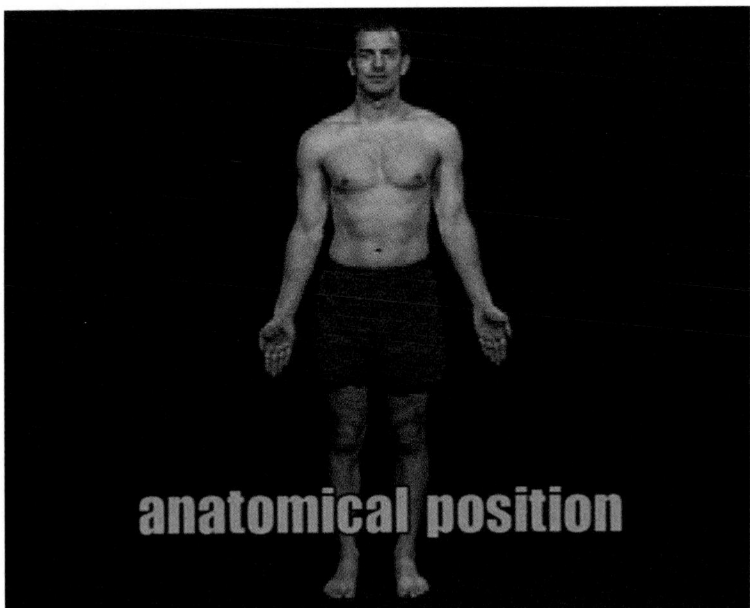
anatomical position

Fig. 2–2

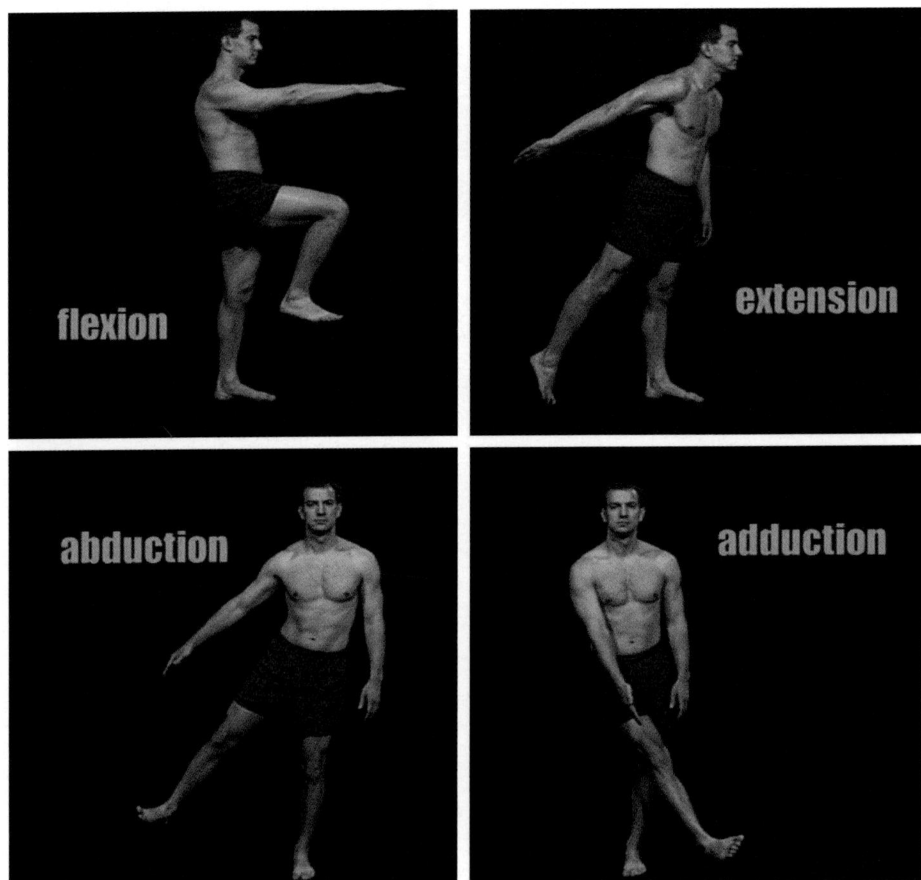
flexion
extension
abduction
adduction

Fig. 2–3

THE EXAMINATION, OVERVIEW

With the patient seated comfortably and appropriately undressed, begin the examination of the **upper extremities**. Inspect for *deformity*, *visible swelling*, *muscle atrophy*, or *abnormal joint range of motion*.

Instruct the patient to open both hands. Observe the dorsal and palmar surfaces and the intrinsic muscles. Assess finger extension by asking the patient to spread the fingers. Next, assess finger flexion by having the patient make a fist. Inspect both fists during supination and pronation of the forearms. Inspect, then extend and flex the wrists. Inspect, then flex and extend the elbows. Inspect the deltoid muscles. Observe shoulder flexion by asking the patient to bring the arms forward and raise them overhead. Observe shoulder internal rotation while having the patient place both hands behind the back. Then assess shoulder external rotation by asking the patient to place both hands behind the head.

Now begin the examination of the **lower extremities**. Inspect for *deformity*, *visible swelling*, *muscle atrophy*, or *abnormal joint range of motion*.

Ask the patient to lie down. Assess hip flexion by grasping the heel and moving the thigh up toward the chest. Return the thigh to a position perpendicular to examination table while holding the shin parallel to the table. Now, move the ankle medially to assess hip external rotation. Move the ankle laterally to assess hip internal rotation. Return the leg to the table. Observe the quadriceps muscles. Inspect the knees. Flex and extend each knee.

Inspect the ankles. Dorsiflex and plantarflex the ankles. Inspect the midfoot and toes. Inspect the plantar surface of both feet.

Now ask the patient to stand. Observe the patient from behind while weight bearing. Note the alignment of the knees. Inspect the calf muscles. Note the alignment of the heels and feet.

Now with the patient standing, begin the examination of the **spine**. Inspect for *deformity* or *abnormal range of motion*. Inspect the cervical spine. Assess neck flexion by instructing the patient to place his chin on the chest. Assess neck extension by asking the patient to look up at the ceiling. Observe right and left rotation by asking the patient to place his chin on each shoulder. Assess lateral flexion (or lateral bending) by asking the patient to incline his ear toward each shoulder. Now, while observing the patient from behind, inspect the thoracic and lumbar spine. Assess thoracolumbar lateral flexion (or lateral bending) by asking the patient to bend to the right and to the left. Observe lumbar flexion by instructing the patient to bend forward at the waist. Assess lumbar extension by having the patient bend backward.

Finally, observe the patient's **gait**. Check for any *limp*, *uneven rhythm*, or *asymmetry*. Observe the swing and stance phases.

THE EXAMINATION, COMPONENT PARTS

Having described the integrated SMSE, lets now take a careful look at each component part.

To begin the examination, the patient should be comfortable, yet appropriately undressed. This usually includes undershorts with/without a gown in men and underwear with a gown in women. Adjusting the gown, whenever necessary, to permit full inspection of each region is very important.

Failure to visualize musculoskeletal structures during the examination because of inadequate exposure represents one of the most common errors made by examiners at all levels of training.

Begin the examination with the upper extremities. Instruct the patient to open both hands while you inspect the dorsal surface for any obvious deformity or visible swelling. Now inspect the palmar surface and note any atrophy of the thenar or hypothenar eminences. Turn the hands over once again with the palms down. Assess finger extension by asking the patient to spread the fingers. Note whether each finger's DIP (distal interphalangeal), PIP (proximal interphalangeal), and MCP (metacarpophalangeal) joints extend fully (Figs. 2–4 through 2–6). Extension of the MCP joints beyond neutral is normal. Assess finger flexion by observing the patient make a fist with each hand. Inspect both the dorsal and palmar

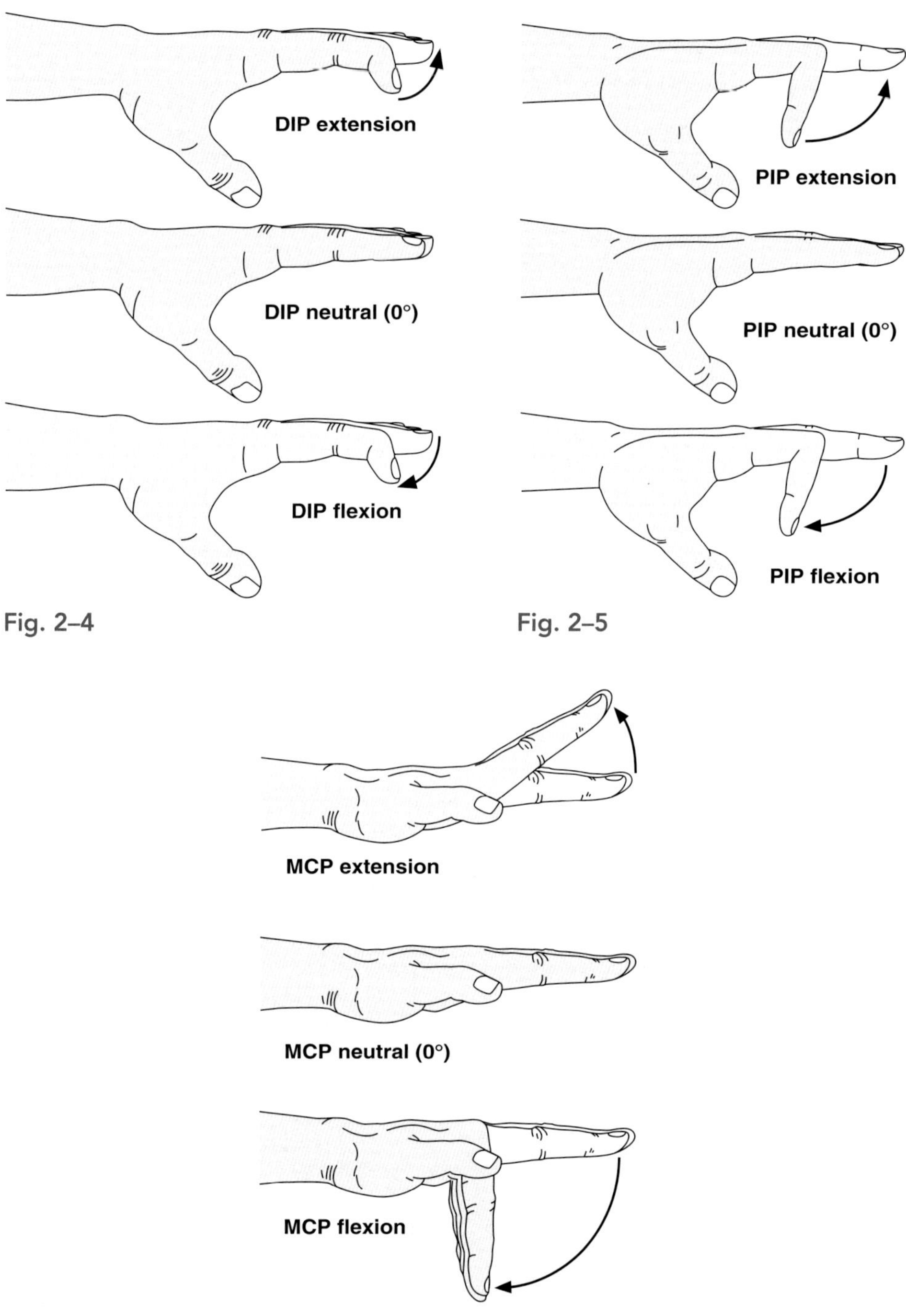

Fig. 2–4

Fig. 2–5

Fig. 2–6

surfaces of each fist to visualize the adequacy of finger flexion (Fig. 2–7A,B). Making a fist is a complex maneuver, involving nearly maximal flexion of all DIP, PIP, and MCP joints (see Figs. 2–4 through 2–6). This permits the tips of digits 2 to 5 to be buried in the palm at the level of the distal palmar crease. Thumb opposition, with partial thumb MCP and IP (interphalangeal) joint flexion, completes the normal fist (Fig. 2–7B). Next, inspect the wrists looking for deformity or visible swelling. Ask the patient to turn both hands over with the palms up. This maneuver permits assessment of both forearm supination and visual inspection of the wrist flexor surface. Then, ask the patient to turn both palms face down. This maneuver permits simultaneous assessment of forearm pronation and visual inspection of the wrist extensor surface. Now, extend and flex each wrist (Fig. 2–8). Take the patient's hand in your dominant

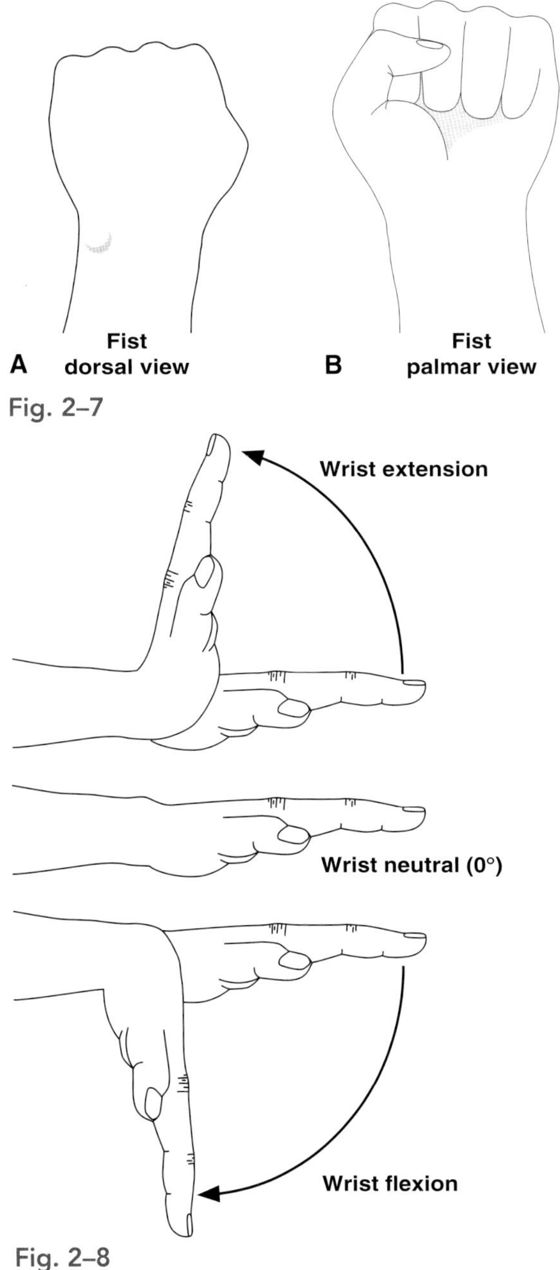

Fig. 2–7

Fig. 2–8

hand, as though you were going to "kiss the hand" (Fig.2–9). This allows you to comfortably move the patient's wrist into full extension using pressure with your index finger against the distal palm (at the level of the metacarpal heads), avoiding unnecessarily squeezing the patient's fingers (Fig. 2–10A). Then, downward pressure with your thumb on the patient's second or third metacarpal allows you to bring the wrist gently into full flexion (Fig. 2–10B). Full wrist extension and flexion should be symmetrical and bring the hand nearly perpendicular to the forearm on each side.

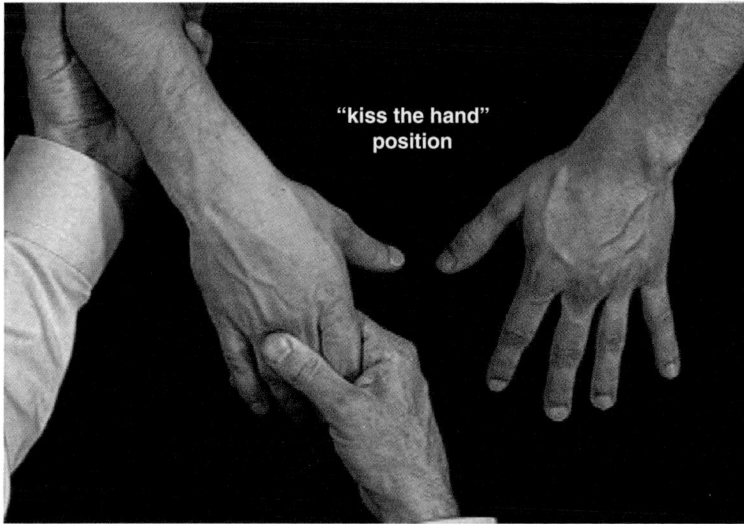

Fig. 2–9

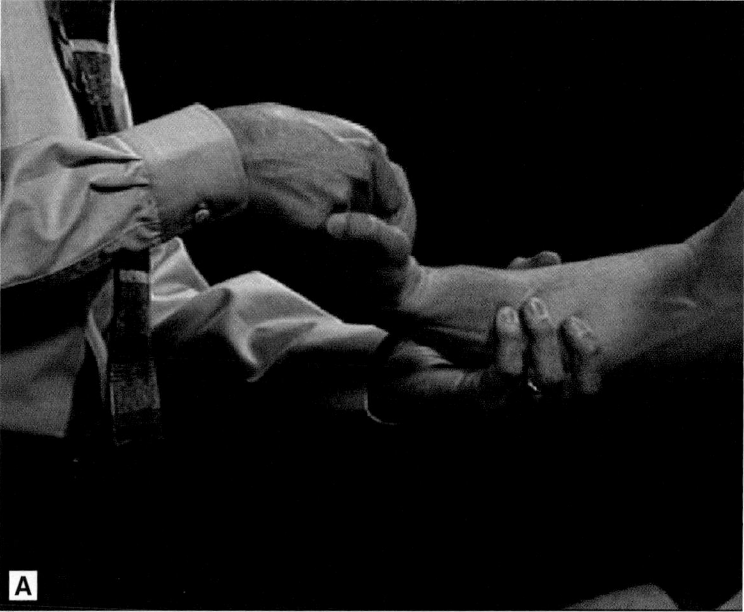

Fig. 2–10

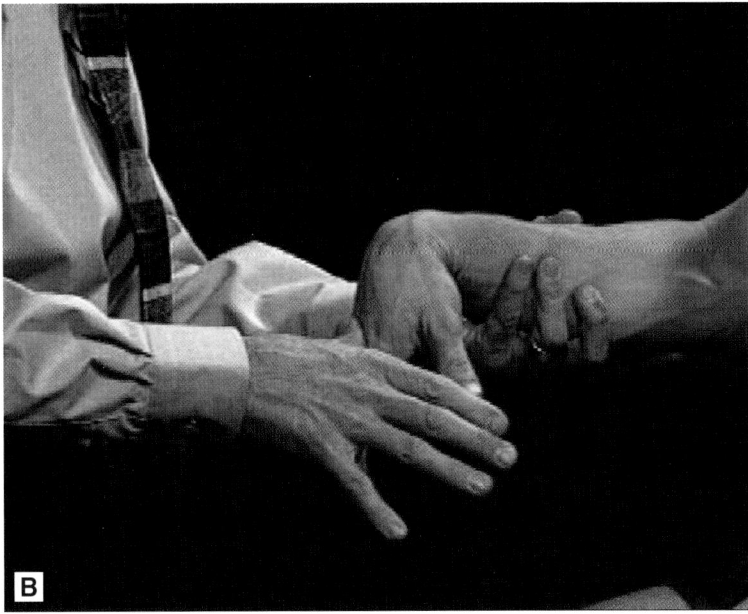

Fig. 2–10

Next, inspect the elbows looking for visible swelling or deformity. Flex and extend the elbows (Fig. 2–11). Full elbow flexion places the proximal forearm against the distal biceps. Full elbow extension returns the joint to the outstretched anatomical position. Place your hand under the olecranon to assist you in detecting a flexion contracture (deficit in full extension).

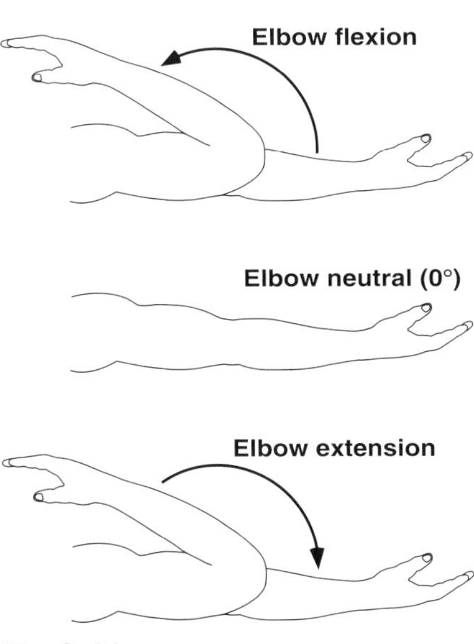

Fig. 2–11

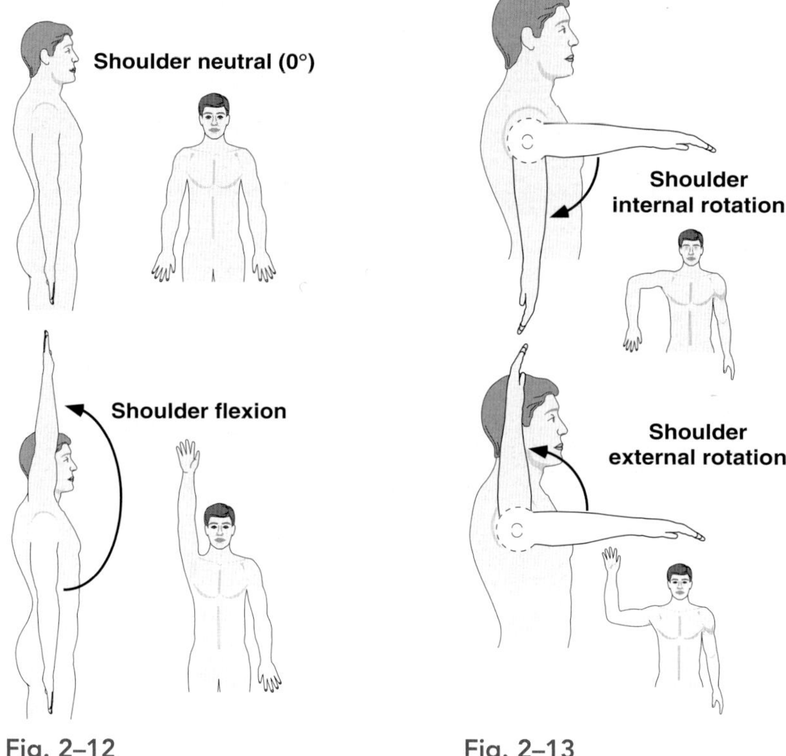

Fig. 2–12

Fig. 2–13

Next, observe the shoulders anteriorly. Inspect the deltoid and pectoral muscles for bulk and symmetry, noting any muscle atrophy. (When testing shoulder function, instructing the patient while demonstrating yourself speeds comprehension and enhances cooperation.)

Assess shoulder flexion (Fig. 2–12) by asking the patient to bring the arms forward and raise them overhead. Normal shoulder flexion brings the arms almost vertical. Observe shoulder internal rotation (Fig. 2–13) by asking the patient to place both hands behind the back (this action also involves some abduction, but the dominant movement is internal rotation).

Next, observe external rotation (see Fig. 2–13) by asking the patient to place both hands behind the head (this action also involves abduction, but primarily requires external rotation). To properly demonstrate external rotation, both arms must be in the plane of the body with the elbows pointed laterally (otherwise, placing both hands behind the head may demonstrate only partial shoulder flexion).

Now, ask the patient to lie supine for the examination of the **lower extremities**.

Assess hip flexion. Grasp the patient's foot with your right hand and position the patient's heel in your palm (Fig. 2–14). This allows comfortable control of the extremity without the need to reposition your grip during the examination. Move the thigh up toward the thorax (Fig. 2–15A). Normal hip flexion brings the anterior thigh nearly to the chest. Next, return the hip to 90° of flexion. Keeping the thigh perpendicular to the examining table while testing hip rotation permits easy visualization of the arcs of movement during external and internal rotation (Fig. 2–15B). Moving the ankle medially assesses hip external rotation. Moving the ankle laterally assesses hip internal rotation. Apply firm but gentle pressure

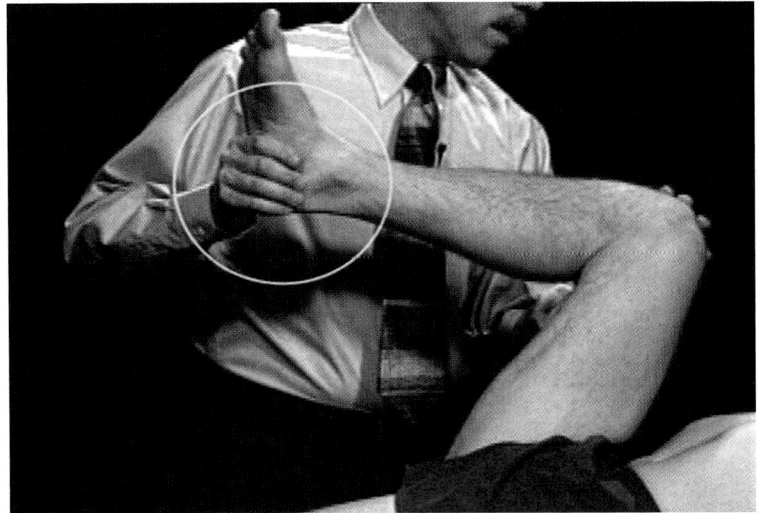

Fig. 2–14

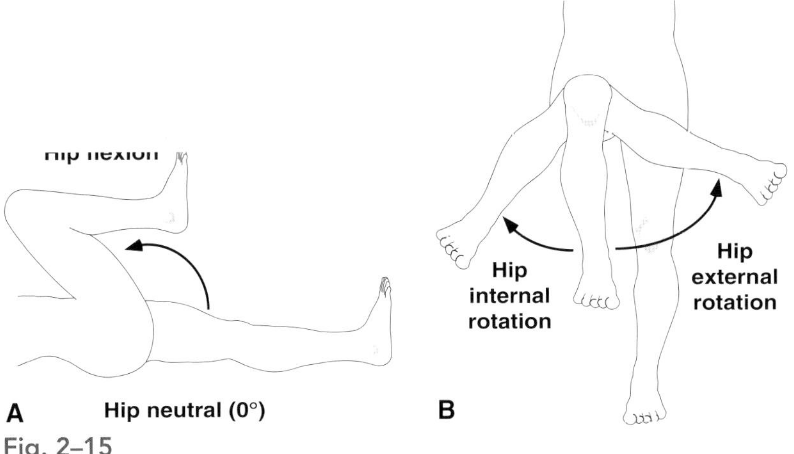

Fig. 2–15

to adequately assess range of motion. Watch the patient's face while performing hip rotation. A change in facial expression may be your first indication that hip range of motion is painful. (*Note: In patients with total hip replacements, be cautious in assessing hip range of motion; flexion, adduction, and internal rotation may dislocate the femoral component.*)

You should provide and adjust a cover sheet during the hip examination to minimize patient exposure (Fig. 2–16).

Begin the examination of the knees by inspecting the quadriceps muscles for bulk and symmetry, noting any muscle atrophy. Next, inspect the knees for any obvious deformity or visible swelling. Flex and extend the knees (Fig. 2–17). Full knee flexion brings the calf muscle against the posterior thigh. Full knee extension returns the joint to the outstretched anatomical position (0 degrees). While holding the leg off the table, look carefully for a flexion contracture (deficit in full extension).

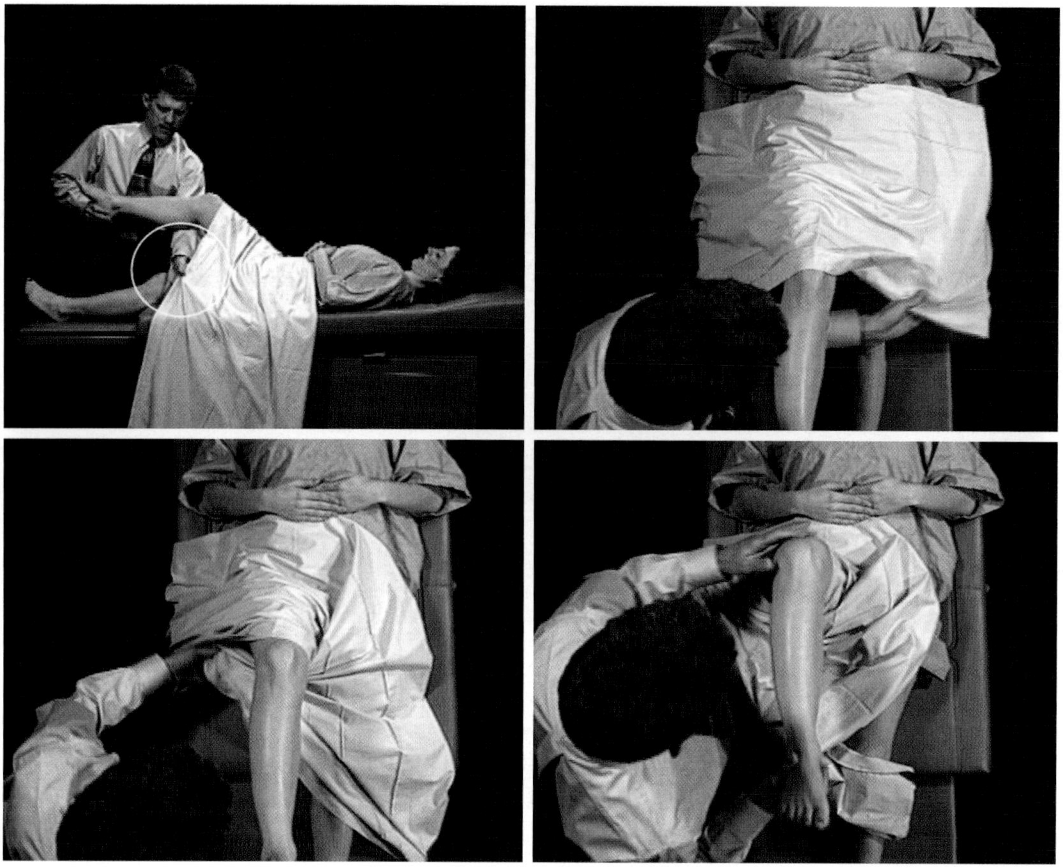

Fig. 2–16

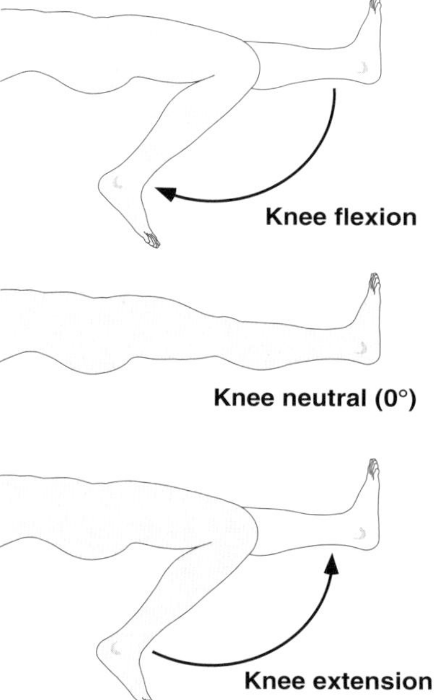

Fig. 2–17

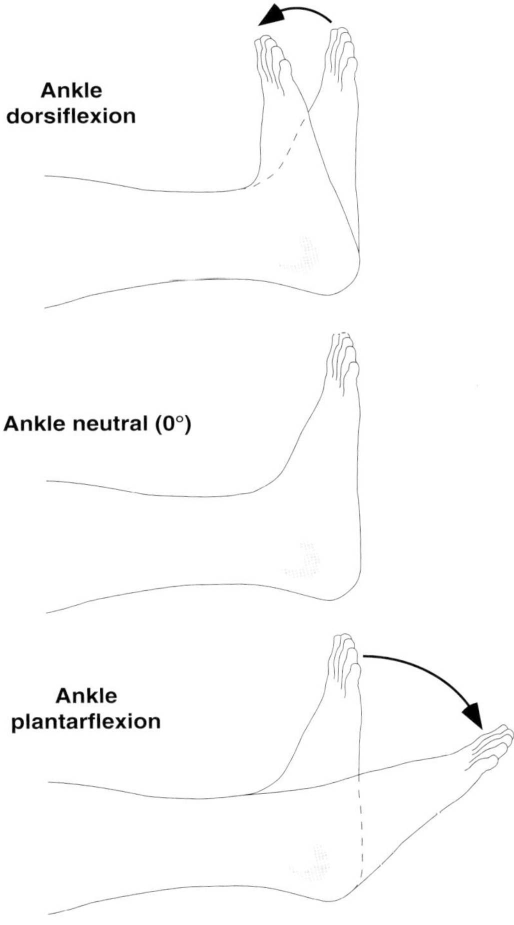

Fig. 2–18

Now inspect the ankles for any obvious deformity or visible swelling. Dorsiflex and plantarflex the ankles (Fig. 2–18). Ankle dorsiflexion brings the foot up in a cephalad direction. Ankle plantarflexion brings the foot down in a plantar direction.

Now, inspect the midfoot and toes for any obvious deformity or visual swelling. Next, inspect the plantar surface of each foot. Note any calluses.

Continue your examination of the **lower extremities** by asking the patient to stand. While observing from behind, note the alignment of the knees during weight bearing (Fig. 2–19).

Inspect the calf muscles for bulk and symmetry noting any muscle atrophy.

Note the alignment of the heels and feet. Inspection of the heels should reveal symmetrical, vertical alignment. Observation of the feet from behind should normally permit visualization of the lateral two or three toes.

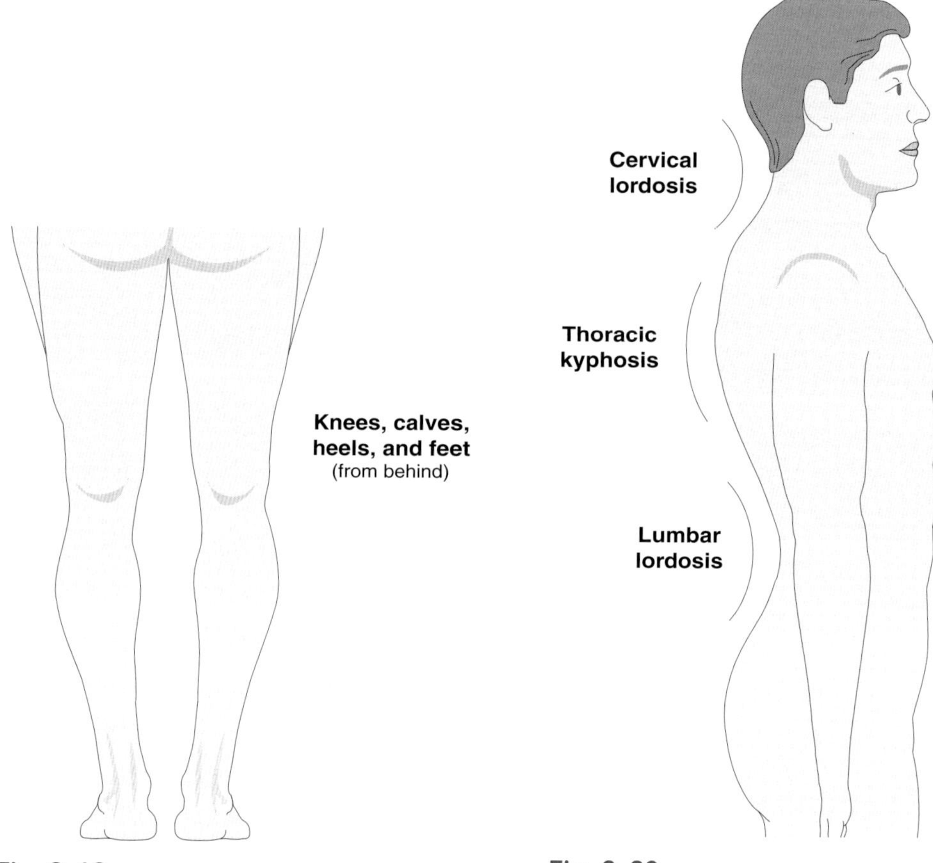

Fig. 2–19

Fig. 2–20

Now, with the patient standing, examine the **spine** (Fig. 2–20).

Observe the alignment of the head and neck. Note any abnormality or deformity.

Assess neck flexion by asking the patient to touch his chin to the chest. (Fig. 2–21A). Assess neck extension by asking the patient to look up at the ceiling (Fig. 2–21B). Observe right and left rotation

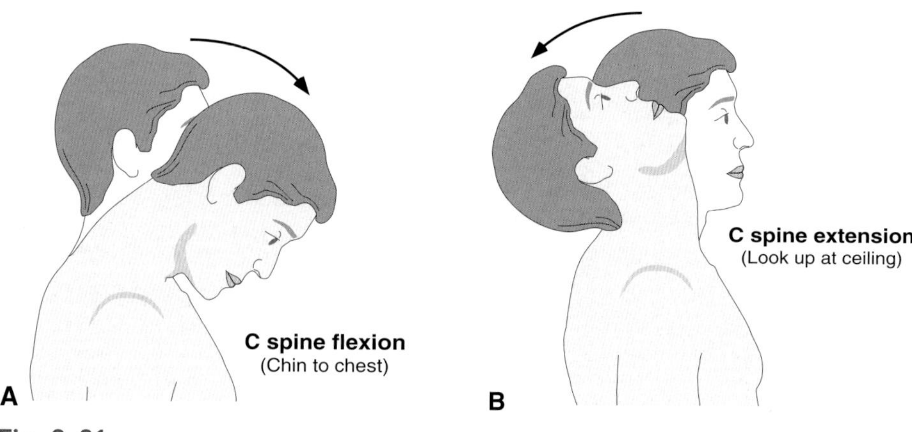

Fig. 2–21

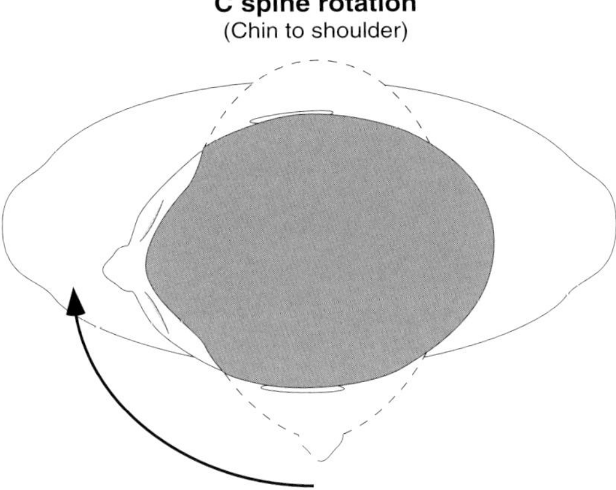

Fig. 2–22

by asking the patient to place his chin on each shoulder (Fig. 2–22). Assess lateral flexion (or lateral bending) by asking the patient to incline his ear toward each shoulder (Fig. 2–23).

Now while observing the patient from behind, inspect the thoracolumbar spine. Note any resting asymmetry or deformity and inspect for the normal resting lumbar lordosis (see Fig. 2–20).

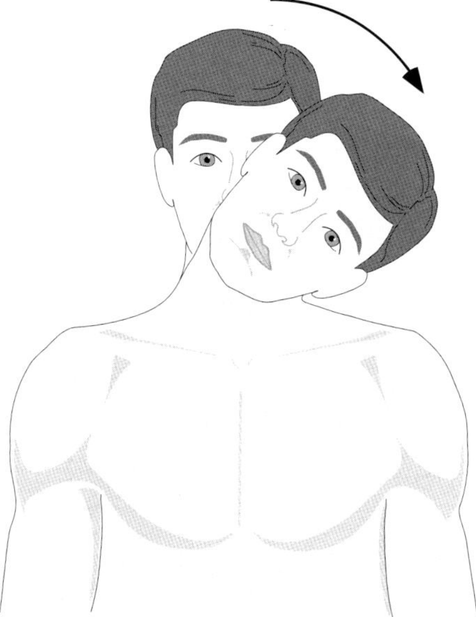

Fig. 2–23

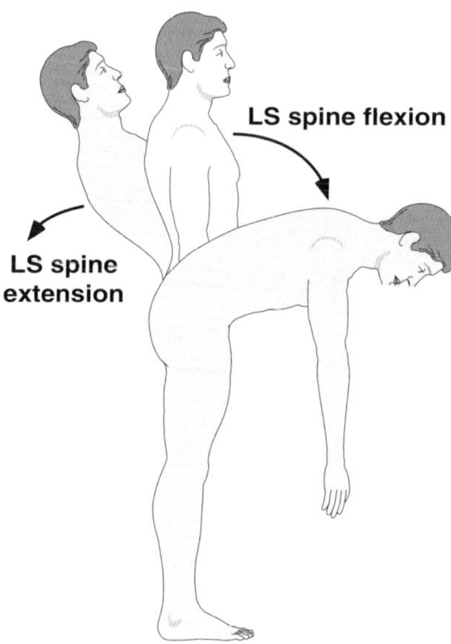

Fig. 2–24

Observe lumbar flexion by instructing the patient to bend forward at the waist and touch the toes (Fig. 2–24). Normal lumbar flexion should involve progressive reversal of the lumbar curvature from lumbar lordosis in the standing position, to flattening of the lordosis in midflexion, to slight lumbar kyphosis at the end of full flexion (Fig. 2–25). Normal lumbar flexion brings the wrists to approximately

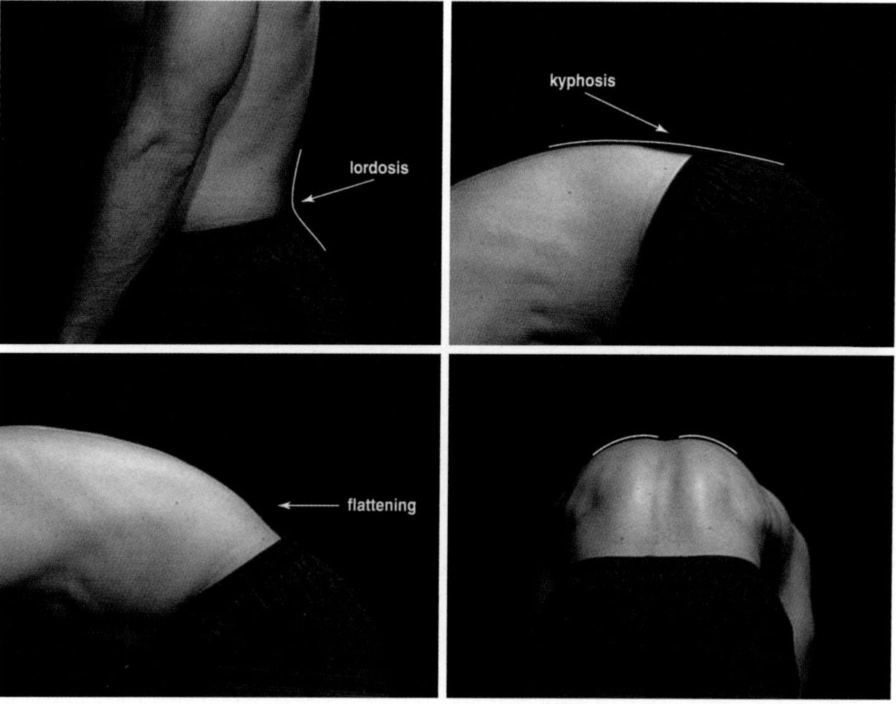

Fig. 2–25

the level of the knees (while hip flexion permits the additional movement involved in toe touching). Observing the patient from behind in full lumbar flexion allows you to inspect for evidence of scoliosis by noting any asymmetry or prominence of the posterior rib cage on either side (see Fig. 2–25).

Assess lumbar extension by asking the patient to bend backward. Simultaneously supporting the low back permits you to help the patient into full extension (see Fig. 2–24).

Next, assess lumbar lateral flexion, (lateral bending) by asking the patient to bend to the right and to the left. Normally, the maneuver brings the fingertips to approximately the level of the knees on each side (Fig. 2–26).

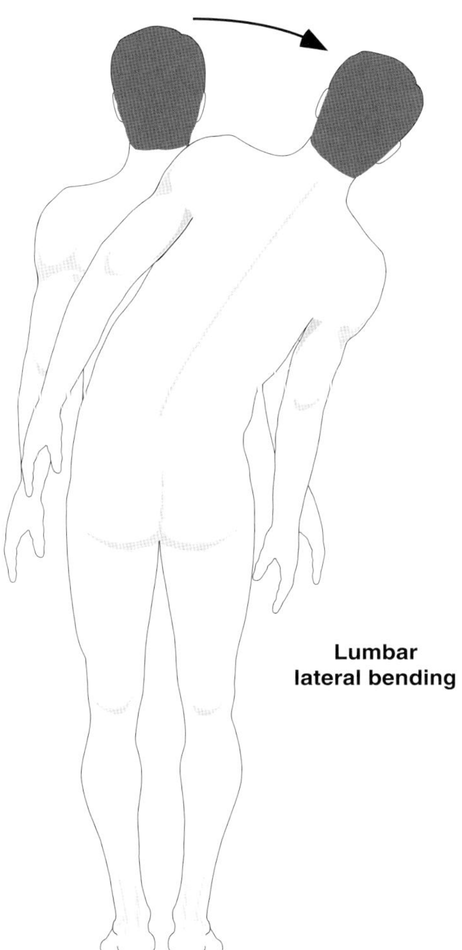

Fig. 2–26

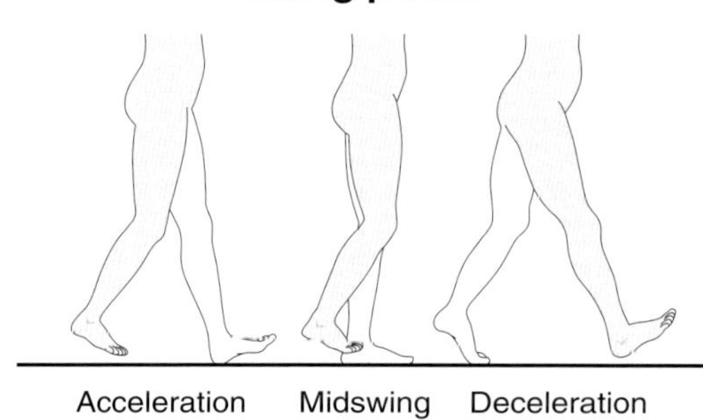

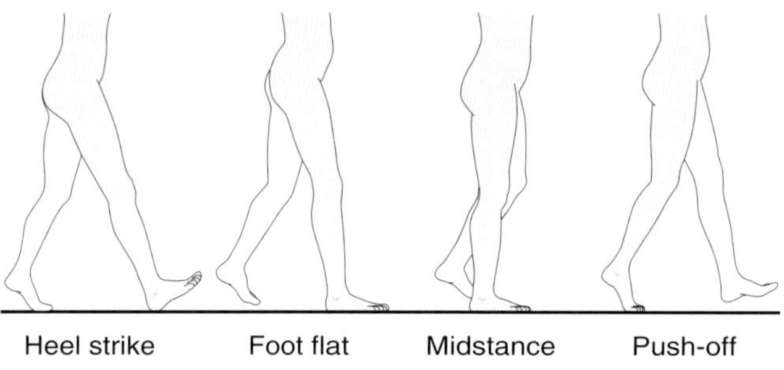

Fig. 2–27

Conclude the examination by observing the patient's **gait**. The normal cyclical movement of walking can be divided into two phases: the swing phase when the foot is swinging forward and the stance phase when the foot is in contact with the ground (Fig. 2–27).

Observe the swing and stance phases while checking for any limp, uneven rhythm, or asymmetry of gait.

SKILL BUILDING

The written material you have just reviewed is designed to give you a conceptual understanding of the examination. Acquiring confidence in the techniques involved and developing a smoothly integrated SMSE will require practice. Set aside some blocks of time with a friend, roommate, or spouse to practice the examination. Once you are comfortable with the techniques involved, you can easily review and practice the order of the examination by yourself (during TV commercials, at the bus stop, during sporting events ... be creative!). The time you invest will pay rich rewards later through the development of excellence in your skills of physical examination.

Using the practice checklist below may make it easier for you to practice the order and content of the examination.

SCREENING MUSCULOSKELETAL EXAMINATION
Practice Checklist

Patient seated

______Inspect dorsal surface hands
______Inspect palmar surface hands
______Spread fingers/make fists
______Inspect fists/supinate and pronate forearms
______Inspect wrists
______Wrist extension
______Wrist flexion
______Inspect elbows
______Elbow flexion
______Elbow extension
______Inspect deltoid muscles
______Shoulder flexion (arms forward, overhead)
______Shoulder internal rotation (hands behind back)
______Shoulder external rotation (hands behind head)

Patient lying down

______Hip flexion (thigh toward chest)
______Hip external rotation (ankle moves medially)
______Hip internal rotation (ankle moves laterally)
______Inspect quadriceps muscles
______Inspect knees
______Knee flexion
______Knee extension
______Inspect ankles
______Ankle dorsiflexion
______Ankle plantarflexion
______Inspect midfoot/toes
______Inspect sole of feet

Patient standing

______Inspect knee alignment/calf muscles and alignment of heels/feet (from behind)
______C spine flexion
______C spine extension
______C spine rotation, right and left
______C spine lateral flexion (side bending), right and left
______LS spine flexion
______LS spine extension
______Lumbar lateral flexion (side bending), right and left
______Observe gait

RECORDING MUSCULOSKELETAL EXAMINATION FINDINGS

A rapid and simple format for recording your screening MS examination is to divide the examination into its four major components: UE (upper extremities), LE (lower extremities), spine, and gait.

UE: fingers, wrists, elbows, and shoulders
LE: hips, knees, ankles, and feet
Spine: cervical, thoracic and lumbosacral
Gait: observation

If your examination is *normal*, you can record these findings as follows:

MS examination: screening UE, LE, spine, and gait normal

If your examination reveals *abnormalities*, note any deformity, visible swelling, muscle atrophy, or altered ROM as follows* (sample patient with primary osteoarthritis and multiple findings):

MS examination
UE: deformity of multiple DIPs; mild visible swelling R 2,4 and L 5 PIPs; subluxation of both first CMCs; thenar atrophy
LE: R hip 90° flex, 40° ER; 10° IR with groin pain at end IR; L hip 120° flex, 60° ER, and 40° IR; valgus deformity of both first MTPs
Spine: C: ↓ mild flex; 40° R and L rotation; ↓ ext
LS: ↓ lat bend/extension with pain at LS junction
Gait: antalgic with short stance phase on right side

CONCLUSION

The screening musculoskeletal examination is an important and useful clinical skill. Practicing this examination and integrating it into your complete physical examination will increase your reliability and speed. In a relatively short time, you will become familiar with the spectrum of normal musculoskeletal function and will appreciate important common abnormalities. While it is not expected that students early in their training will know what additional evaluation may be needed to further define such abnormalities, it is important that you be able to recognize and record these findings.

A rapid yet thorough musculoskeletal examination performed in an organized, sequential fashion represents the backbone of physical diagnosis of musculoskeletal problems. The screening musculoskeletal examination is the first step in acquiring this skill and provides the foundation for learning additional musculoskeletal examination skills at a later point in your training.

---

*bilat = bilateral; ER = external rotation; ext = extension; flex = flexion; IR = internal rotation; lat = lateral.

3

The General Musculoskeletal Examination

INTRODUCTION

The *general musculoskeletal examination* (GMSE) is designed to build directly on the sequence and techniques taught in the screening musculoskeletal examination (SMSE). It is intended to provide a comprehensive assessment of joint inflammation through the use of palpation and will enable you to recognize the important physical finding of joint swelling, essential to diagnosing arthritis. While the skills involved are more complex than those of the SMSE, the proper techniques of joint palpation can be mastered on normal individuals.

With practice, a systematic and thorough GMSE can be performed in ~6 to 8 minutes. Furthermore, the GMSE provides the foundation for learning more detailed, regional musculoskeletal examinations (RMSE) at a later point in your training.

CLINICAL UTILITY

The GMSE is clinically useful as the initial examination in individuals with *generalized musculoskeletal complaints (possible arthritis or connective tissue disease)* and in individuals with apparently *local or regional musculoskeletal complaints found to have additional abnormalities on the SMSE.*

OBJECTIVES

This instructional program will enable you to identify the *location of the joint line* and expected areas of *visible and palpable swelling* of major peripheral small and large joints. It will develop your skill in *joint palpation* and permit you to identify the location of clinically important *bursae* as well as *fibromyalgia tender points*. Most importantly, it will prepare you to perform a fully integrated GMSE.

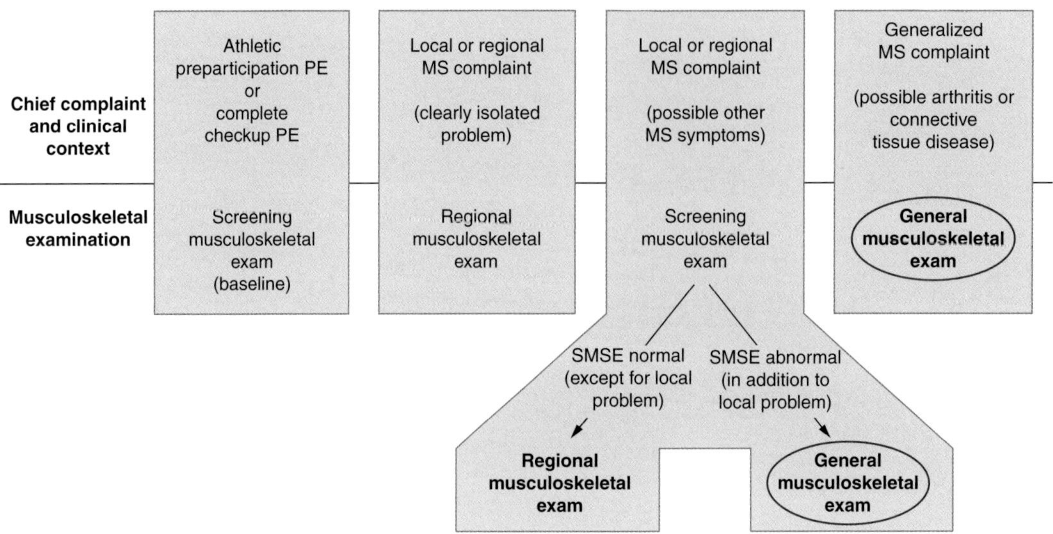

ESSENTIAL CONCEPTS

Categories of Abnormality The six basic categories of abnormality you will assess with the general examination include

1. Deformity
2. Visible swelling
3. Muscle atrophy
4. Tenderness, warmth, and palpable swelling (bony enlargement or synovial swelling)
5. Abnormalities of range of motion
6. Abnormalities of gait

Symmetry A central axial spine, paired peripheral joints, and symmetric musculature provide the basis for essential side-to-side comparison during the musculoskeletal examination. Recognizing asymmetry is extremely important and may provide your first clue in diagnosing an abnormality.

Active and Passive Range of Motion Both active and passive range of motion are used to assess joint function in the screening and general musculoskeletal examinations. The combined use of passive as well as active range of motion minimizes the need for patient instruction and this maximizes the speed and efficiency of the examination (Fig. 3–1A, B).

Whenever joint movement is anticipated to be painful, it is best to first observe active range of motion (patient-initiated movement) to appreciate the degree of pain and dysfunction before gently attempting passive range of motion (examiner-initiated manipulation).

Importance of Objective Findings An essential feature of the GMSE is the use of joint palpation to assess for the presence of objective abnormalities.

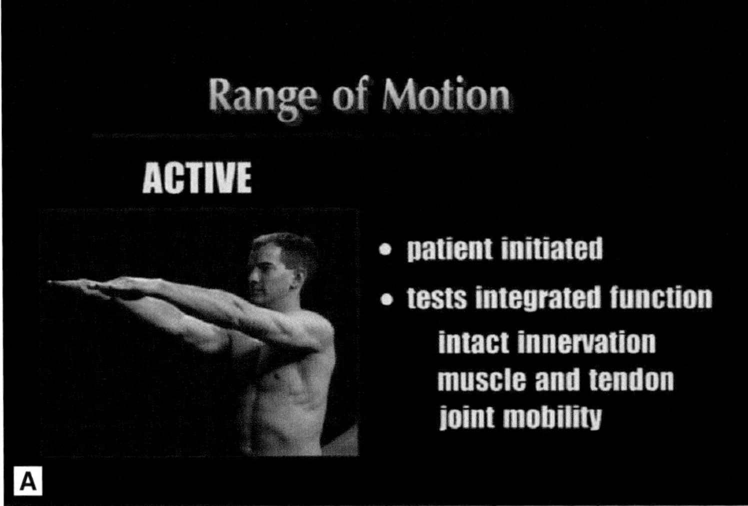

Fig. 3–1

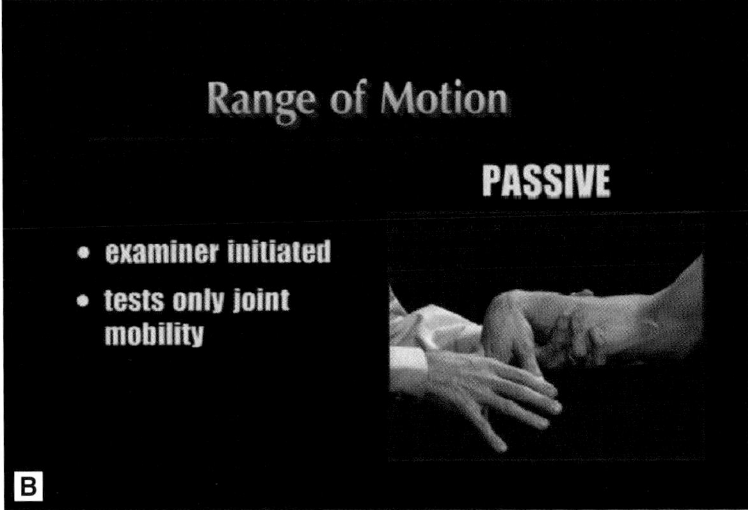

Fig. 3–1

Joint tenderness alone is subjective (joint tenderness ≠ arthritis). Tenderness must be correlated with the finding of objective, visible, or palpable abnormality for a diagnosis of arthritis to be made.

Joint redness (erythema) is an objective abnormality and depends on the acuity and severity of the underlying inflammation. When present, significant erythema may suggest the possibility of infection or crystalline arthritis. *The vast majority of objectively swollen, abnormal joints you will see in clinical practice will not be red.*

Joint warmth (heat) is also an objective finding and depends on the acuity and severity of the underlying inflammation. Clinically important chronic inflammation is often cool to palpation.

Joint swelling is also an objective finding and is an extremely important and definitive clinical sign. Swelling due to synovial fluid (joint effusion) or swollen synovial tissue (thickened joint membrane), called synovitis, and swelling due to bony enlargement (osteophytes) are extremely important physical findings indicating the presence of arthritis.

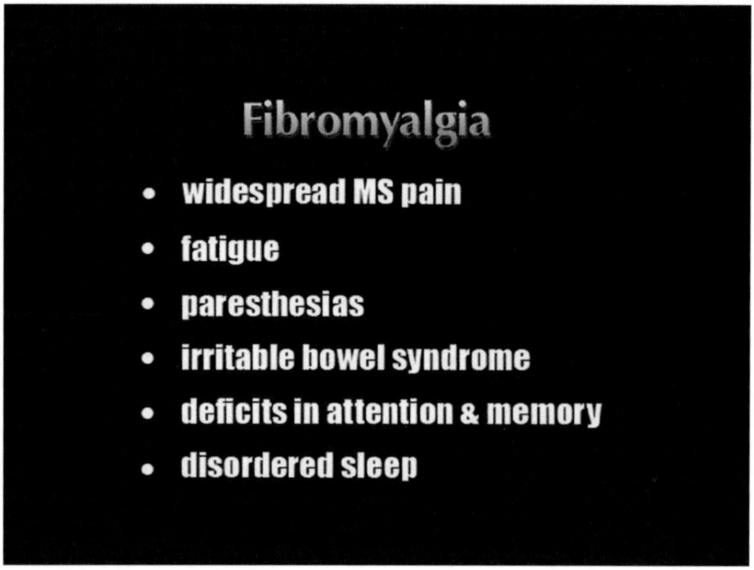

Fibromyalgia

- widespread MS pain
- fatigue
- paresthesias
- irritable bowel syndrome
- deficits in attention & memory
- disordered sleep

Fig. 3–2

Diffuse Musculoskeletal Pain In patients presenting with musculoskeletal pain, it is frequently important to assess for **regional** or **widespread tenderness**. Establishing the patient's level of tenderness and pain threshold is very important in understanding the problem and establishing an appropriate diagnosis and management strategy.

Fibromyalgia is a common medical problem, reported in up to 4% of the population. The 1990 American College of Rheumatology (ACR) classification criteria for fibromyalgia include widespread musculoskeletal pain plus the presence of 11 of 18 tender points on physical examination. While these criteria have been helpful in standardizing research on fibromyalgia, they were never intended to be rigidly applied to individual patients. A spectrum of regional or widespread tenderness and pain combined with variable combinations of tender points may be seen in patients who clearly have clinical features of fibromyalgia, yet don't meet these strict criteria (the 2010 ACR classification criteria for fibromyalgia no longer include the requirement for tender points). A history of widespread musculoskeletal pain, fatigue, paresthesias, irritable bowel symptoms, deficits in attention and memory, and disordered sleep all suggest possible fibromyalgia syndrome (Fig. 3–2).

A properly performed fibromyalgia tender point examination allows the clinician to assess the patient's pain threshold in a variety of locations in a standardized manner. Individuals with fibromyalgia may not only be tender at these discrete sites, but may also have widespread tenderness throughout the body. Women characteristically have more tender points on examination than men (Fig. 3–3).

Finding remarkable **tender points** in the absence of objective swelling on GMSE is further confirmation that a clinically important generalized pain problem is present, suggesting a diagnosis of fibromyalgia rather than arthritis.

With this background, you are now ready to learn the integrated GMSE.

THE EXAMINATION, OVERVIEW

With the patient seated comfortably and appropriately undressed, begin the examination of the **upper extremities**. *Inspect for deformity, visible swelling, or muscle atrophy; palpate for joint swelling; and assess range of motion.*

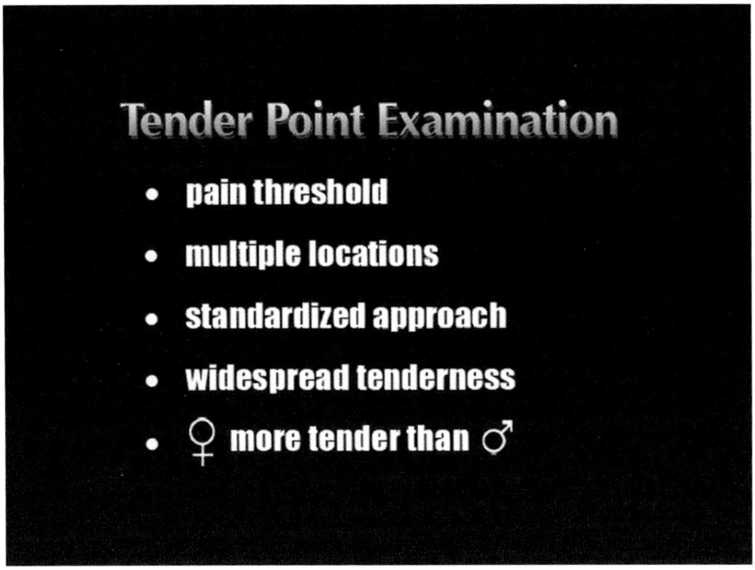

Tender Point Examination

- pain threshold
- multiple locations
- standardized approach
- widespread tenderness
- ♀ more tender than ♂

Fig. 3–3

Instruct the patient to open both hands. Observe the dorsal and palmar surfaces and the intrinsic muscles. Assess finger extension by asking the patient to spread the fingers. Next, assess finger flexion by having the patient make a fist. Inspect both fists during pronation and supination of the forearms. Palpate the DIP (distal interphalangeal) joints, followed by the PIP (proximal interphalangeal) joints, followed by the MCP (metacarpophalangeal) joints of both hands. Palpate the thumb, IP (interphalangeal), MCP, and first CMC (carpometacarpal) joints. Inspect and palpate, then extend and flex each wrist. Inspect and palpate the olecranon region of each elbow. Palpate the elbow at the lateral joint line, then flex and extend each elbow. Inspect and palpate the sternoclavicular (SC) and acromioclavicular (AC) joints. Inspect the deltoid muscles and deltopectoral groove. Observe shoulder flexion by asking the patient to bring the arms forward and raise them overhead. Observe shoulder internal rotation (IR) by having the patient place both hands behind the back. Then, observe shoulder external rotation (ER) by having the patient place both hands behind the head.

Now ask the patient to lie down for the examination of the **lower extremities**. *Inspect for deformity, visible swelling, or muscle atrophy; palpate for joint swelling; and assess range of motion.* Palpate the greater trochanters. Assess hip flexion by grasping the heel and moving the thigh up toward the chest. Return the hip to 90° of flexion while holding the knee at 90° of flexion. Now, move the ankle medially to assess hip external rotation (ER) and move the ankle laterally to assess hip internal rotation (IR). Inspect the quadriceps muscles. Inspect the knees. Look for the presence of a joint effusion by checking for a "bulge sign" (or "fluid wave") at each knee. Compress the patella to check for pain or crepitus at the patellofemoral joint. Flex and extend each knee.

Inspect the ankles. Check dorsiflexion, plantar flexion, and subtalar motion at each ankle. Palpate the posterior calcaneus (Achilles insertion) and plantar calcaneus (plantar fascia insertion) at each heel. Inspect the midfoot, forefoot, and toes. Palpate MTP (metatarsophalangeal) joints 5 through 2 of each foot. Next, palpate the IP and MTP joints of each great toe. Inspect the PIP and DIP joints of the toes. Inspect the sole of each foot.

Now ask the patient to stand. Observe the patient from behind while weight bearing. Note the alignment of the knees. Inspect the calf muscles. Note the alignment of the heels and feet.

Now with the patient standing, begin the examination of the **spine**. *Inspect for deformity or abnormal range of motion.* Inspect the cervical spine. Assess neck flexion by instructing the patient to place his chin on the chest. Assess neck extension by asking the patient to look up at the ceiling. Observe right and left rotation by asking the patient to place his chin on each shoulder. Assess lateral flexion (lateral bending) by asking the patient to incline his ear toward each shoulder.

Now, while observing the patient from behind, inspect the thoracolumbar spine. Note any resting asymmetry or deformity and inspect for the normal resting lumbar lordosis. Observe lumbar flexion by instructing the patient to bend forward at the waist. Assess lumbar extension by having the patient bend backward. Assess thoracolumbar lateral flexion (lateral bending) by asking the patient to bend to the right and to the left.

Finally, observe the patient's **gait**. *Check for any limp, uneven rhythm, or asymmetry.* Observe the swing and stance phases.

If appropriate, check for paired fibromyalgia tender points.

If appropriate, perform a neurovascular assessment.

THE EXAMINATION, COMPONENT PARTS

To begin the examination, the patient should be comfortable, yet *appropriately undressed*. This usually includes undershorts with or without a gown in men and underwear with a gown in woman. Adjusting the gown whenever necessary to permit full visualization of each region is very important.

Failure to visualize musculoskeletal structures during the examination because of inadequate exposure represents one of the most common errors made by examiners at all levels of training.

Begin the examination with the **upper extremities**. Instruct the patient to open both **hands**. Inspect the dorsal surface for any obvious deformity or visible swelling (Fig. 3–4A). Inspect the palmar surface

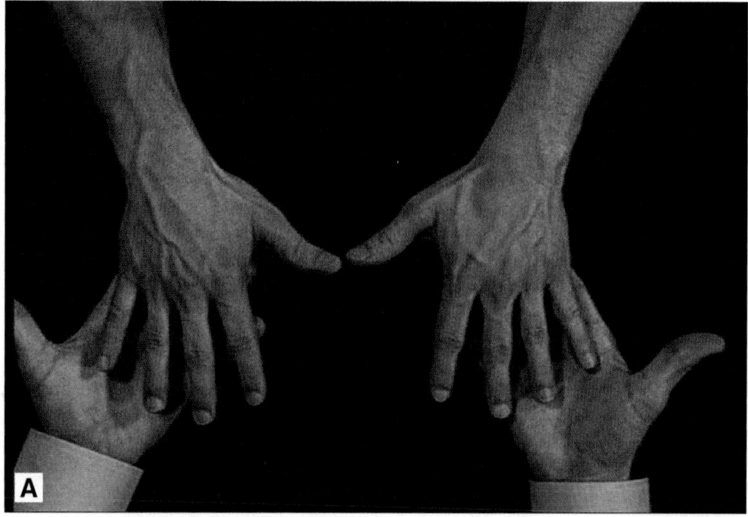

Fig. 3–4

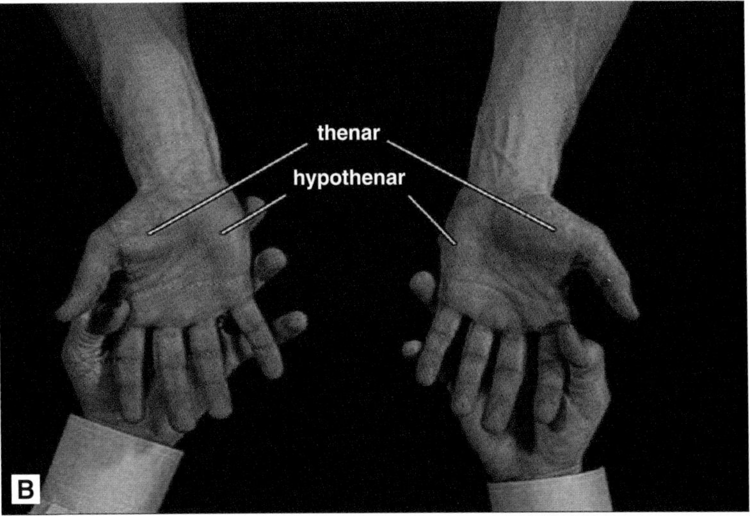

Fig. 3–4

and note any atrophy of the thenar or hypothenar eminences (Fig. 3–4B). Turn the hands over once again with the palms down. Next, rapidly assess integrated hand function: check finger extension by asking patient to spread the fingers. Note whether each finger's DIP, PIP, and MCP joints extend fully (Fig. 3–5A). Extension of the MCP joints beyond neutral is normal (Fig. 3–5B).

Assess finger flexion by observing the patient make a fist with each hand. Inspect the dorsal surface of each fist. Then, ask the patient to turn both fists over while you inspect the palmar surface to see that the tips of digits 2 to 5 are buried in the palm at the level of the distal palmar crease. Having the patient actively expose both surfaces of each fist allows you also to assess pronation and supination of the forearms.

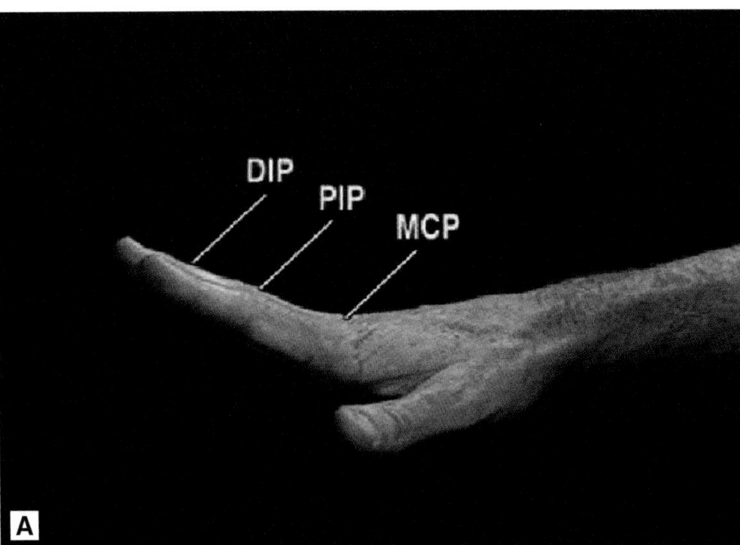

Fig. 3–5

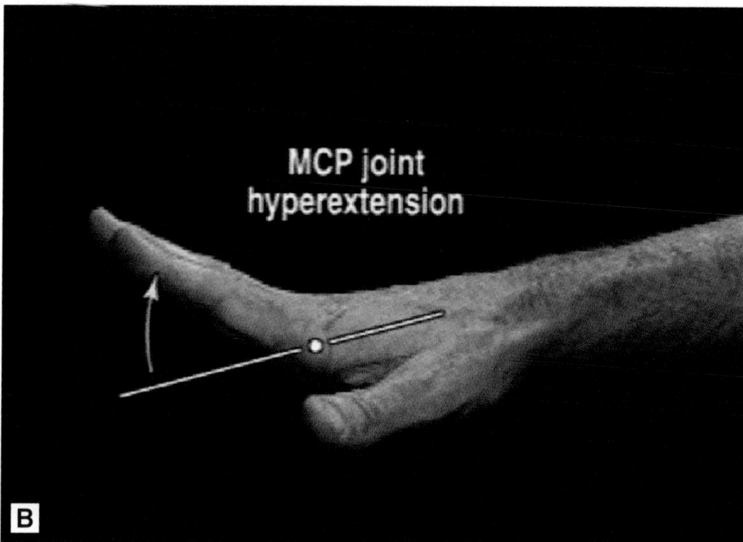

Fig. 3–5

Next, palpate the DIP, PIP, and MCP joints to assess for tenderness, warmth, or palpable swelling.

(Note: A systematic approach to palpating the finger joints is important. We suggest starting with digit 5, then 4, 3, and 2 of one hand followed by digit 5, then 4, 3, and 2 of the other, with thumbs assessed subsequently. This will facilitate side-to-side comparison in an orderly sequence.)

Palpate the **DIP joints** of digits 5 through 2 of each hand (Fig. 3–6). Place the thumb of your dominant hand on the dorsal surface and the index finger of your dominant hand on the palmar surface of the DIP joint. Next, bring your nondominant hand over the dorsal surface of the patient's hand and simultaneously compress the medial and lateral margins of the DIP joint between your nondominant thumb and index finger (Fig. 3–7). Applying firm but gentle pressure with one thumb and index finger

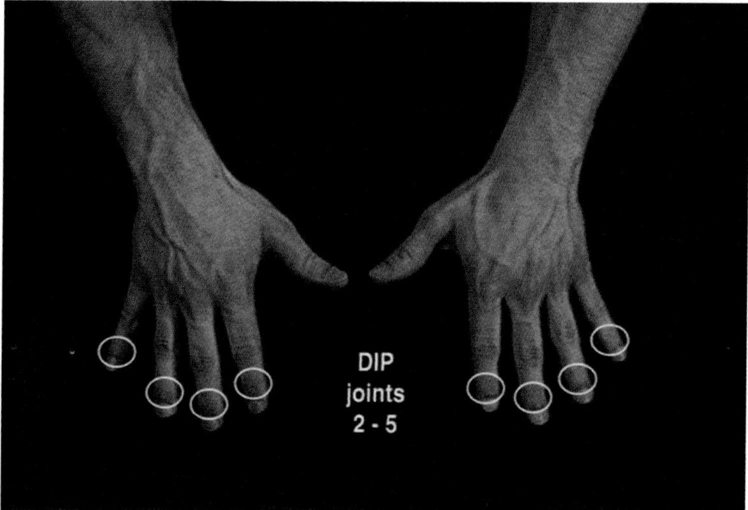

Fig. 3–6

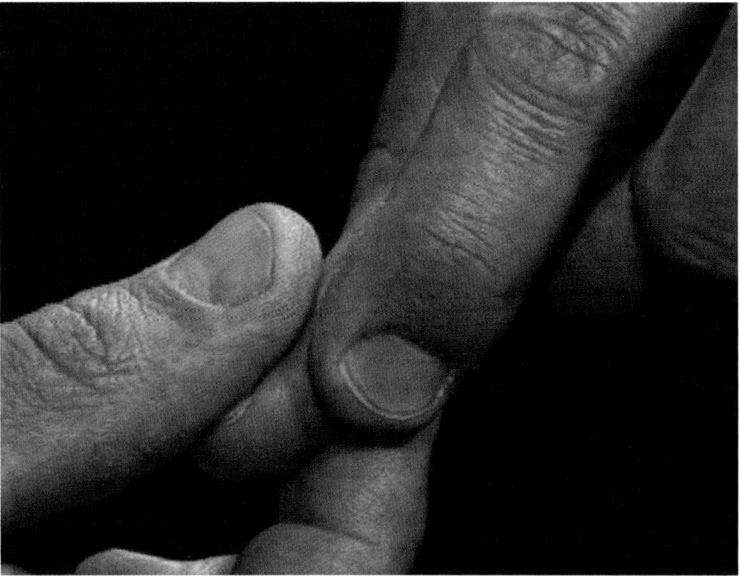

Fig. 3–7

will compress any swollen synovial membrane or synovial fluid toward the opposite joint margin where your other thumb and index finger can feel the distention. Applying gentle pressure in an alternating fashion allows *subjective* assessment of whether or not the joint is tender and *objective* assessment of whether bony (osteophytic) or synovial swelling (synovitis) is present. Although the DIP joint line itself cannot be felt, the normal joint is nontender with minimal skin and subcutaneous tissue present between your examining fingers and normal bony margins (Fig. 3–8A, B).

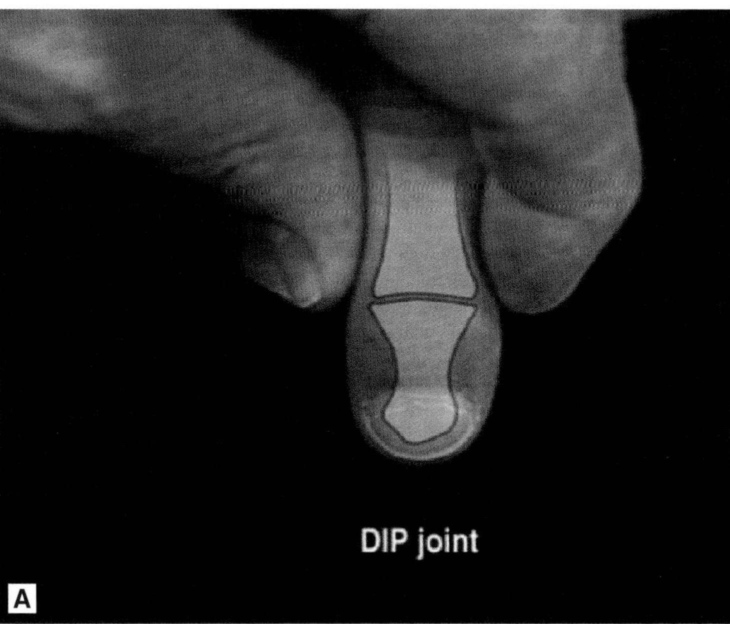

Fig. 3–8

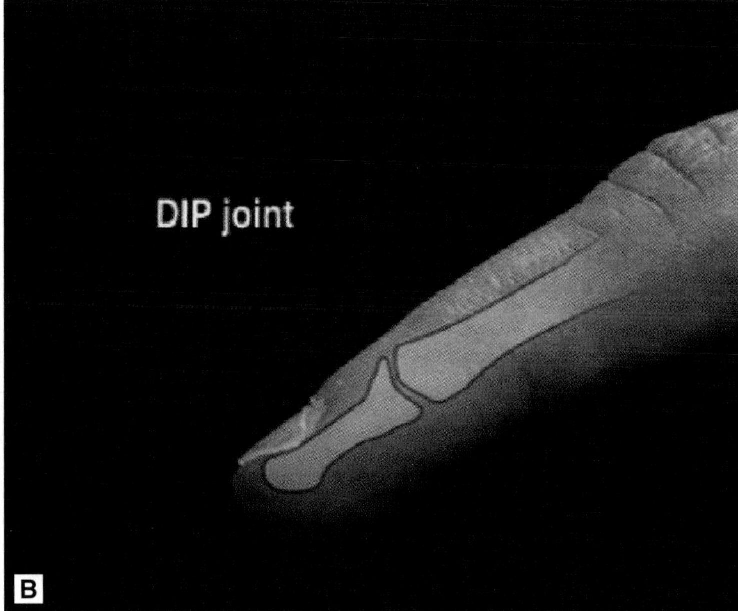

Fig. 3–8

Now palpate the **PIP joints** of digits 5 through 2 of each hand. The technique for palpating the PIP joints is identical to that used in assessing the DIP joints (Fig. 3–9A, B).

Note that the joint line of the PIP joints (unlike the DIP joints) is usually palpable. The normal PIP joint line can be felt as a narrow, distinct depression running perpendicular to the axis of the finger

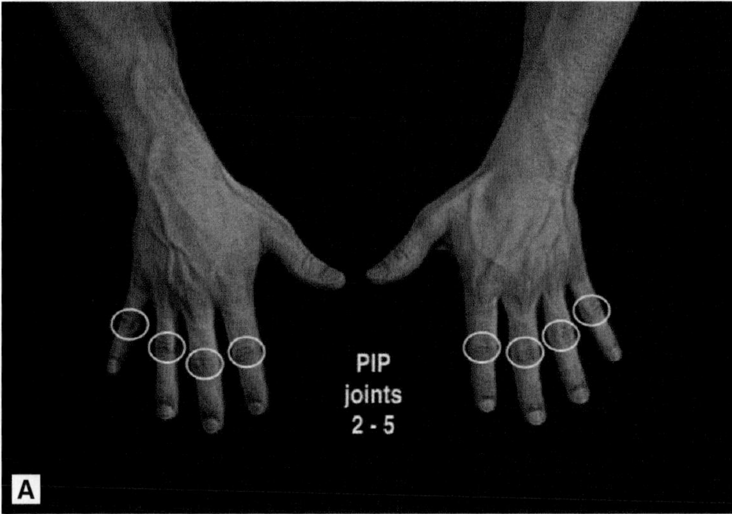

Fig. 3–9

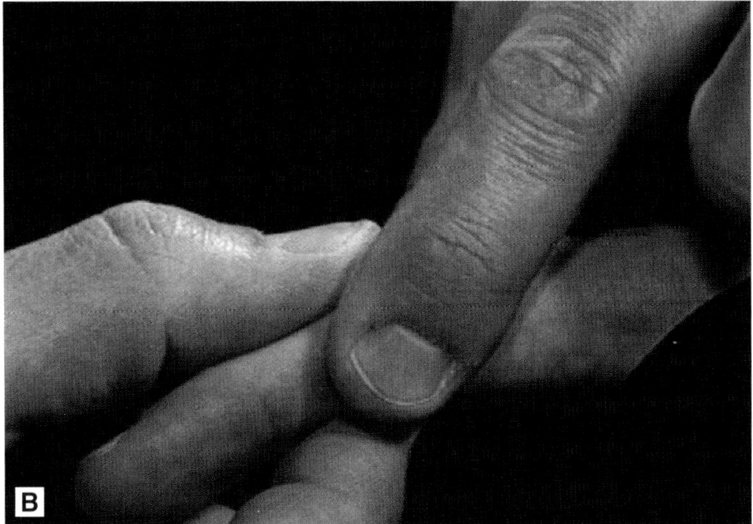

Fig. 3–9

(Fig. 3–10A). Palpating the joint in partial flexion helps open the joint space beneath your palpating thumb (Fig.3–10B). Remember, the distal member of each finger joint swings under the proximal member; therefore, the joint line at each interphalangeal joint is more distal than you might initially think.

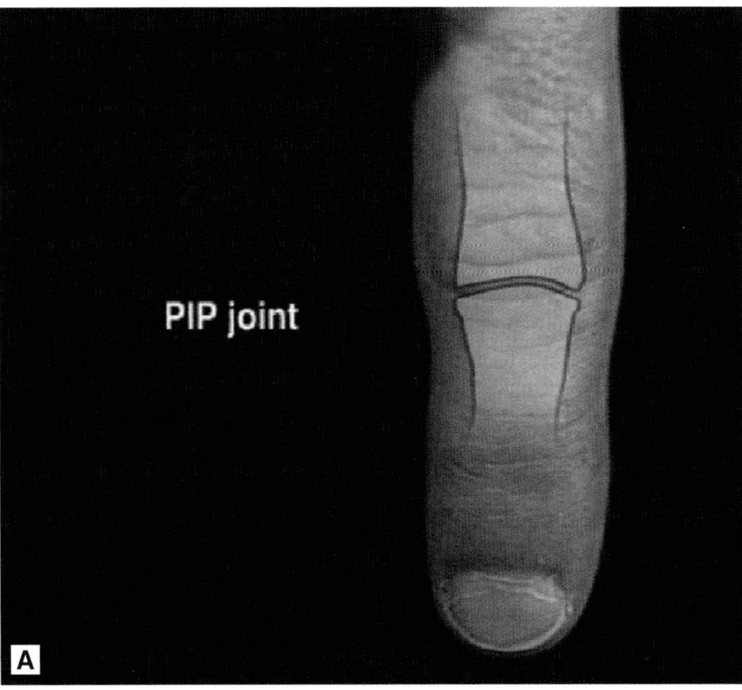

Fig. 3–10

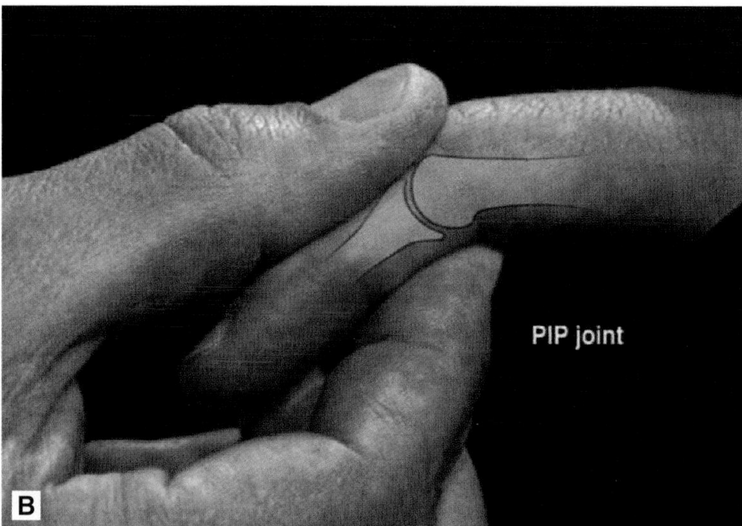

Fig. 3–10

Next palpate the **MCP joints** of digits 5 through 2 of each hand. Like the DIP and PIP joints, the MCP joints are best palpated in flexion. The patient's hand should be relaxed with the palm down. Support the patient's palm with your second through fourth fingers while using your fifth fingers to keep the patient's fingers in flexion (Fig. 3–11A). Use your thumbs to palpate the anterior joint line on either side of the extensor tendon (Fig. 3–11B). Small oscillating movements of your palpating thumbs perpendicular to the joint line will allow you to appreciate the normal definition of the metacarpal head and anterior surface of the plateau of the proximal phalanx (Fig. 3–11C).

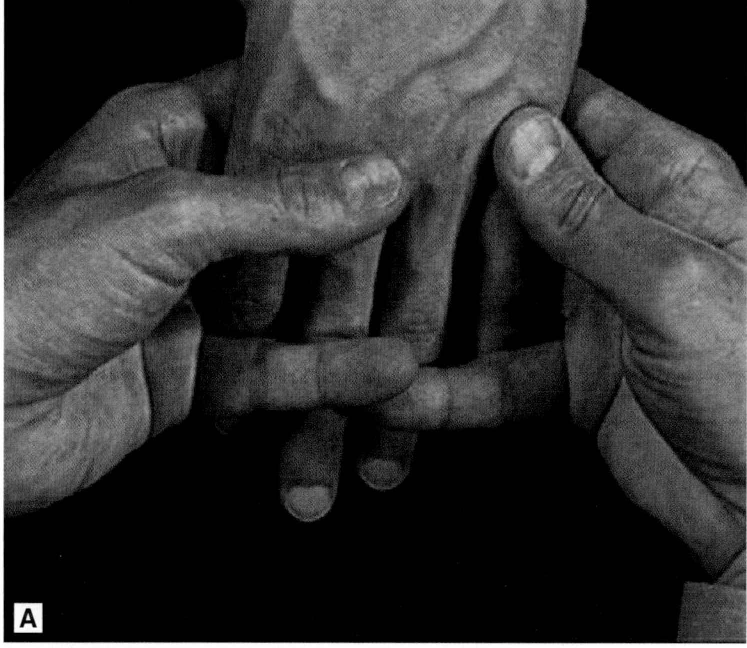

Fig. 3–11

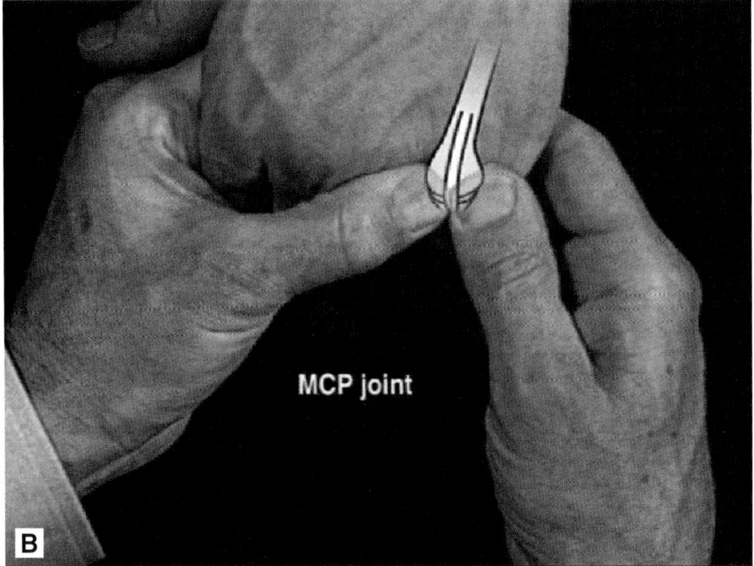

Fig. 3–11

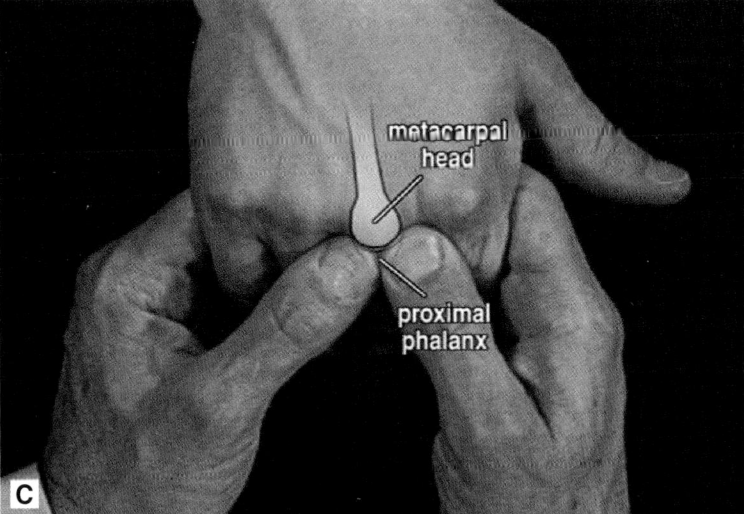

Fig. 3–11

Now, examine each **thumb**. Take the patient's hands in your hands to make a side-to-side comparison. Inspect for visible swelling or deformity. Palpate the IP (interphalangeal) joint using your nondominant thumb and index finger for lateral compression and your dominant thumb and index finger in the dorsal and palmar position. (Like the DIP joints of digits 2 through 5, it is not possible to normally feel the joint line of the thumb IP joint.) Next, grasp the patient's thumb with your second through fourth fingers while you gently flex the MCP joint (Fig. 3–12A). This will open the joint space, permitting you to readily palpate the MCP joint line with your thumb (Fig. 3–12B).

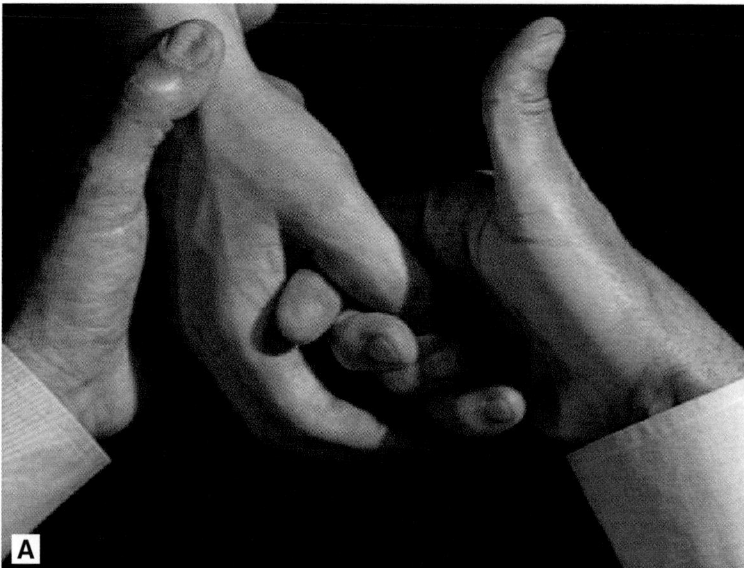

Fig. 3–12

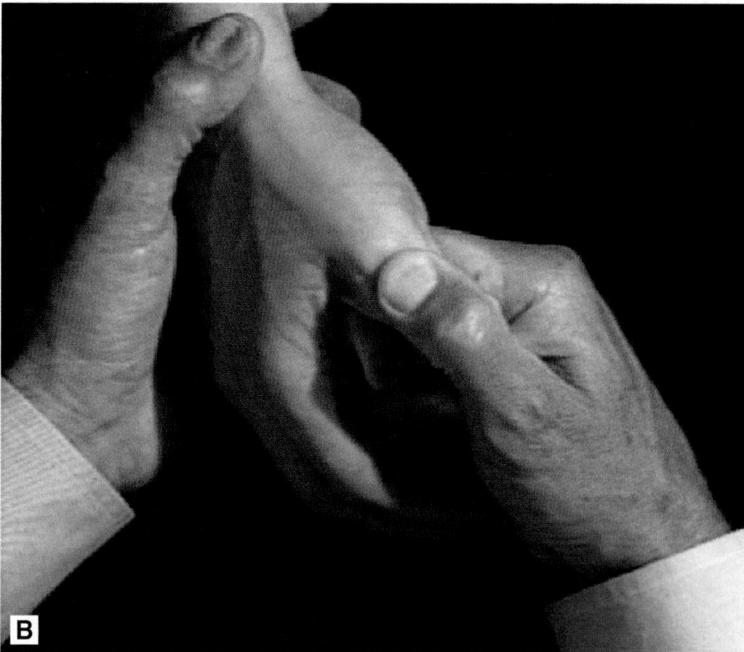

Fig. 3–12

Next palpate the **first carpometacarpal** (first CMC) joint, where the thumb articulates with the wrist at the trapezium (Fig. 3–13A). Place your nondominant thumb directly over the anatomic snuff box at the base of the patient's thumb (Fig. 3–13B). Use your other hand to gently but firmly rotate the patient's first metacarpal on the trapezium. Note any discomfort or palpable crepitus. (Palpation of the first CMC joint line itself is difficult, but this technique effectively allows assessment of whether pain or crepitus is present.)

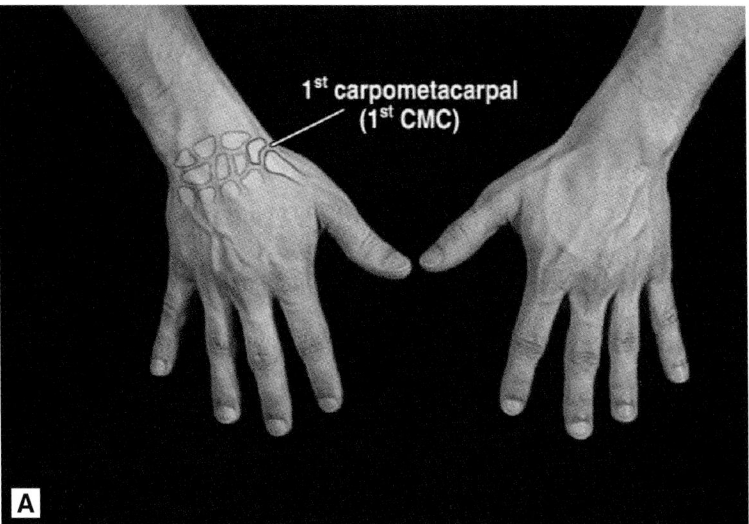

Fig. 3–13

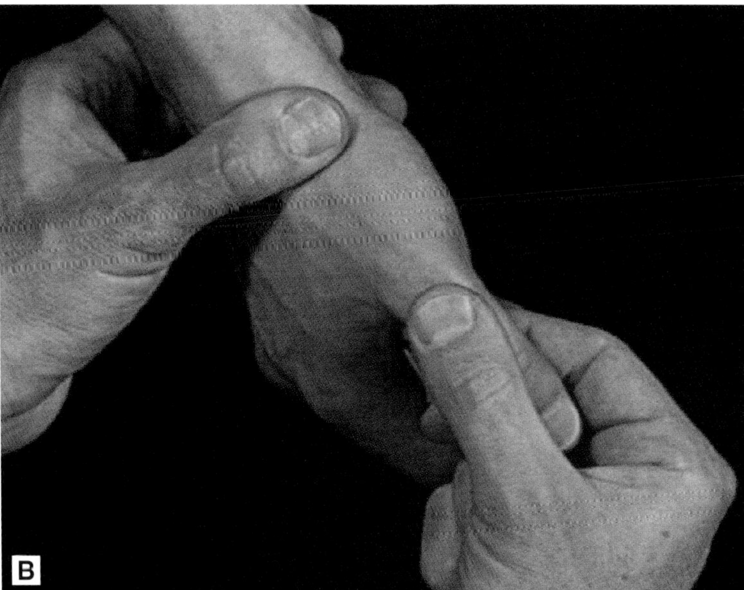

Fig. 3–13

Abnormalities at the DIP, PIP, and MCP joints include visible swelling or deformity, palpable synovial membrane swelling, and/or joint fluid accumulation (both called "synovitis") and palpable hard tissue swelling (bony proliferation or osteophyte formation). All are objective findings of abnormality and provide important diagnostic information.

Next inspect the **wrists** looking for deformity or visible swelling. Palpate the wrist dorsally by placing both thumbs along the joint line while supporting the patient's palm with the remaining fingers of your hands (Fig. 3–14A). Gently rocking the patient's wrist passively in small arcs of flexion and extension allows palpation of the dorsal surface under your examining thumbs. Synovial swelling and tenosynovitis suspected visually can be confirmed by palpation using this technique. Now, extend and flex each wrist. Take the patient's hand in your dominant hand, as though you were going to "kiss the hand" (Fig. 3–14B). This allows you to comfortably move the patient's hand into full extension using

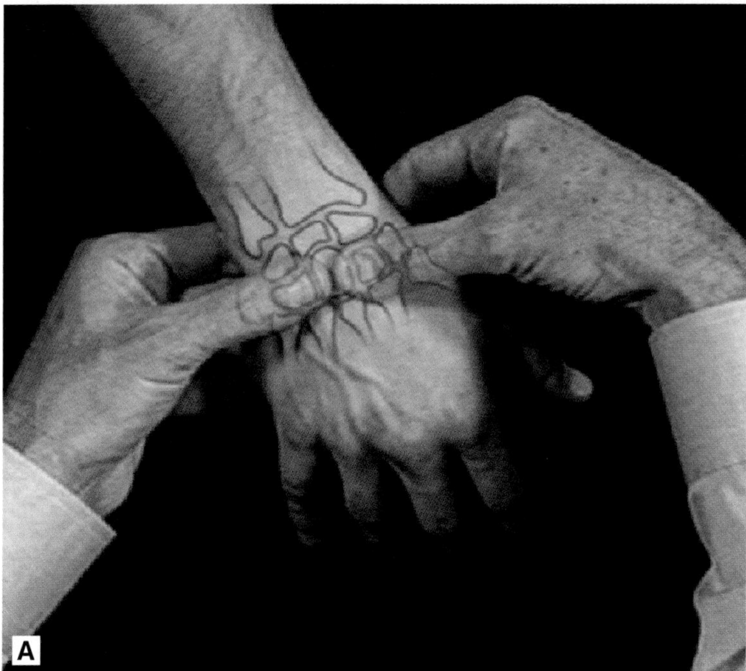

Fig. 3–14

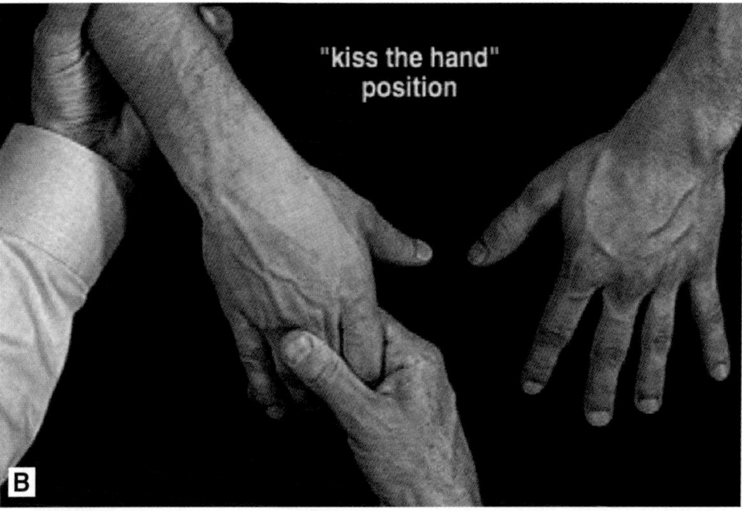

Fig. 3–14

pressure with your index finger against the distal palm (against the patient's second to fifth metacarpal heads) and avoids unnecessarily squeezing the patient's fingers (Fig. 3–15A). Next, downward pressure with your thumb on the patient's second or third metacarpal allows you to bring the wrist gently into full flexion (Fig. 3–15B). Full wrist extension and flexion should be symmetrical and bring the hand nearly perpendicular to the forearm on each side.

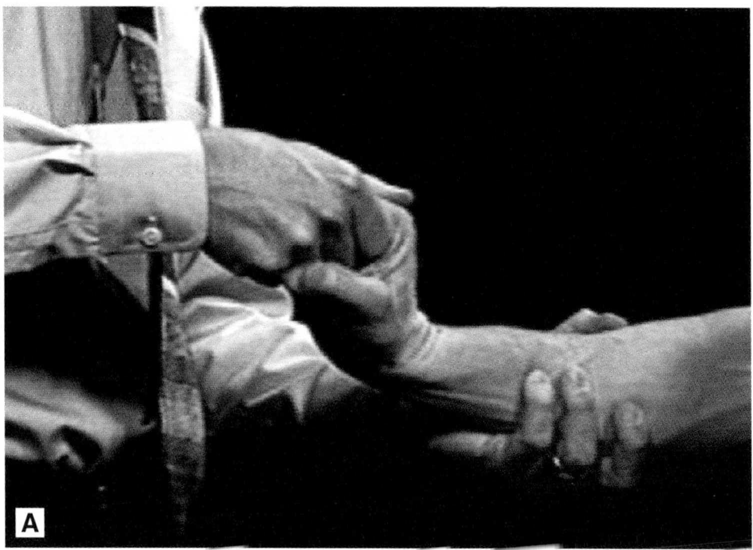

Fig. 3–15

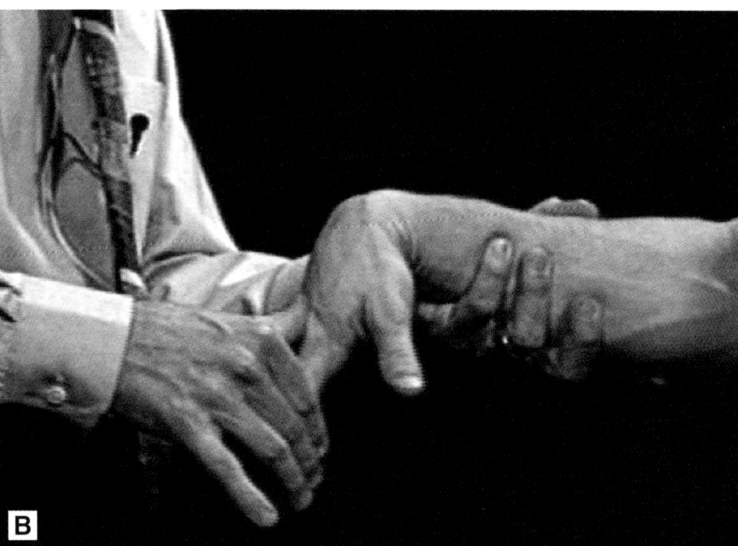

Fig. 3–15

Following your examination of the wrist, assume a loose "handshake" position with the patient while you examine the **elbows** (Fig. 3–16A). Inspect for any obvious swelling or deformity. Next, slide your other hand along the forearm to the olecranon surface. Note any subcutaneous nodules or palpable swelling of the olecranon bursa (Fig. 3–16B). Swelling of the olecranon bursa presents

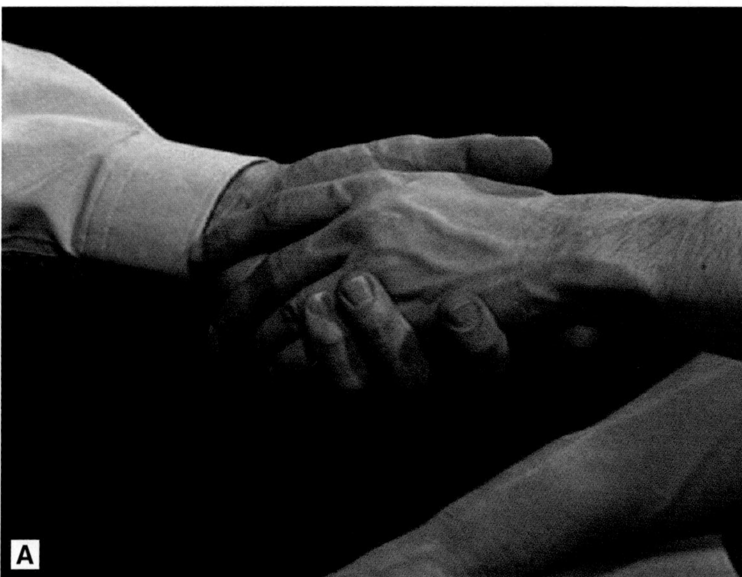

Fig. 3–16

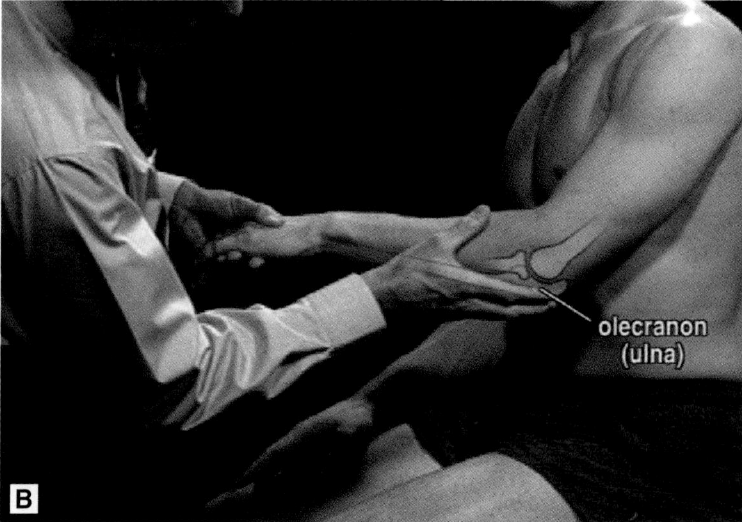

Fig. 3–16

itself as visible and/or palpable distention directly overlying the olecranon. Next, identify the normal small depression present between the olecranon and the lateral epicondyle, especially visible during full extension (Fig. 3–17A, B). This depression is the first area to be obliterated by an elbow effusion. Next, use your examining thumb to palpate the lateral epicondyle. Then, slide your thumb slightly distally while you gently pronate and supinate the forearm with your other hand, still in the

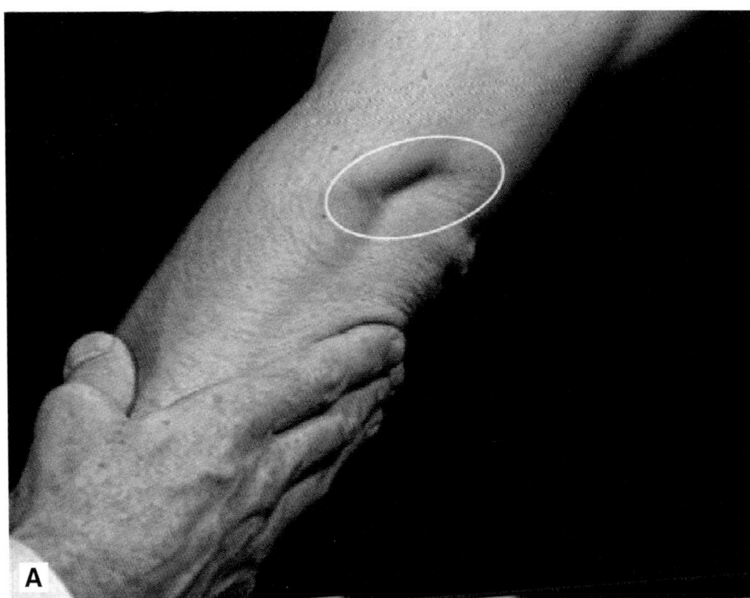

Fig. 3–17

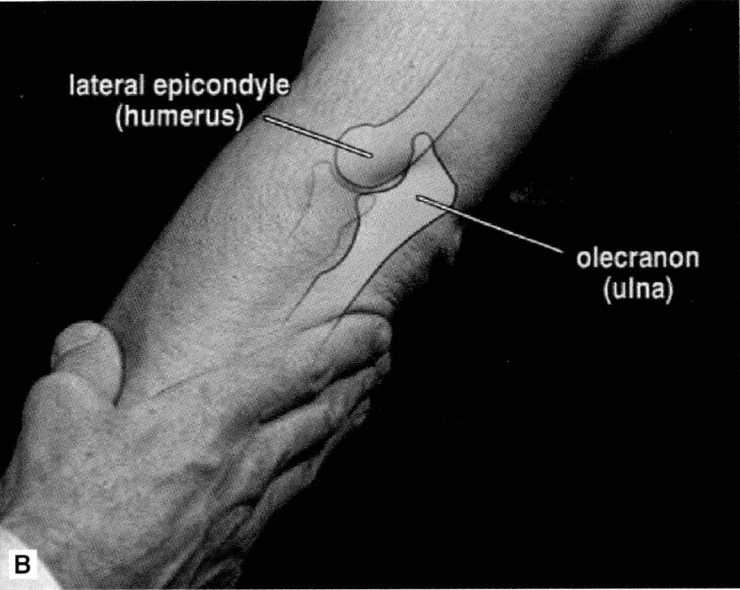

Fig. 3–17

"handshake" position. You can now feel the patient's radial head, moving under your palpating thumb (Fig. 3–18A). The joint space between the lateral epicondyle and radial head should now be readily appreciable with only skin and subcutaneous tissue between your thumb and the joint line itself. Next, continue palpating the lateral joint line while you bring the elbow into full extension (Fig. 3–18B).

Synovial swelling of the elbow joint results in progressive obliteration of the normal small lateral depression and a "boggy" or thickened feel to the usually well-defined joint line between the lateral epicondyle and radial head. Furthermore, synovial distention may produce a visible or palpable bulge in the space between the lateral epicondyle and olecranon when the elbow is moved into full extension. Palpable swelling (frequently combined with the patient's hesitation to permit full elbow extension due to pain) confirms the presence of synovial swelling and/or fluid within the elbow joint.

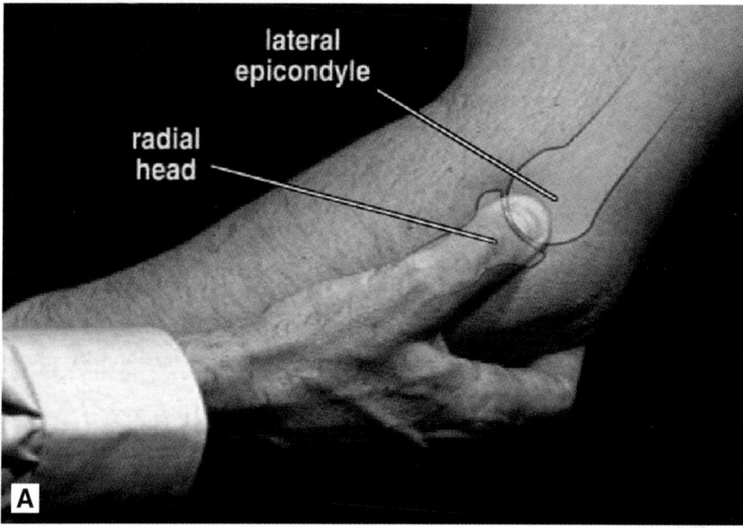

Fig. 3–18

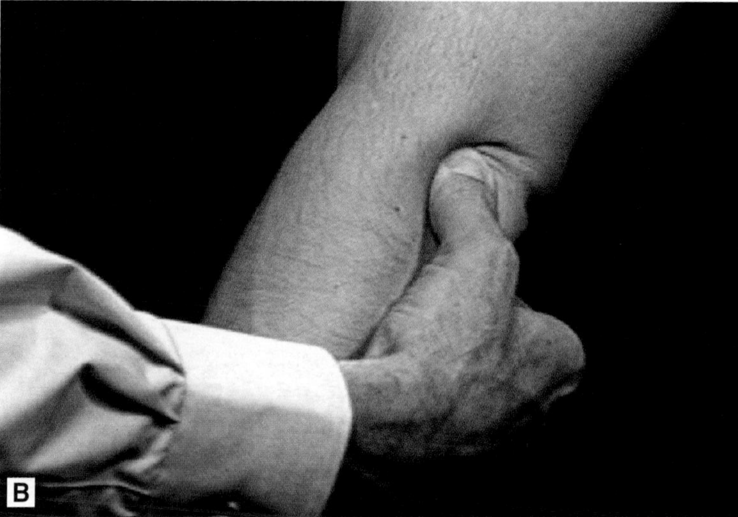

Fig. 3–18

Next, flex and extend each elbow. Full elbow flexion places the proximal forearm against the distal biceps. Elbow extension returns the joint to the outstretched anatomical position. Place your hand under the olecranon to assist you in detecting a flexion contracture (deficit in full extension).

Next observe the **shoulders**. Inspect the sternoclavicular (SC) joints for visible swelling or asymmetry. Palpate the jugular notch with your index or middle finger, then slide slightly laterally to feel the SC joint line. The joint is subcutaneous and the bony margins of the proximal end of the clavicle and superolateral manubrium are normally easily palpable (Fig. 3–19A). Next, inspect the acromioclavicular (AC) joints for asymmetry or visible swelling. Palpate the AC joint by applying pressure with your index and middle fingers to the top of the shoulder, ~2 cm medial to the lateral edge of the acromion (Fig. 3–19B). The joint line itself is often difficult to feel, but palpation allows at least subjective assessment of joint tenderness.

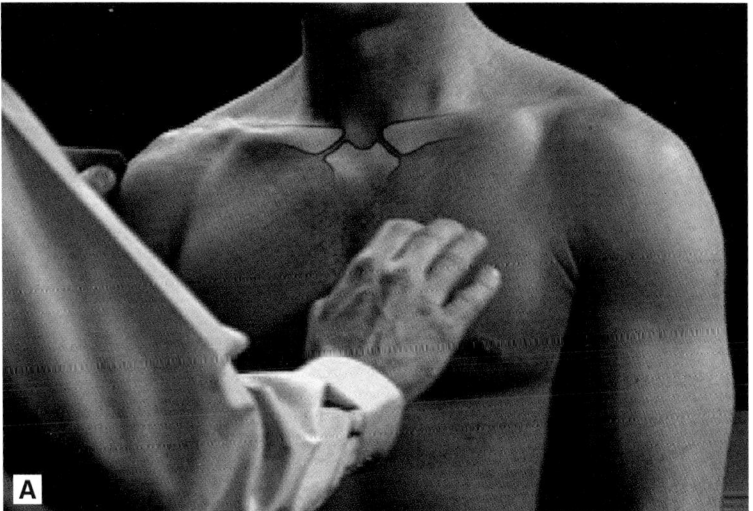

Fig. 3–19

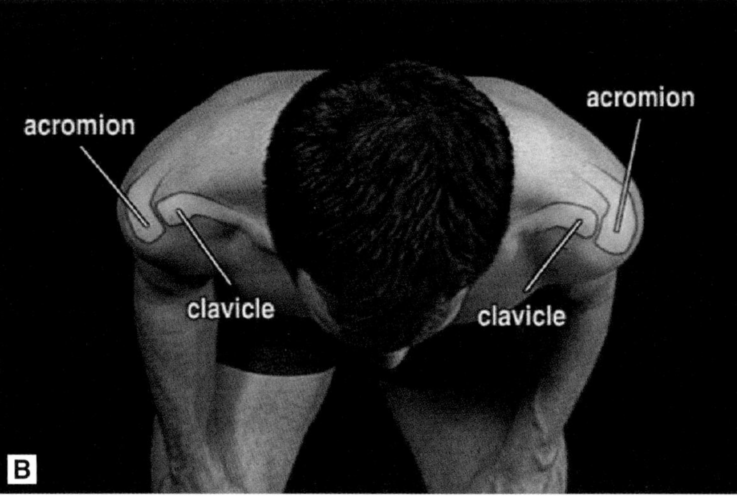

Fig. 3–19

Next, inspect the deltoid and pectoral muscles for any atrophy or asymmetry. Look for the normal deltopectoral groove. If a shoulder effusion is present, the deltopectoral groove may be effaced with (sometimes subtle) swelling anteriorly, an uncommon but helpful sign.

Now assess shoulder flexion by asking the patient to bring the arms forward and raise them overhead. Normal shoulder flexion brings the arms almost fully vertical. Observe shoulder internal rotation by asking the patient to place both hands behind the back. While this motion also involves abduction, the dominant movement is internal rotation.

Next, observe external rotation by asking the patient to place both hands behind the head. While this motion also involves abduction, it primarily requires external rotation. To properly demonstrate external rotation, both arms must be in the plane of the body with the elbows pointed laterally (Fig. 3–20).

If all active shoulder range of motion is painless and full, no further evaluation is necessary. However, if the patient has specific shoulder symptoms (pain or limited range of motion), a more detailed examination (RMSE) of the shoulder may be required.

Now ask the patient to lie supine for the examination of the lower extremities and begin your examination of the **hips**. While standing on the patient's right side, place your thumbs on the superior anterior iliac spines on each side. Your remaining fingers, directed posteriorly toward the examination table, now lie over each greater trochanter (Fig. 3–21A). Check for possible

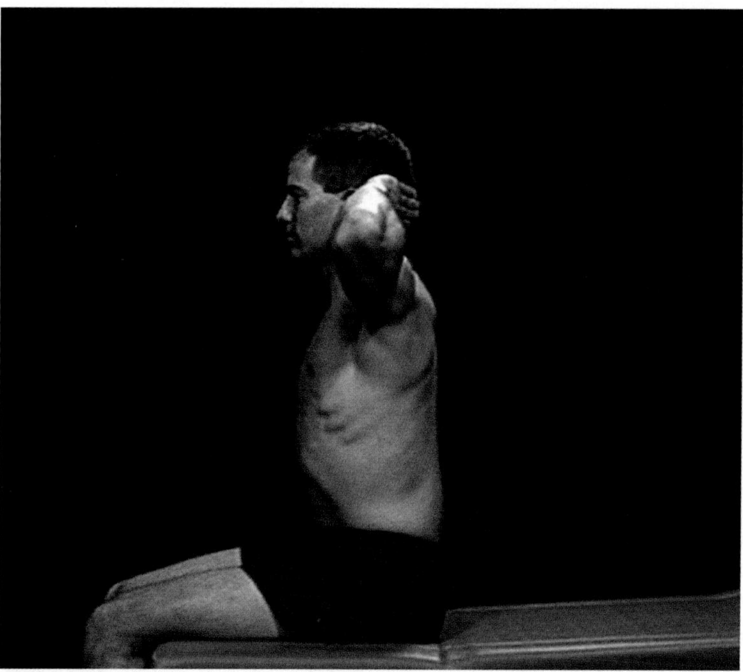

Fig. 3–20

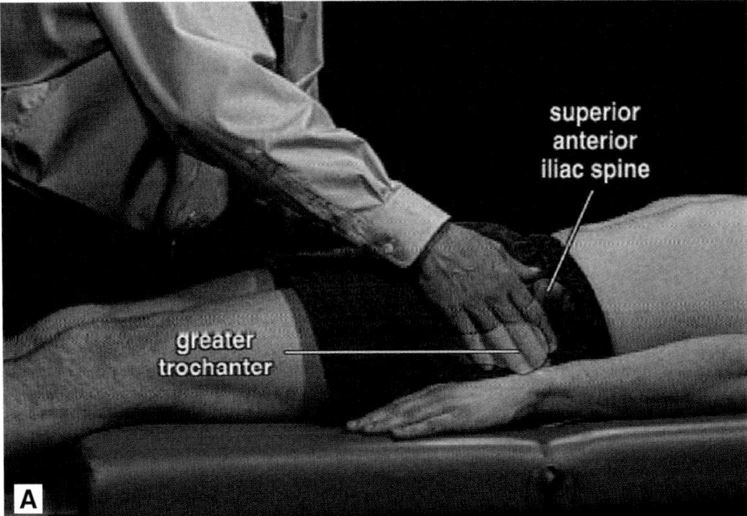

Fig. 3–21

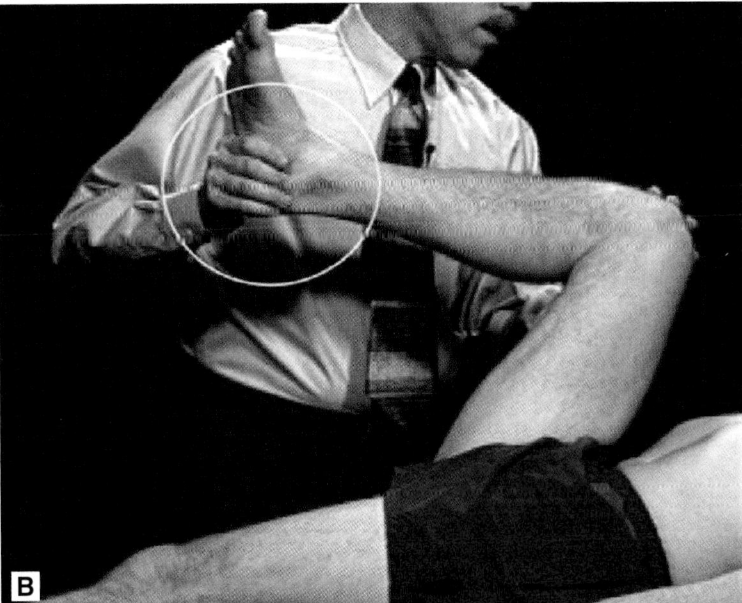

Fig. 3–21

trochanteric bursitis by applying firm pressure to the superior and lateral regions of the trochanter. Note any tenderness. Next, check hip range of motion. Grasp the patient's foot with your right hand and position the patient's heel in your palm (Fig. 3–21B). This allows comfortable control of the extremity without the need to reposition your grip during the hip examination. Assess hip flexion by moving the thigh up toward the thorax. Normal hip flexion brings the anterior thigh nearly to the chest (Fig. 3–22A). Return the hip to 90° of flexion (Fig. 3–22B). Keeping the thigh perpendicular to the examining table while testing hip rotation permits easy visualization of the arcs of movement. Moving the ankle medially assesses hip external rotation (Fig 3–23A). Moving the ankle laterally assesses hip internal rotation (Fig. 3–23B). Apply firm but gentle pressure to adequately assess range of motion.

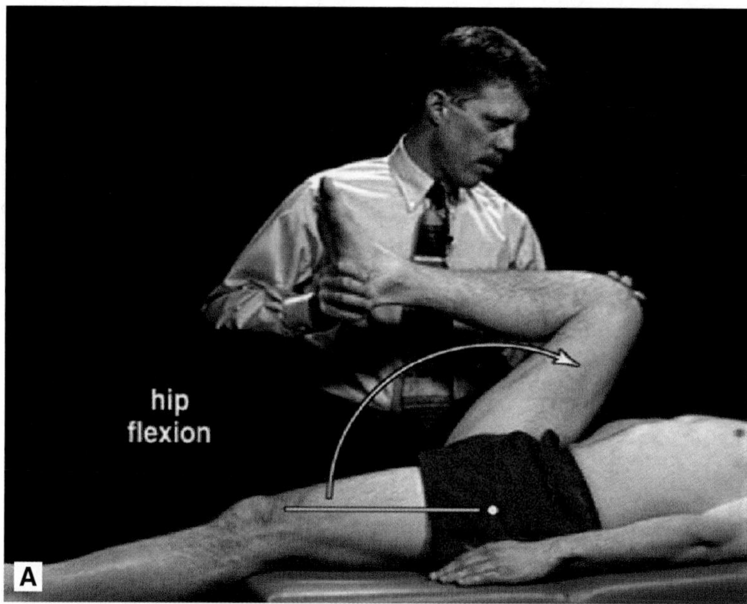

Fig. 3–22

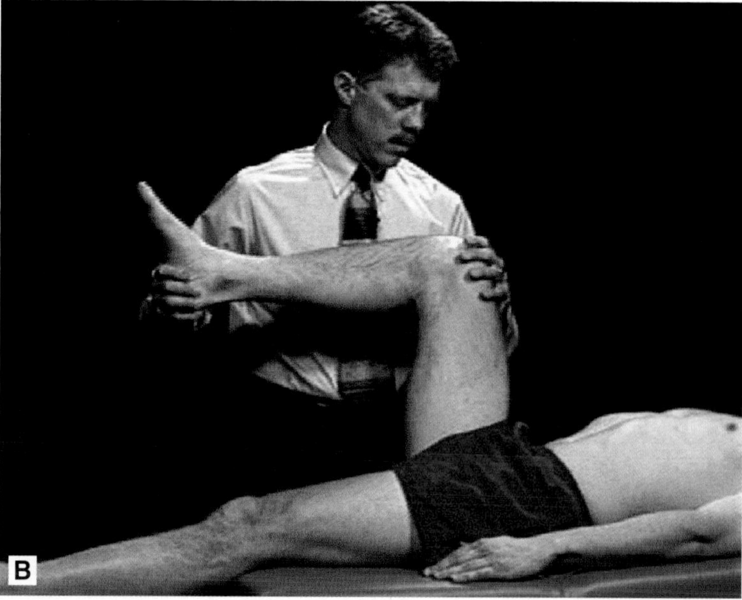

Fig. 3–22

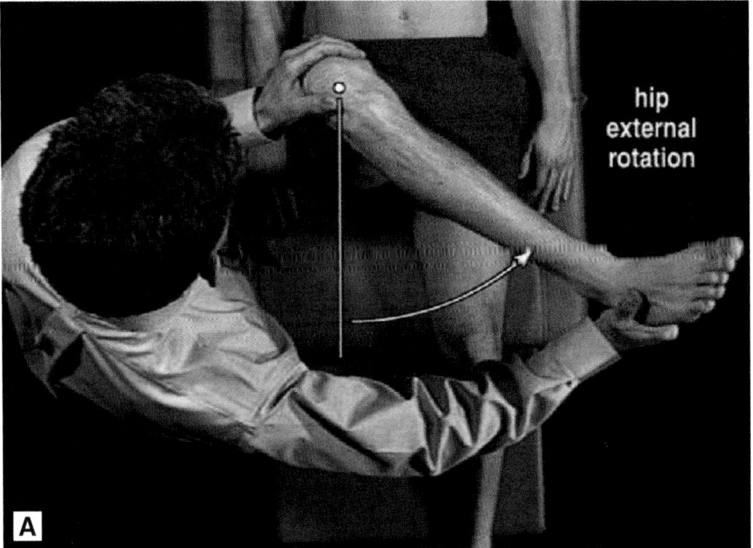

Fig. 3–23

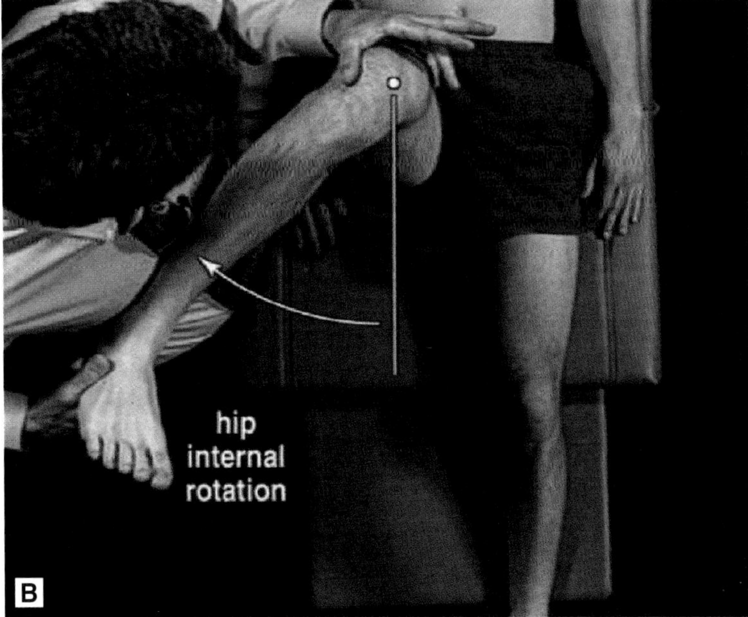

Fig. 3–23

Watch the patient's face while you perform hip rotation. A change in facial expression may be your first indication that hip range of motion is painful.

(*Note: In patients with total hip replacements, be cautious in assessing hip range of motion; flexion, adduction, and internal rotation may dislocate the femoral component.*)

During the hip examination, you can adjust a cover sheet to minimize patient exposure. Grasp the patient's heel and begin moving the thigh up toward the chest. With your left hand, reach under the patient's knee and grasp the sheet (Fig. 3–24A, B) and draw it across the perineum as you complete hip flexion (Fig. 3–25A, B).

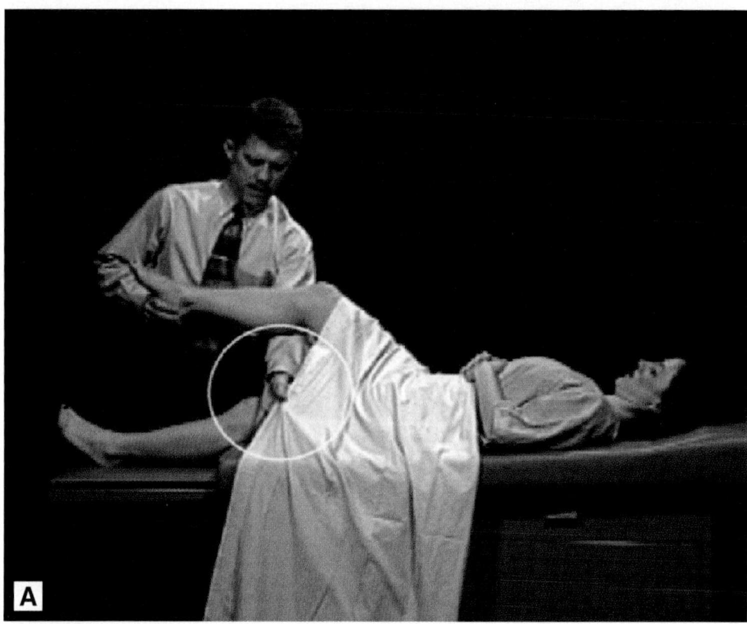

Fig. 3–24

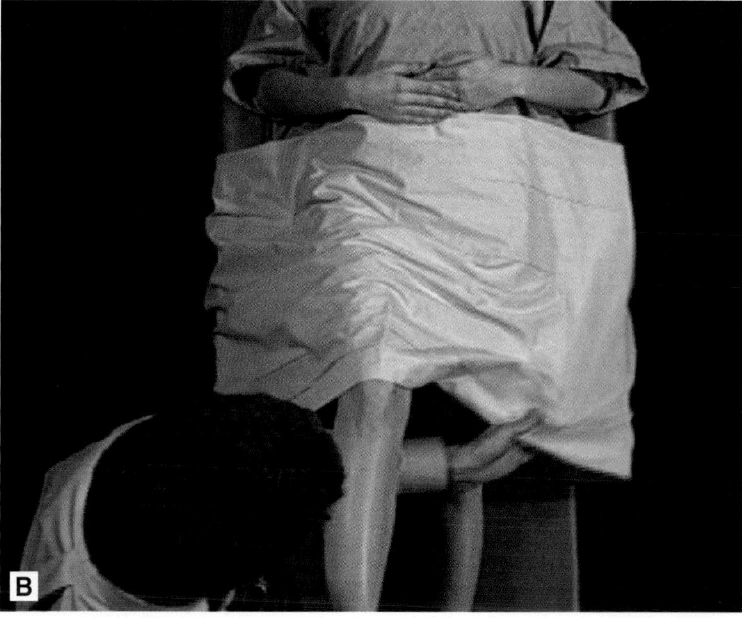

Fig. 3–24

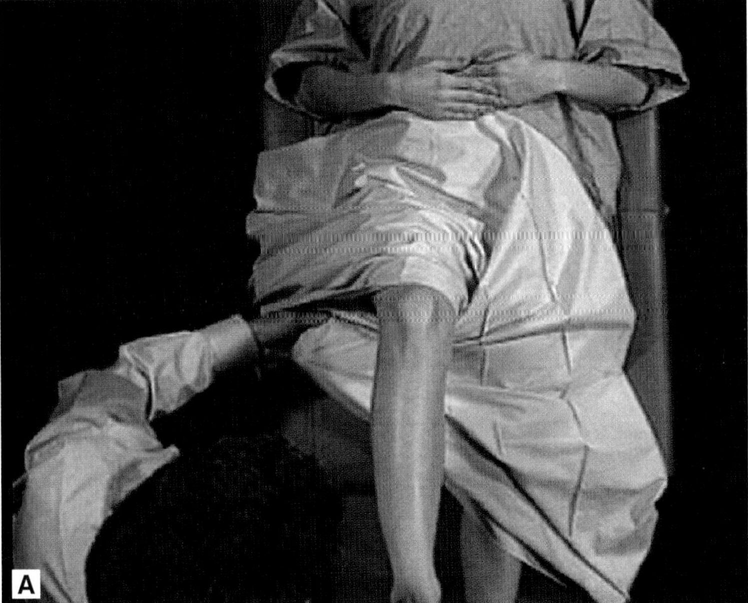

Fig. 3–25

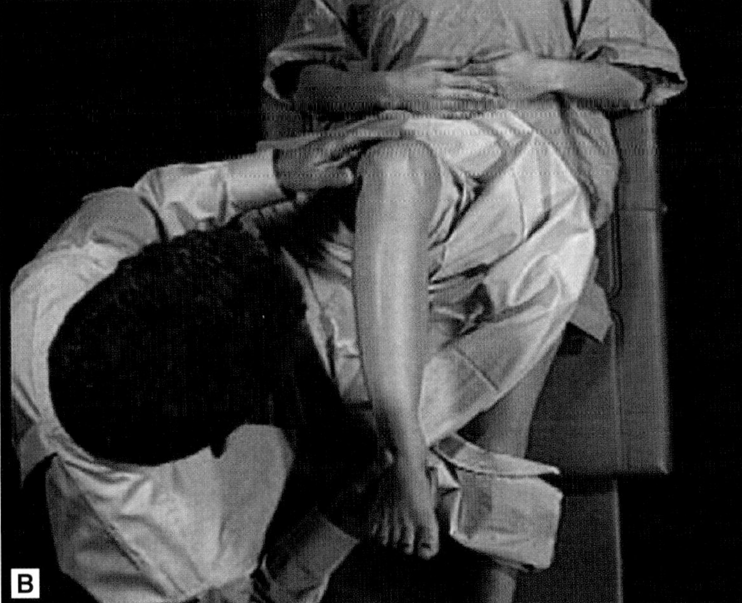

Fig. 3–25

Begin your examination of the **knees** by inspecting the quadriceps muscles for bulk and symmetry. Note any muscle atrophy. With the legs fully extended and the quadriceps muscles relaxed, inspect the knees and note any obvious deformity or visible swelling. Examine the prepatellar bursae. Swelling of the prepatellar bursa presents as visible or palpable distention directly in front of the patella. Note the soft tissue prominence below the patella on either side of the patellar tendon. This is the normal infrapatellar fat pad, usually more prominent in women (Fig. 3–26A, B).

Next, inspect the knee joint for any evidence of an effusion. Locate the normal depression that lies between the medial edge of the patella and the medial femoral epicondyle on the inner aspect of each knee. This depression is the first area to be obliterated by a knee effusion.

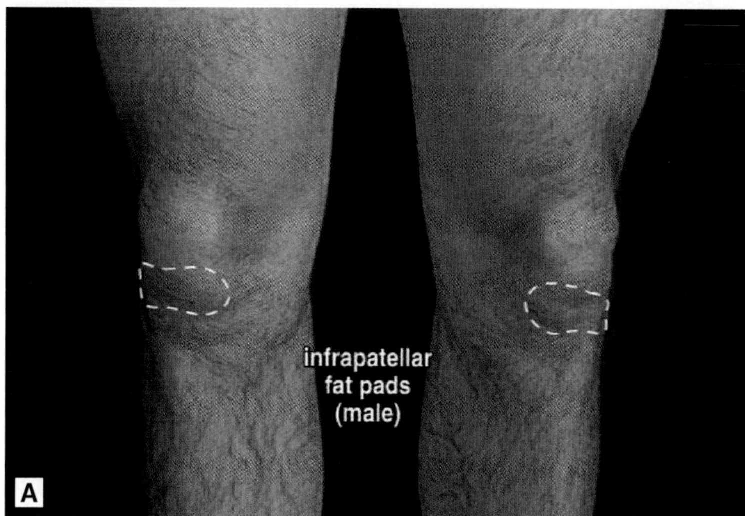

Fig. 3–26

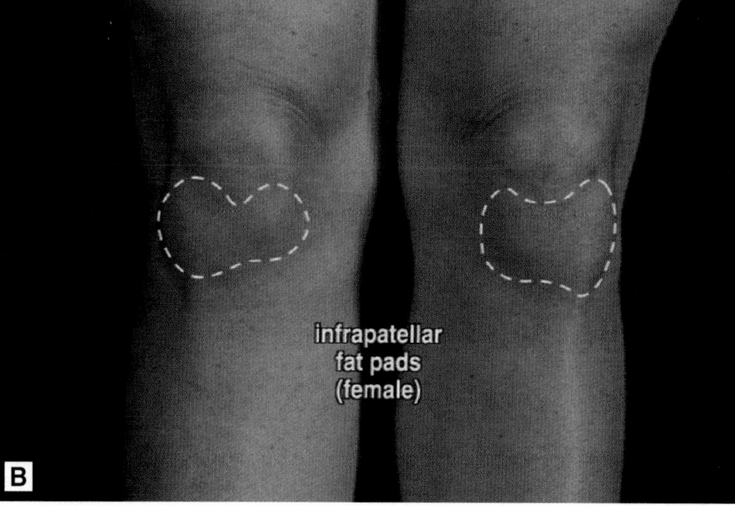

Fig. 3–26

SMALL EFFUSIONS

A small volume of synovial fluid will tend to pool medially, causing a slight bulge to develop where there was previously a normal concavity (Fig. 3–27A). A suspected small effusion can be readily confirmed by testing for a "bulge sign" (also known as a "fluid wave").

To check for a fluid wave in the patient's left knee, remain standing on the right side of the examination table and place the ring and little fingers of your right hand on the tibial tubercle. Place your right thumb on the medial aspect of the knee just below the level of the patella (Fig. 3–27B) and sweep your thumb in a cephalad and lateral direction, pushing any movable fluid from the medial sulcus of the joint into

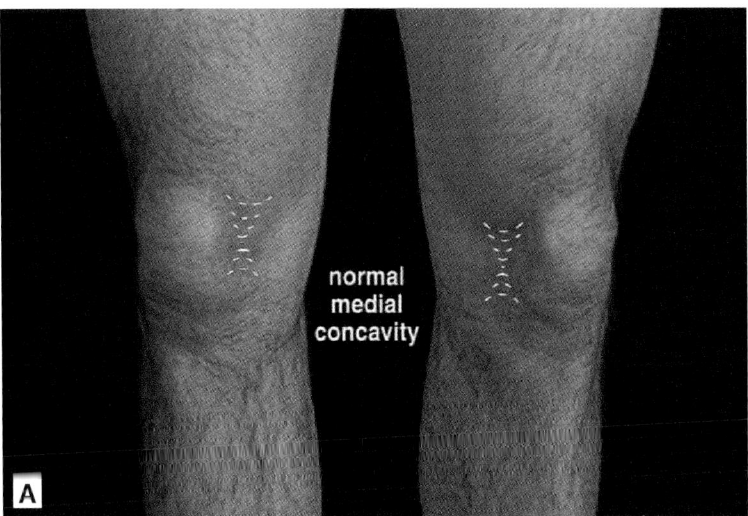

Fig. 3–27

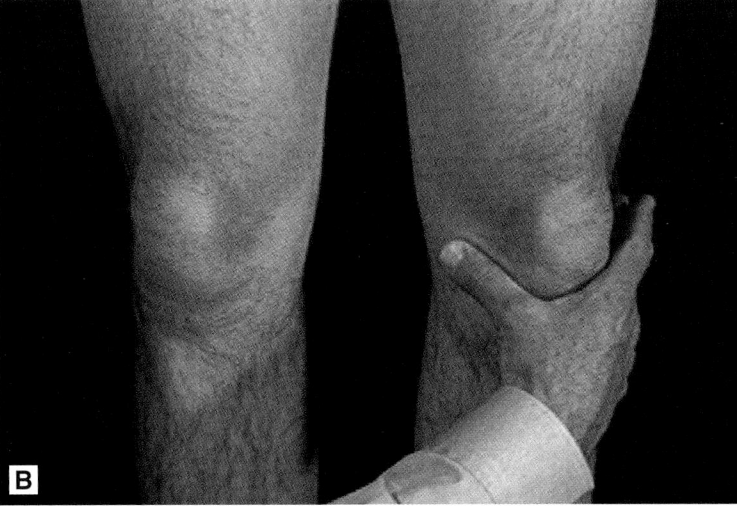

Fig. 3–27

the superolateral suprapatellar pouch (Fig. 3–28A). Your right ring and little fingers provide an excellent fulcrum against the tibial tubercle, as you sweep your right thumb in a superolateral direction. Keep your index finger fully extended (your thumb and index fingers forming a backward "L") to prevent inadvertently compressing the area into which you are attempting to move the joint fluid (Fig. 3–28A, B). Any fluid that has been moved to the opposite side of the joint will accumulate in the space which lies between the superior pole of the patella and the distal vastus lateralis (Fig. 3–28B). This area, the lateral "suprapatellar

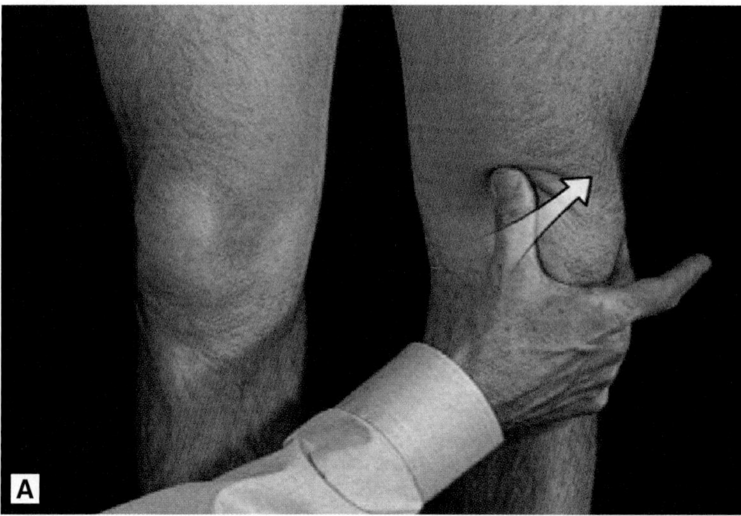

Fig. 3–28

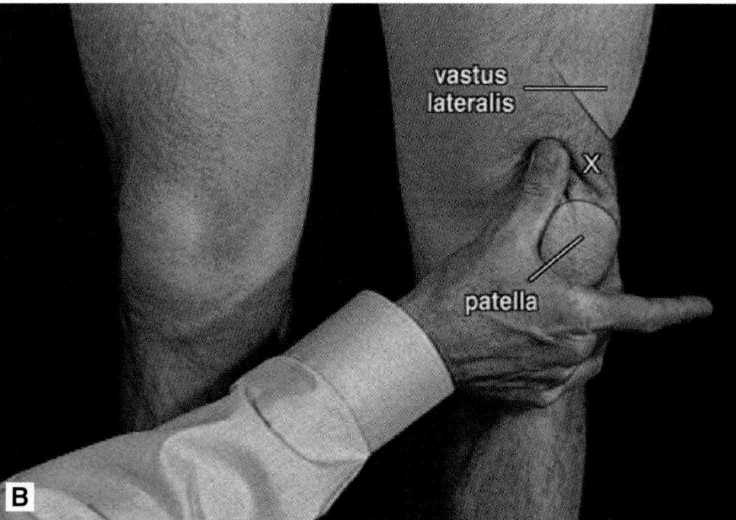

Fig. 3–28

pouch," can now be compressed using your right hand with your fingers fully extended (Fig. 3–29A), driving any fluid back across the joint, causing a visible bulge on the medial side (Fig. 3–29B).

To check for a fluid wave in the patient's right knee, remain standing on the patient's right side. Beginning just below the level of the patella, use your right or left hand with your fingers fully extended

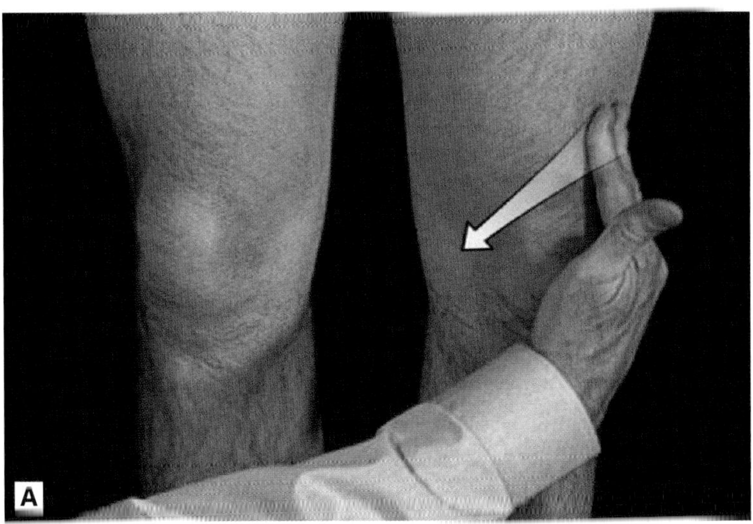

Fig. 3–29

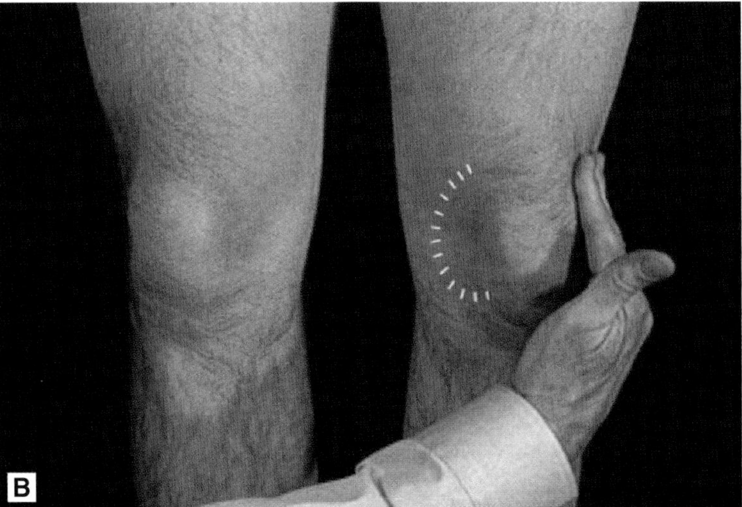

Fig. 3–29

to sweep the medial sulcus of the right knee in a cephalad and lateral direction (Fig. 3–30A). Fluid at the medial joint line will now be compressed and driven into the lateral suprapatellar pouch (Fig. 3–30B). Now use the flattened back of your right hand and compress the lateral suprapatellar pouch (Fig. 3–31A). Any fluid will now be driven back across the knee and appear as a bulge on the medial side (Fig. 3–31B). (Although it is possible to obtain a "bulge sign" using other methods, this technique is easy to perform and yields consistent results.)

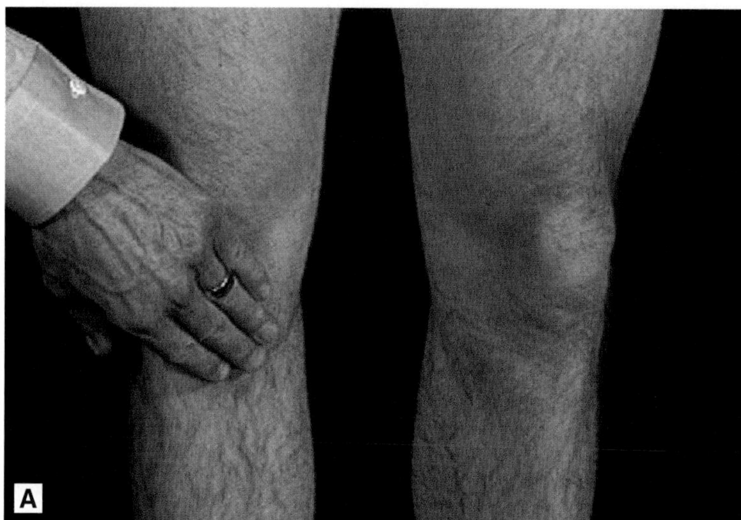

Fig. 3–30

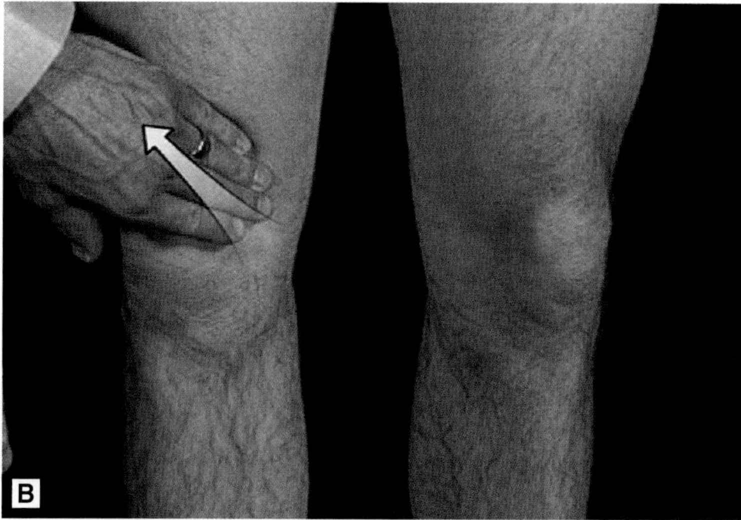

Fig. 3–30

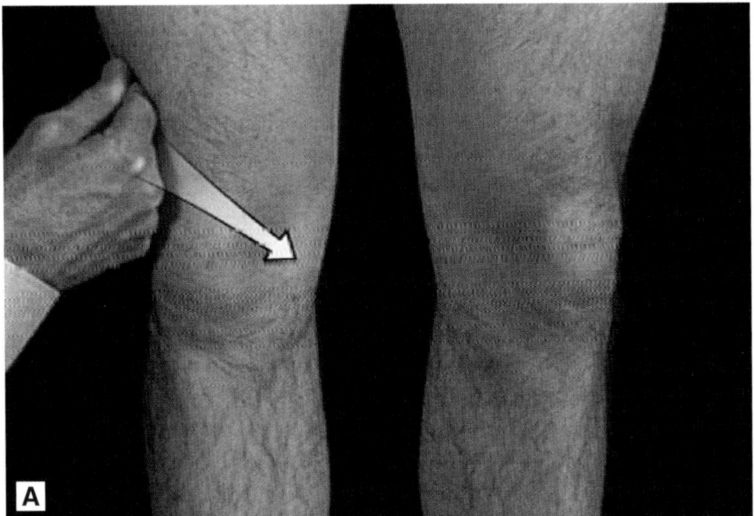

Fig. 3–31

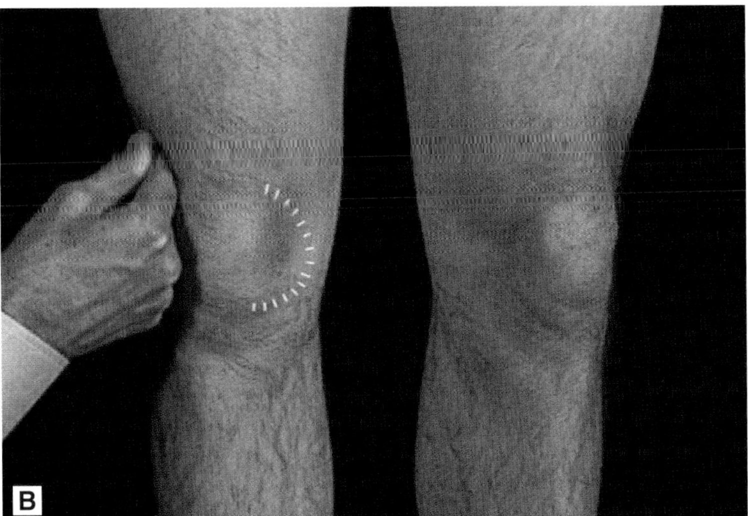

Fig. 3–31

MODERATE EFFUSIONS

The presence of a moderate knee effusion causes not only loss of the normal concavity at the medial joint line but also a visible bulge superolaterally (Fig. 3–32A). This bulge, in the "bare area" distal to the vastus lateralis, develops as fluid accumulates in the lateral suprapatellar pouch (Fig. 3–32B).

If a moderate effusion is suspected on visual inspection, you can confirm it by gently compressing the suprapatellar pouch with your left hand as you slide it inferiorly toward the patella. This will drive

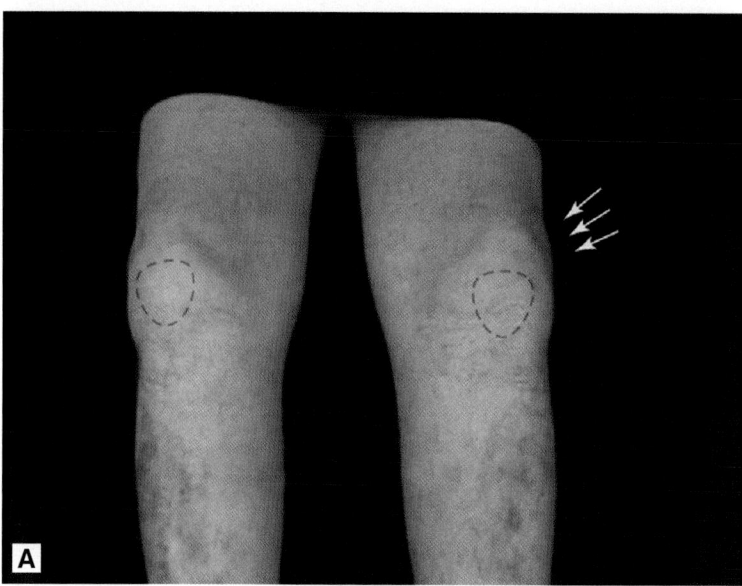

Fig. 3–32

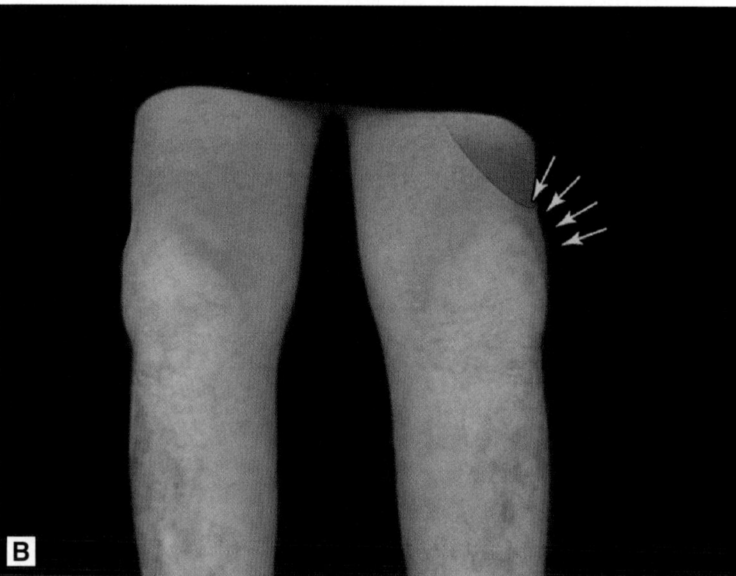

Fig. 3–32

any joint fluid centrally, beneath the patella, causing the patella to "float" above the intercondylar groove (Fig. 3–33A). With your left hand compressing the suprapatellar pouch medially, laterally, and superiorly, use your right index and middle fingers to apply several rapid, downward compressions to the patella (Fig. 3–33B). When sufficient fluid is present, you will feel a tapping or clicking sensation at the end of patellar compression, as the patella bounces off the femur. This is called a "patellar tap" or "ballotable patella" (Fig. 3–33C). This technique is performed in the same manner on both the right and left knees.

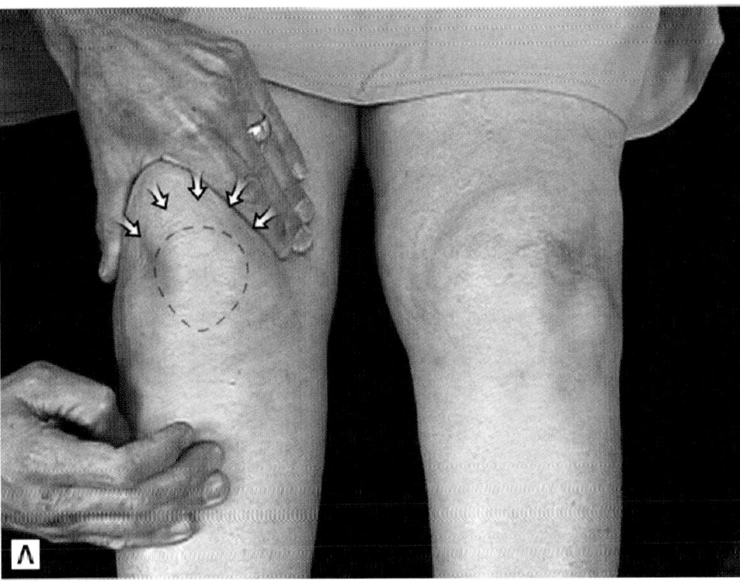

Fig. 3–33

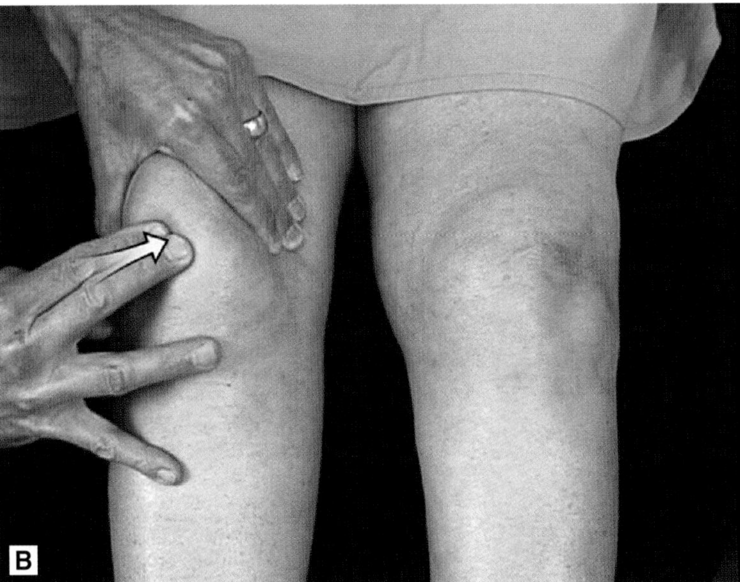

Fig. 3–33

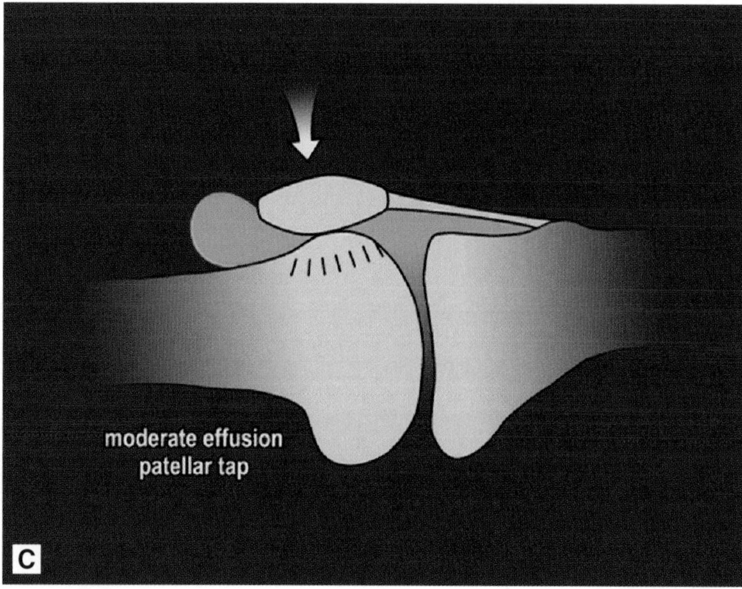

Fig. 3–33

LARGE EFFUSIONS

If a large knee effusion is present, it is usually most obvious on visual inspection. As expected, a large volume of synovial fluid will first cause loss of the normal concavity at the medial side of the knee, followed by a visible bulge superolaterally. In addition, however, a large knee effusion will cause visible distention of the *entire* suprapatellar pouch with visible and palpable bulging medially, superolaterally, and superiorly (Fig. 3–34A, B). Such gross distention usually makes it difficult to detect a fluid wave or even a ballotable patella with such a large, tense volume of fluid.

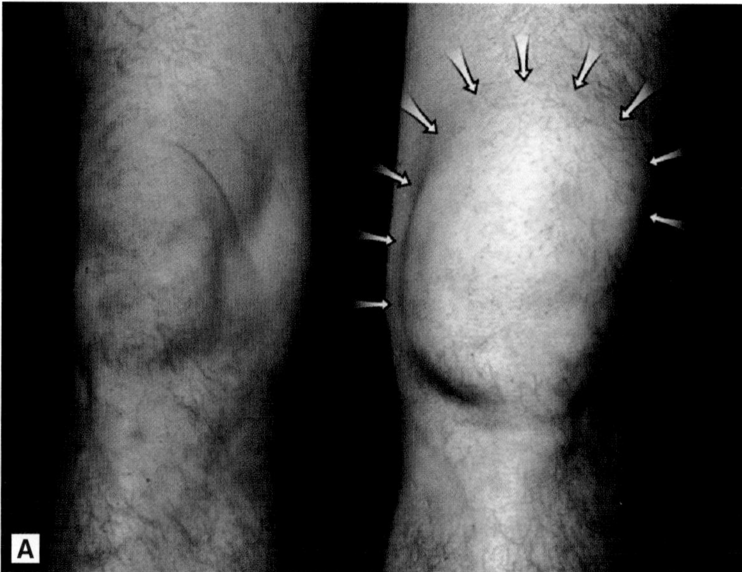

Fig. 3–34

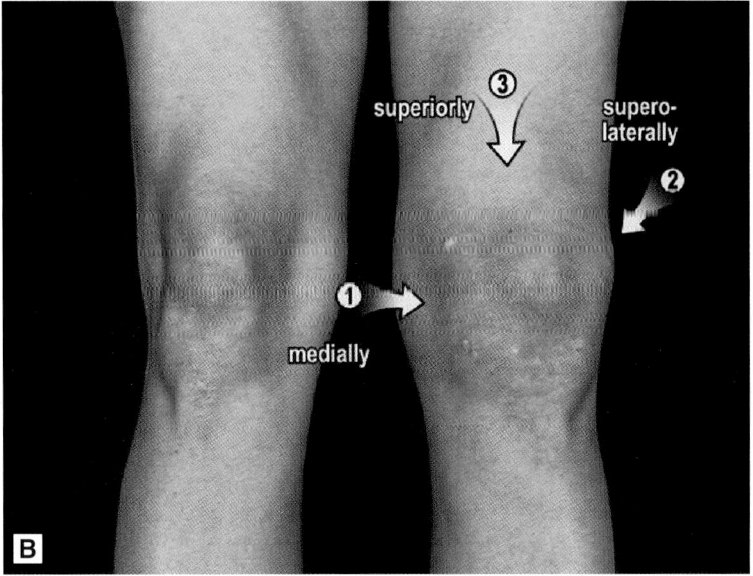

Fig. 3–34

Next, check the patellofemoral joint. Apply downward pressure on the patella, gently rocking it in the femoral groove (Fig. 3–35A). Note any tenderness or crepitus.

Now, check knee range of motion. Place your left hand over the patella while flexing and extending each knee (Fig. 3–35B). Note any patellofemoral crepitus. Full knee flexion brings the calf muscle against the posterior thigh. Full extension returns the joint to the outstretched anatomical position. While holding the leg off the table, look carefully for a flexion contracture (deficit in full extension).

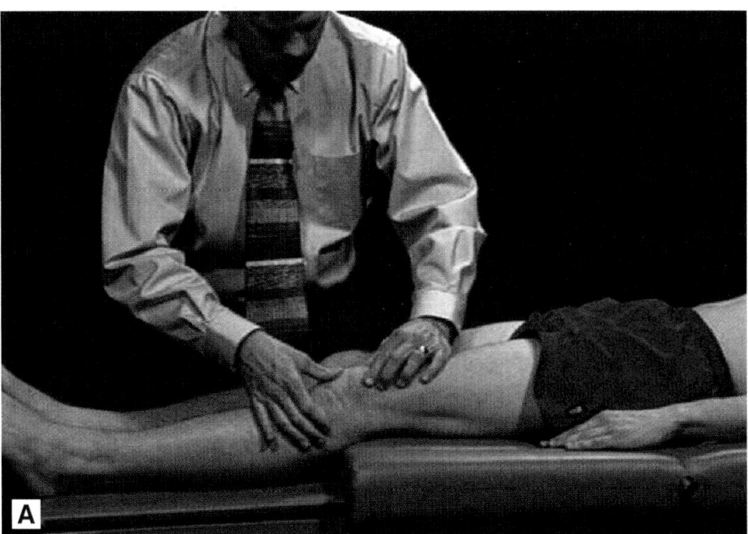

Fig. 3–35

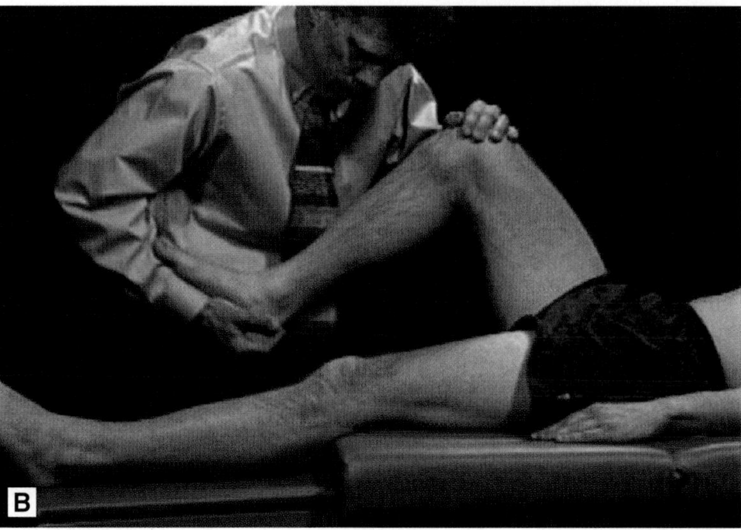

Fig. 3–35

If no effusion is present and range of motion is painless and full, no further evaluation may be necessary. However, if the patient has specific knee symptoms (pain or limited range of motion), a more detailed examination (RMSE) of the knee may be required.

Now inspect each **ankle** for any obvious deformity or visible swelling. Begin by inspecting and comparing each medial malleolus, lateral malleolus, and the anterior joint line for evidence of visible swelling (Fig. 3–36). Next, assess tibiotalar motion by checking ankle dorsiflexion and plantarflexion. Dorsiflex the ankle by applying pressure to the sole of the forefoot, bringing the foot up in a cephalad direction. Plantarflex the ankle by applying gentle pressure to bring the foot down in a plantar direction.

Now bring the ankle into the neutral position (0 degrees, with the foot perpendicular to the tibia). Grasp the heel with your right hand (Fig. 3–37A), supporting the sole of the foot against your forearm

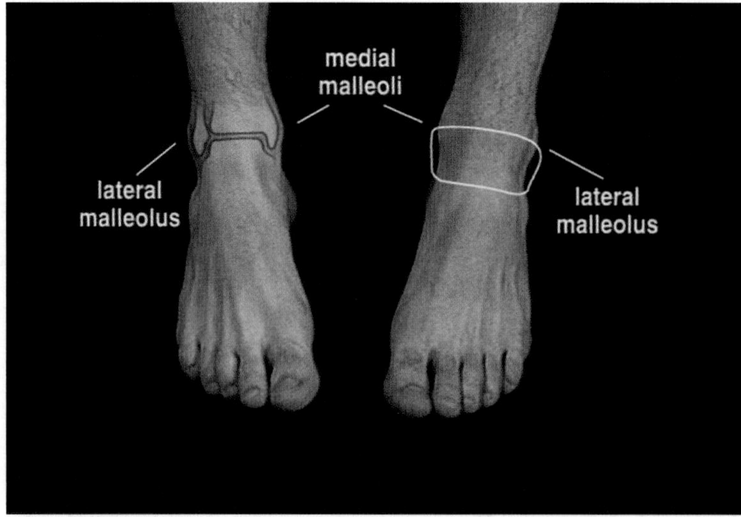

Fig. 3–36

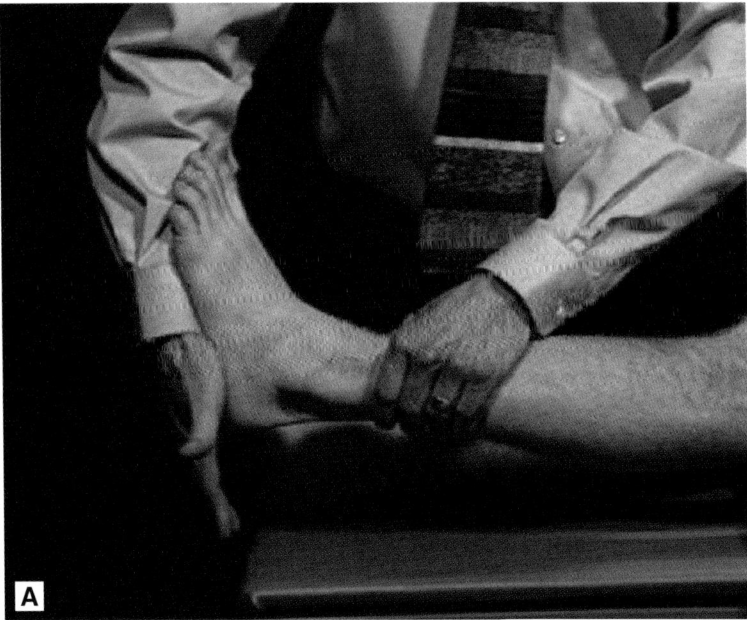

Fig. 3–37

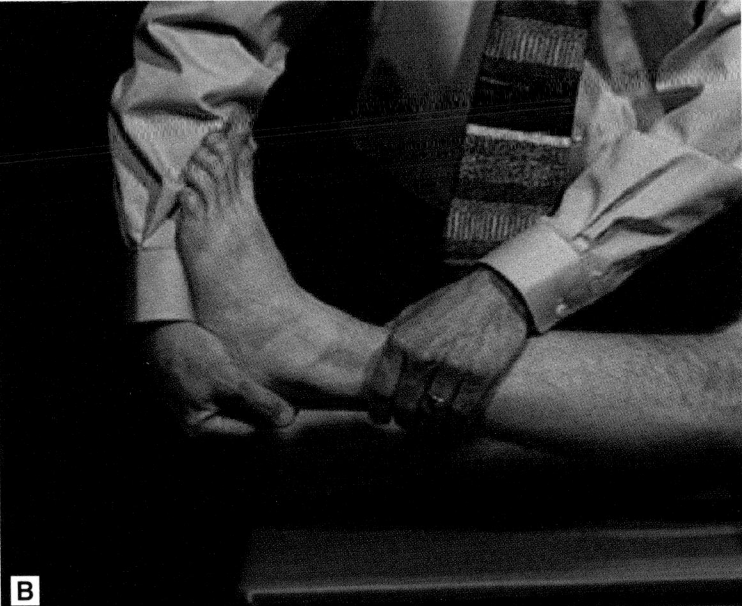

Fig. 3–37

(Fig. 3–37B). Test subtalar (talocalcaneal) motion by gently inverting (heel in) and everting (heel out) the heel (Fig. 3–38).

Now palpate the Achilles tendon and plantar fascia at each heel to assess for tenderness. Palpate the insertion site of the Achilles tendon by applying pressure with your index and middle fingers over the

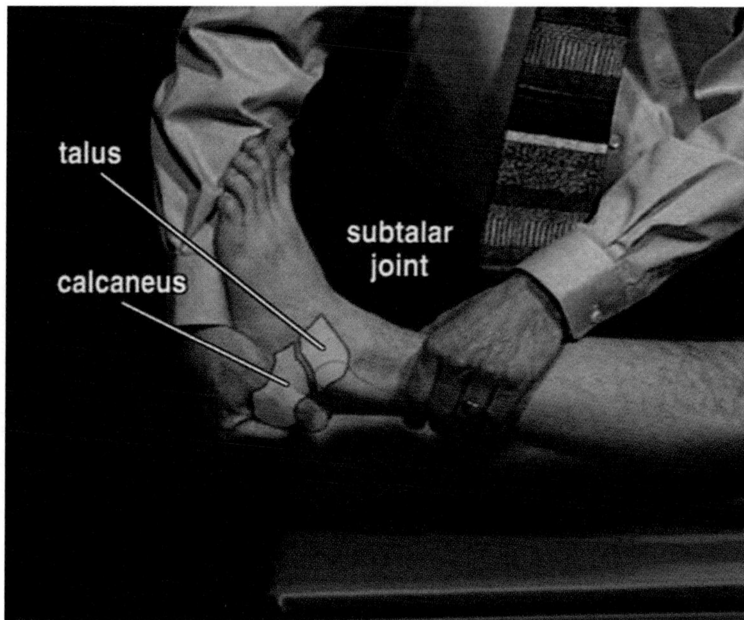

Fig. 3–38

posterior calcaneus (Fig. 3–39A). Palpate the insertion of the plantar fascia by applying pressure to the medial aspect of the plantar calcaneus on the sole of the foot (Fig. 3–39B).

Next, inspect each **midfoot**. The tarsometatarsal joints of the midfoot connect the hind foot to the forefoot (Fig. 3–40). Note any asymmetry or visible swelling.

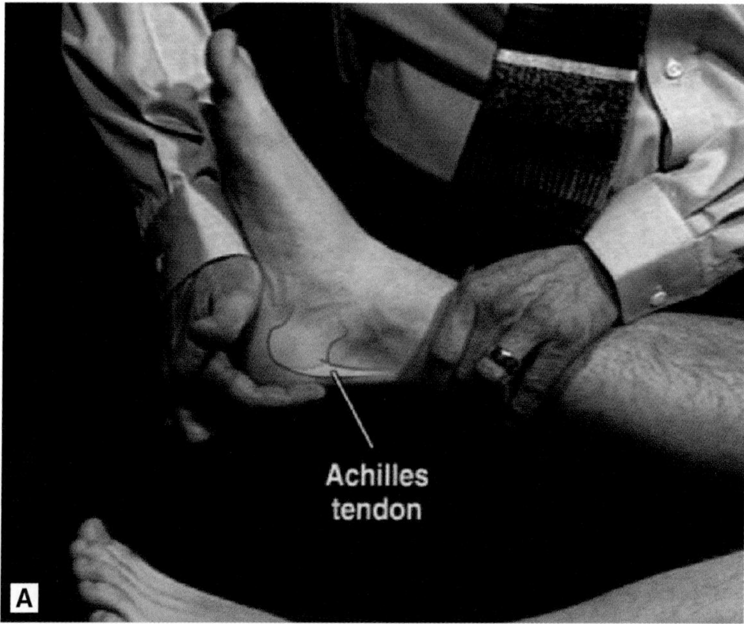

Fig. 3–39

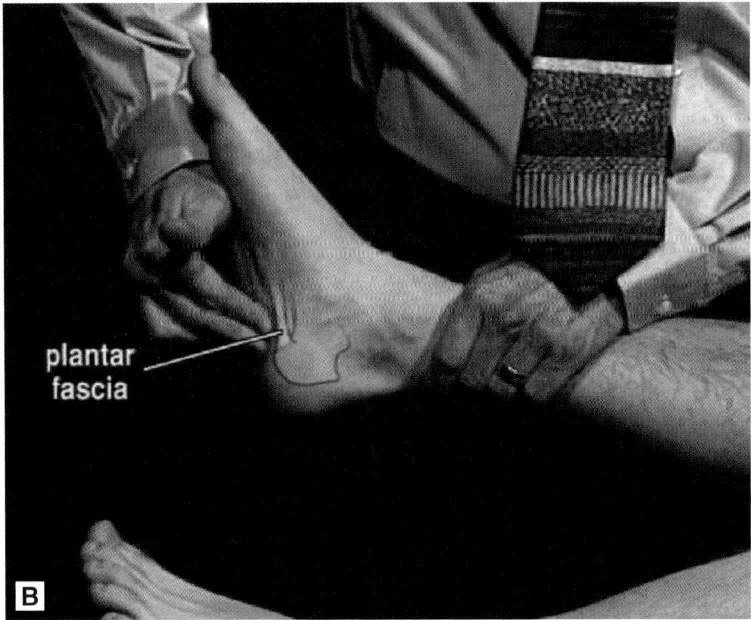

Fig. 3–39

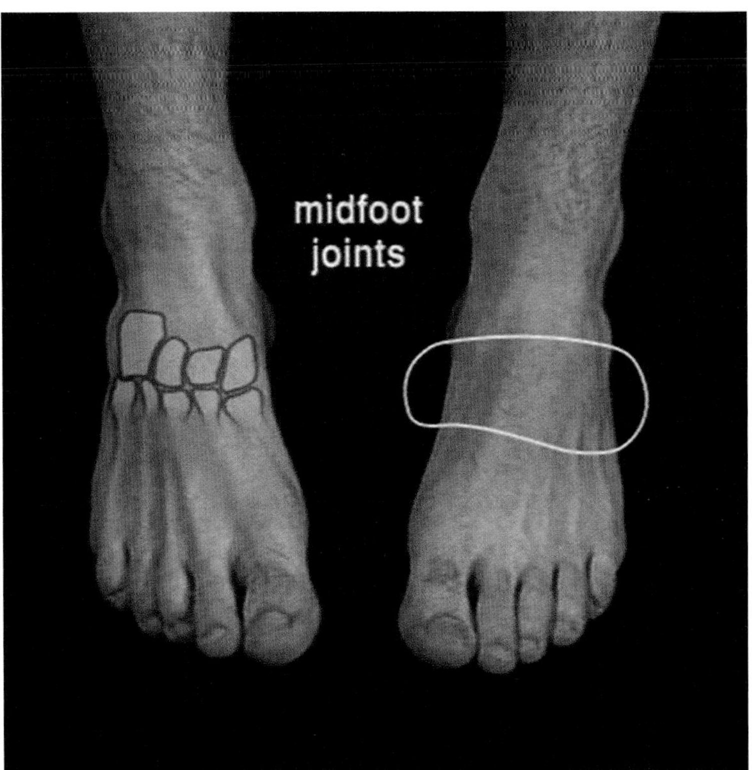

Fig. 3–40

Now inspect each **forefoot**. Note the dorsal surface just proximal to the web space of each toe (Fig. 3–41A). These normal shallow depressions may be absent if there is MTP joint synovitis, since this region directly overlies the metatarsophalangeal joints (Fig. 3–41B).

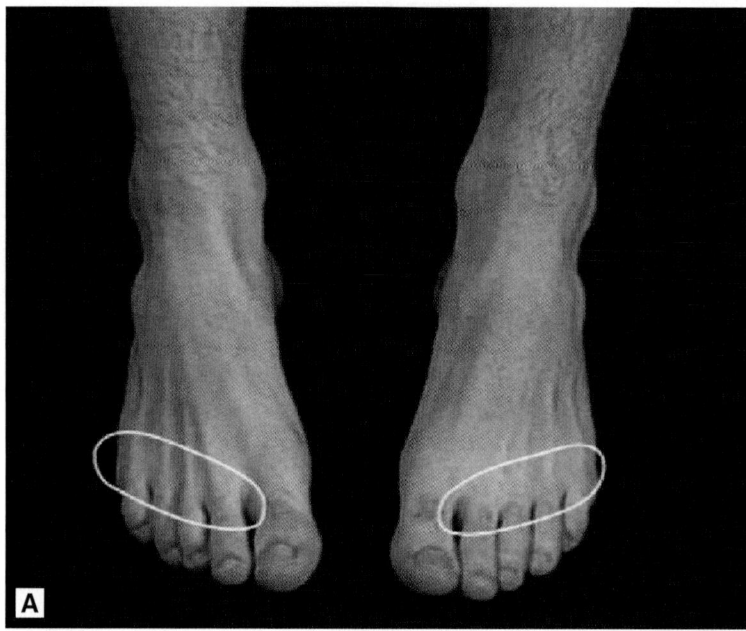

Fig. 3–41

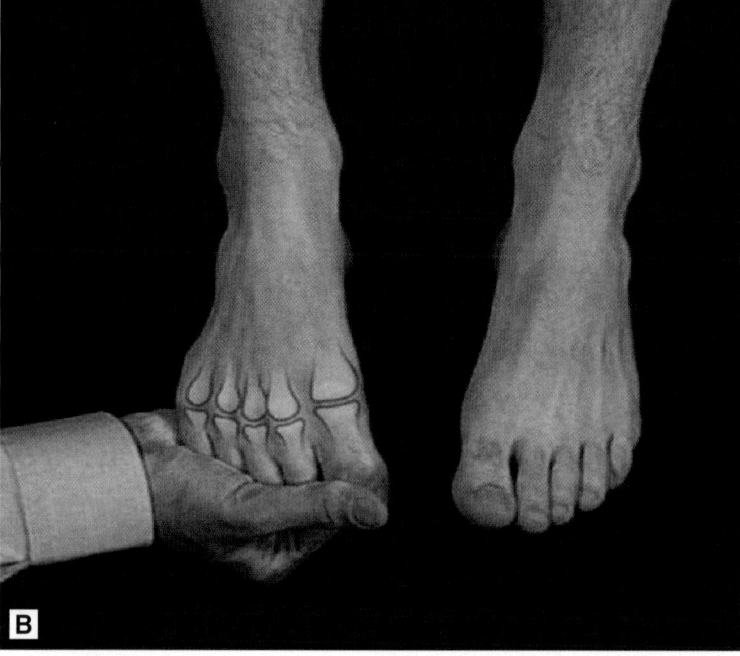

Fig. 3–41

Standing at the patient's right side, palpate the MTP joints of toes 5 through 2 on each foot.

Begin with the fifth toe. Using your index finger, apply firm pressure to the sole of the foot beneath each metatarsal head. This pressure will move each toe into plantar flexion, opening the joint space dorsally. Position your thumb to one side of the extensor tendon and identify the metatarsal head. While applying firm pressure on plantar side of the MT head with your index finger, move your thumb distally, sliding off the MT head, and your thumb will now be directly over the joint line (Fig. 3–42A). MTP joints can usually be felt dorsally as distinct, small depressions running perpendicular to the axis of the toes (Fig. 3–42B, C).

MTP joint synovitis usually results in a boggy or "squishy" feeling beneath your examining thumb, as the inflamed synovial membrane obscures the normally distinct bony margins dorsally. Occasionally,

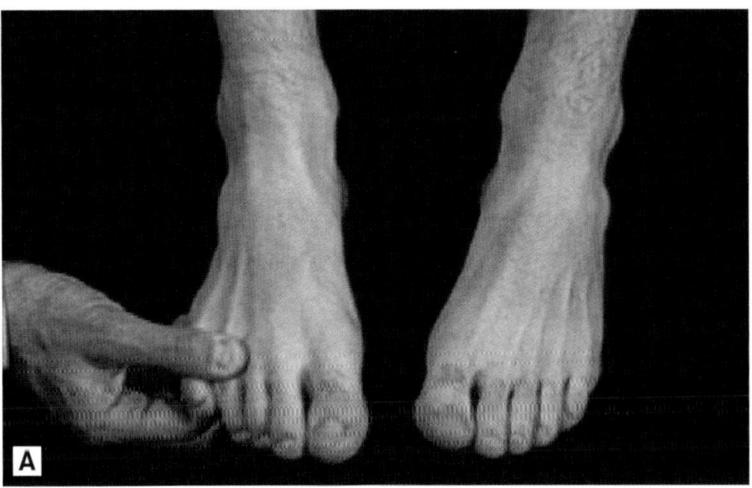

Fig. 3–42

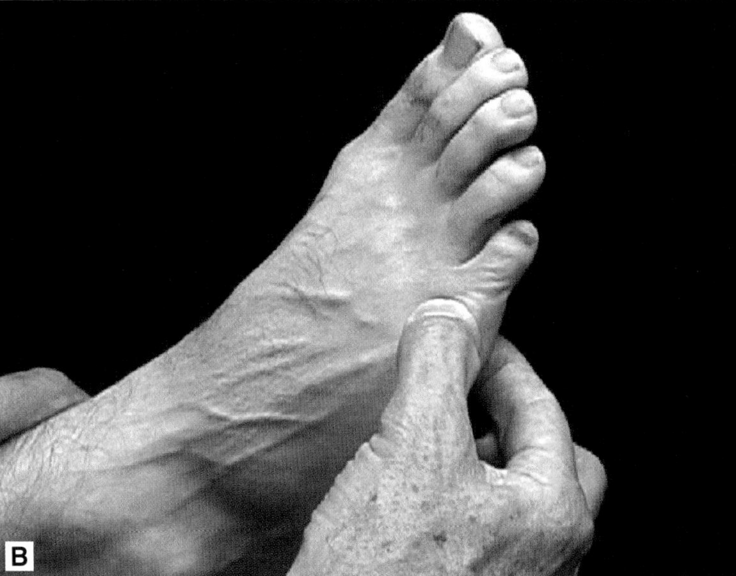

Fig. 3–42

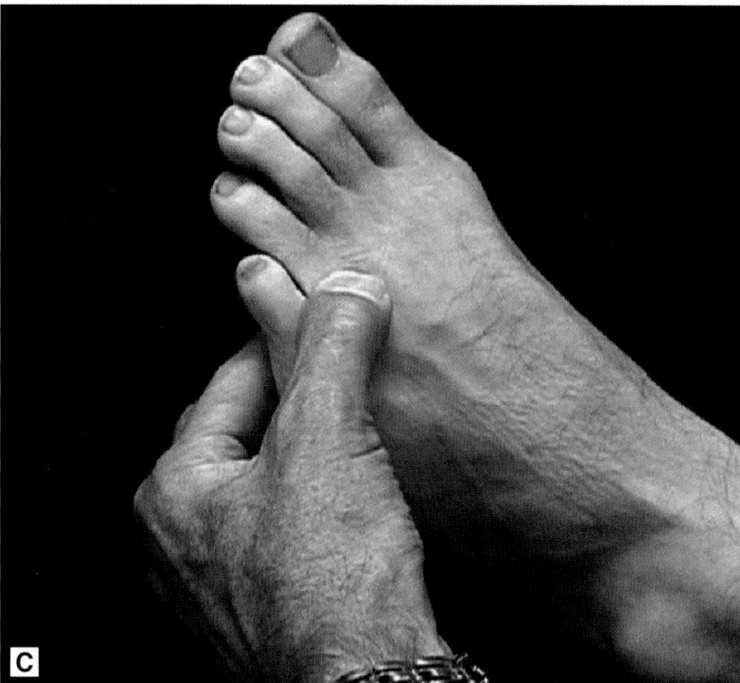

Fig. 3–42

despite proper technique, you will not be able to feel distinct MTP joint lines in normal patients, but there should be no bogginess beneath our thumb.

Use your right thumb and index finger to palpate the right forefoot and your left thumb and index finger to palpate the left forefoot.

(*Note: A systematic approach to palpating the finger joints is important. We suggest starting with digit 5, then 4, 3, and 2 of one hand followed by digit 5, then 4, 3, and 2 of the other. This will facilitate side-to-side comparison in an orderly sequence.*)

Next, palpate the MTP and IP joints of each **great toe**. Bringing the first MTP joint into slight flexion facilitates palpating the joint line (Fig. 3–43A).

The first MTP joint line itself lies distal to the bony prominence of the first metatarsal head (Fig. 3–43B). Palpating the first MTP joint can be facilitated by pulling on the great toe, in the plane of the foot. Palpate the great toe IP joint using your thumb and index finger (similar to the technique used for palpating the IP joint of the thumb).

Next, inspect the DIP and PIP joints of toes 2 through 5. Look for deformity, visible swelling, or asymmetry and compare side to side. Normally, there is a slight flaring of toes 2 through 5 from proximal to distal. Swelling of the DIP or PIP joints can result in disruption of this normal contour (for example, sausage digits). These abnormalities are easily overlooked unless careful visual inspection is performed. If any abnormality is suspected, briefly palpate those DIP and PIP joints.

Now, inspect the plantar surface of each foot, noting any calluses or ulcers.

Continue your examination of the lower extremities by asking the patient to stand. While observing from behind, note the alignment of knees during weight bearing. Inspect the calf muscles for bulk and symmetry, noting any muscle atrophy.

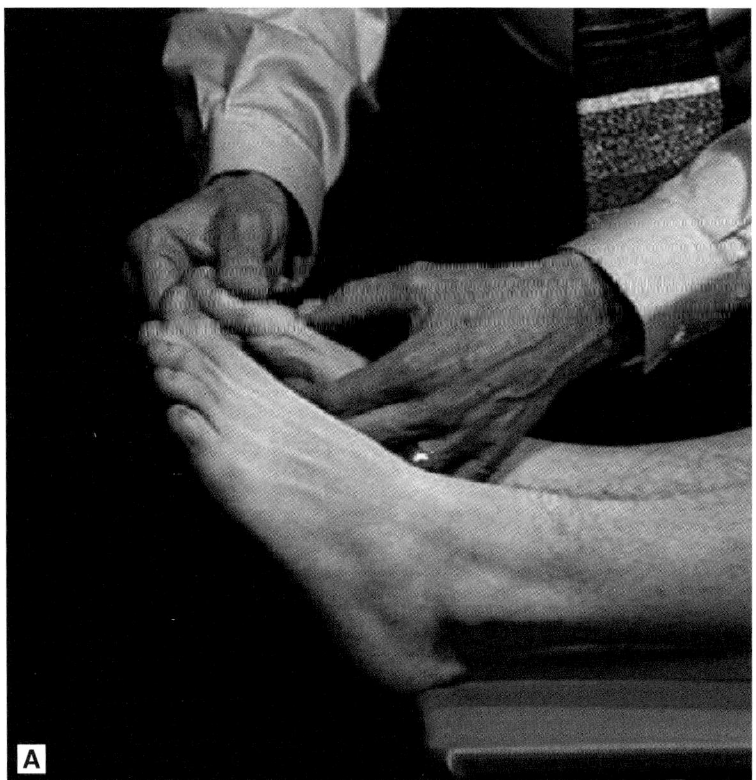

Fig. 3–43

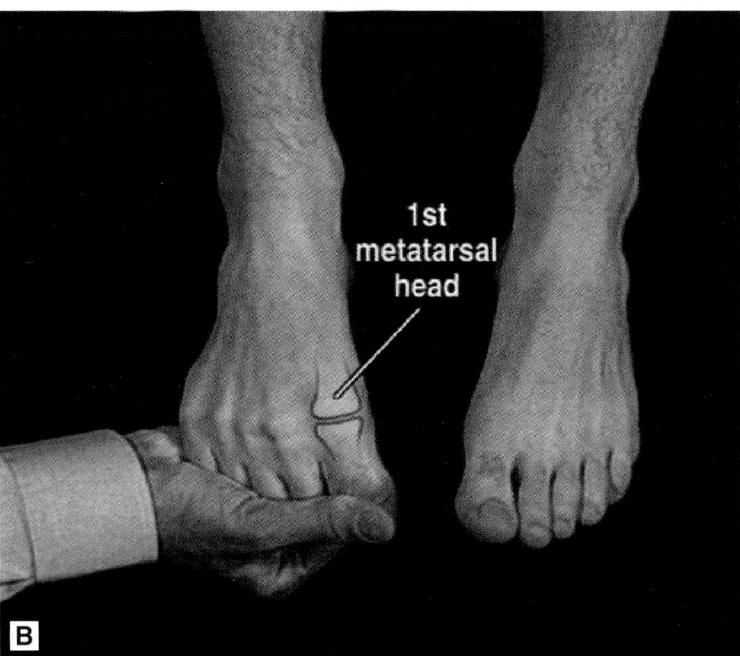

Fig. 3–43

Now, note the alignment of the heels and feet. Inspection of the heels should reveal symmetrical, vertical alignment. Observation of the feet from behind should normally permit visualization of the lateral toes 2 through 3.

Now, with the patient standing examine the **spine**.

Observe the alignment of the head and **neck** and note any abnormality. Assess neck flexion by asking the patient to touch his chin to the chest (Fig. 3–44A).

Assess neck extension by asking the patient to look up at the ceiling (Fig. 3–44B).

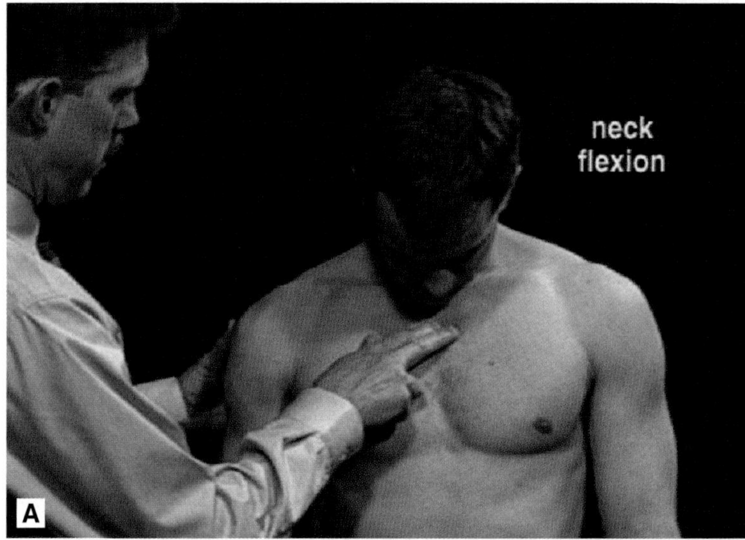

Fig. 3–44

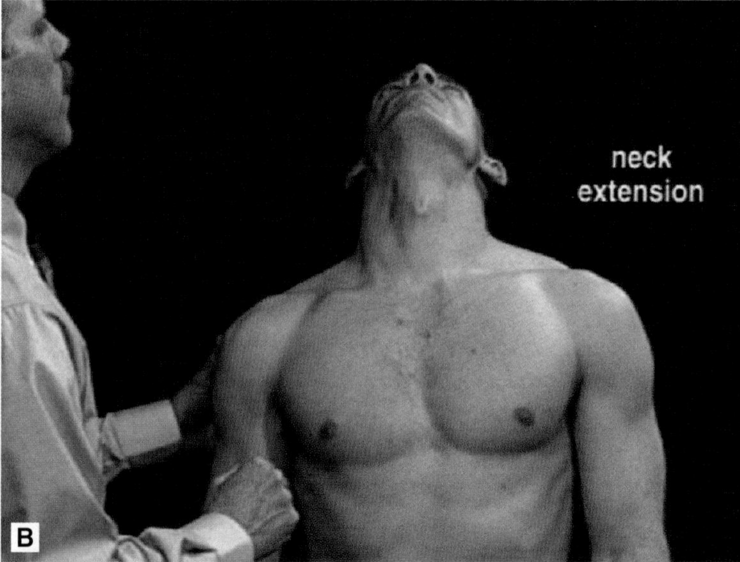

Fig. 3–44

Observe right and left rotation by asking the patient to place his chin on each shoulder (Fig. 3–45A). Assess lateral flexion (lateral bending) by asking the patient to incline his ear toward each shoulder (Fig. 3–45B).

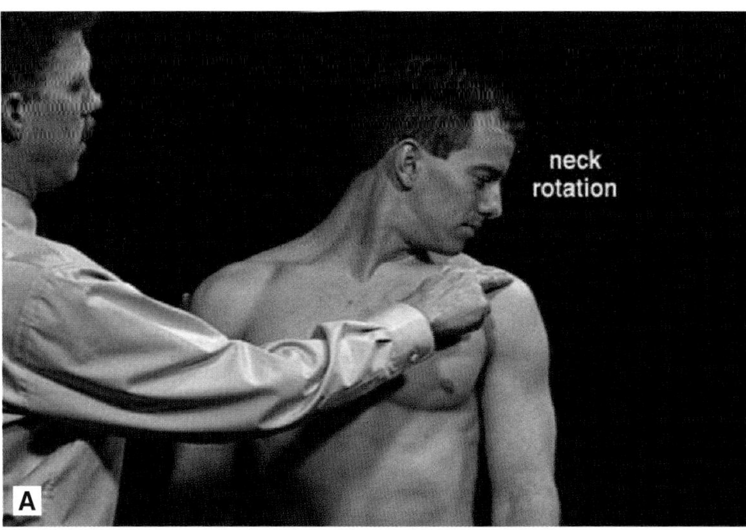

Fig. 3–45

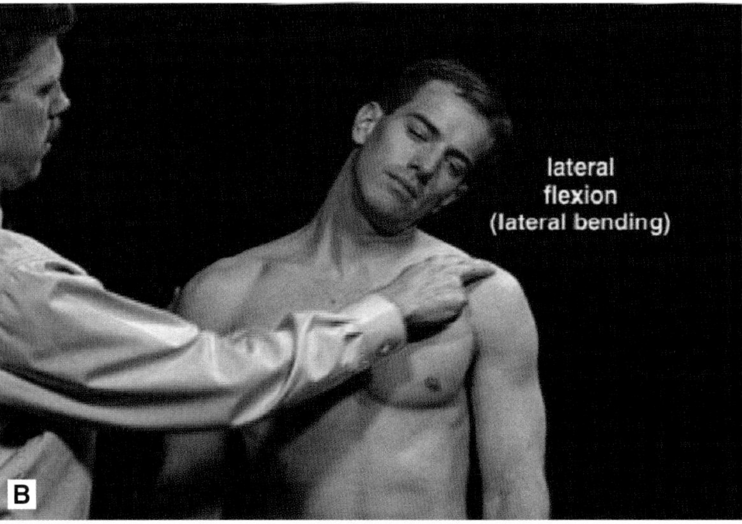

Fig. 3–45

Now while observing the patient from behind, inspect the **thoracolumbar** spine. Note any resting asymmetry or deformity and inspect for the normal resting lumbar lordosis (Fig. 3–46A).

Observe **lumbar** flexion by instructing the patient to bend forward at the waist and touch the toes. Normal lumbar flexion should involve progressive reversal of the lumbar curvature from lumbar lordosis in the standing position, to flattening of the lordosis in midflexion (Fig. 3–46B), to slight lumbar kyphosis

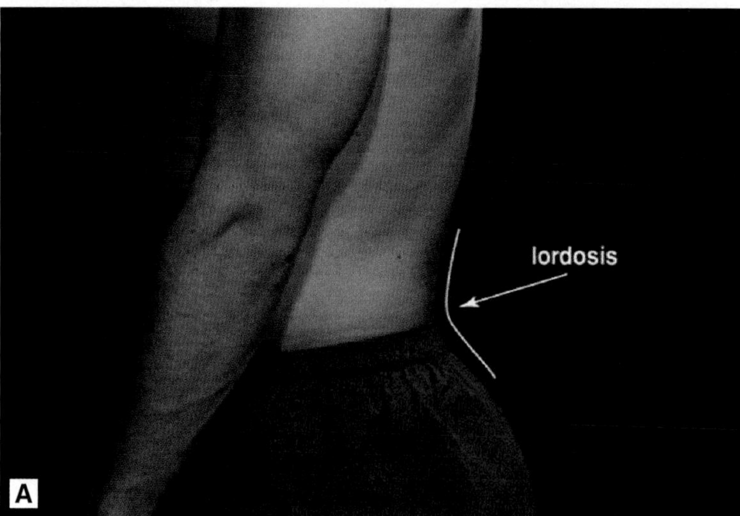

Fig. 3–46

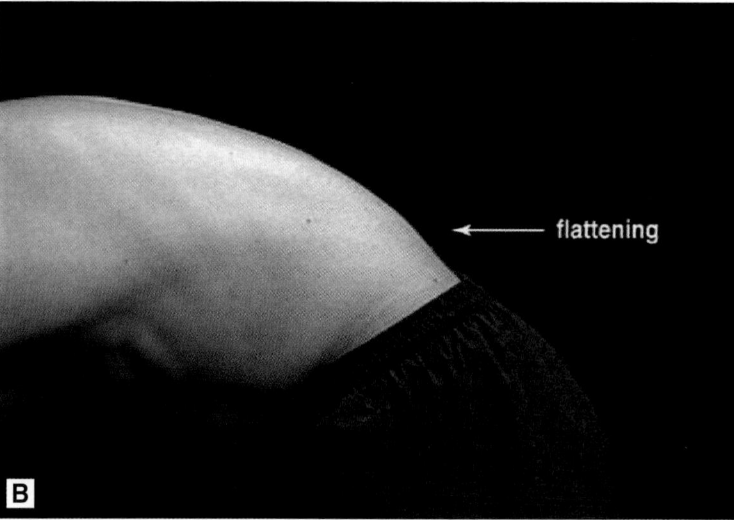

Fig. 3–47

at the end of full flexion (Fig. 3–47A). (Normal lumbar flexion brings the wrists to approximately the level of the knees, while hip flexion permits the additional movement involved in toe touching.)

Observing the patient from behind in full lumbar flexion allows you to inspect for evidence of scoliosis by noting any asymmetry or prominence of the posterior rib cage on either side (caused by the significant rotatory component of scoliosis usually present) (Fig. 3–47B).

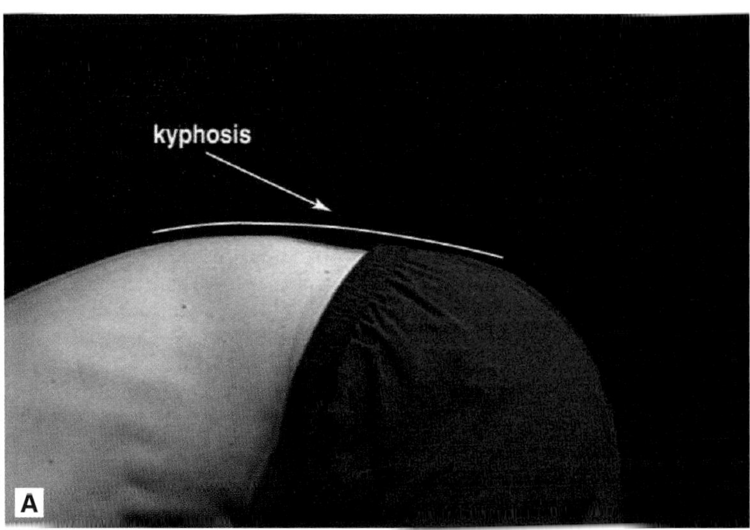

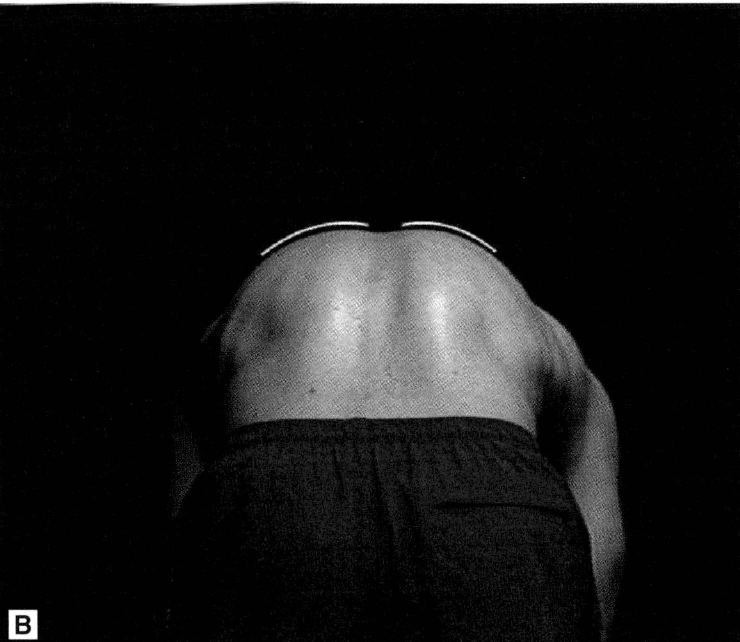

Fig. 3–47

Assess lumbar extension by asking the patient to bend backward. Simultaneously supporting one shoulder and the low back permits you to help the patient into full extension (Fig. 3–48A). Assess lumbar lateral flexion (lateral bending) by asking the patient to bend to the right and to the left (Fig. 3–48B). (Normally this maneuver brings the fingertips to approximately the level of the knees on each side.)

Next observe the patient's **gait**. The normal cyclical movement of walking can be divided into two phases: the swing phase, when the foot is swinging forward, and the stance phase, when the foot is in contact with the ground. Observe these phases while checking for any limp, uneven rhythm, or asymmetry of gait (Fig. 3–49).

Next, if appropriate in patients presenting with diffuse musculoskeletal pain or suspected fibromyalgia, evaluate the patient for the presence or absence of paired soft tissue fibromyalgia **tender points** (Fig. 3–50).

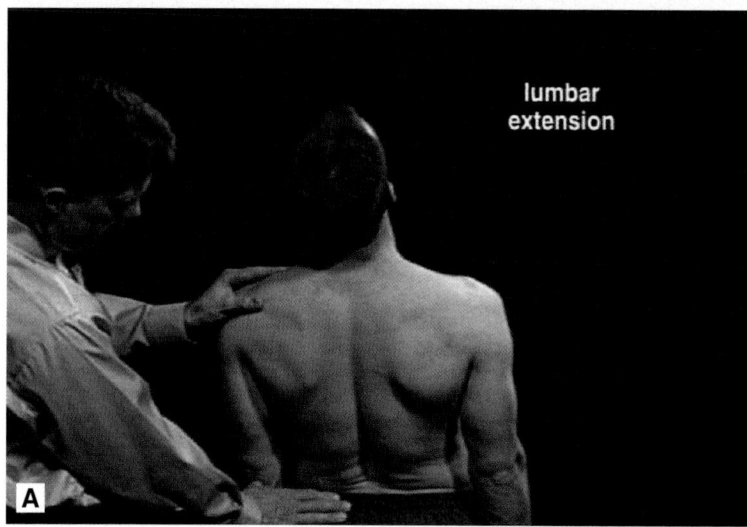

Fig. 3–48

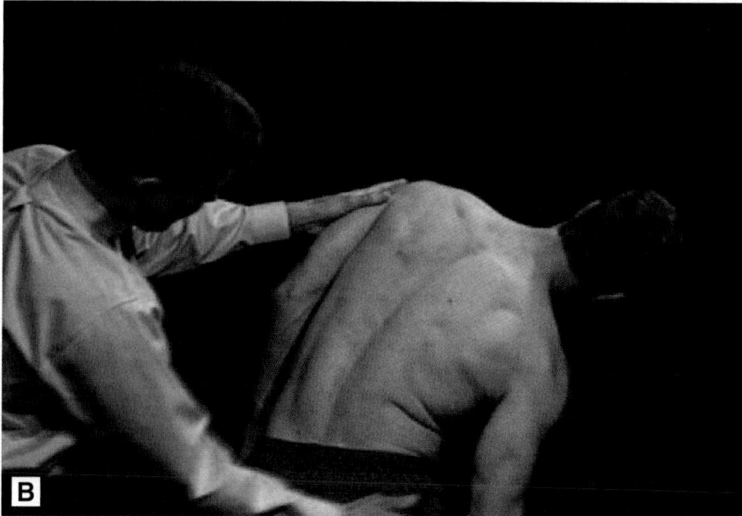

Fig. 3–48

Stance phase

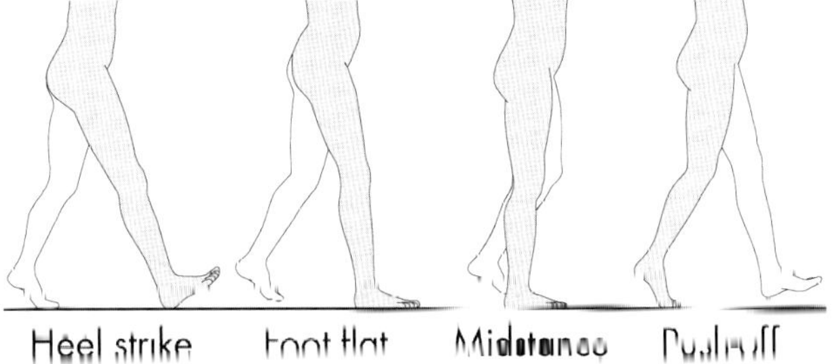

Heel strike

Swing phase

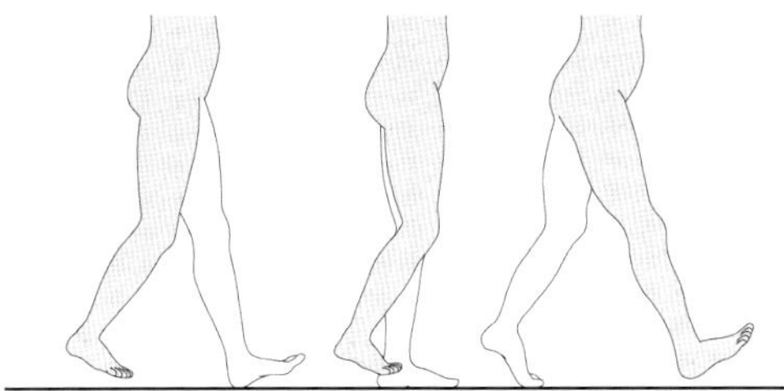

Acceleration Midswing Deceleration

Fig. 3–49

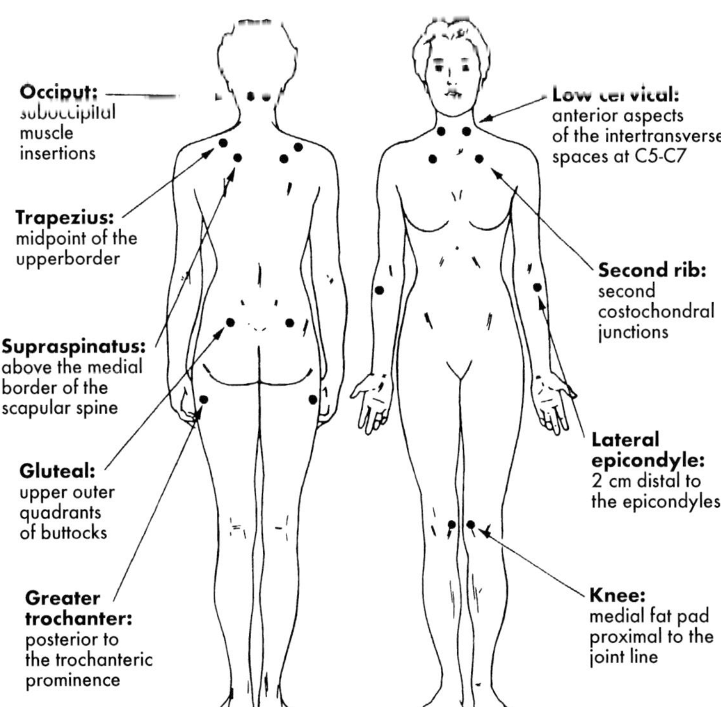

Fig. 3–50. The location of the nine paired tender points that comprise the 1990 ACR criteria for fibromyalgia. Primer on the Rheumatic Diseases, 12 ed. 2001:188. *(Reprinted with permission of the Arthritis Foundation 1330 W. Peachtree St. Atlanta, GA 30309.)*

The assessment for fibromyalgia tender points can be organized in a brief, sequential, and efficient manner as follows: Begin your assessment by establishing the patient's overall pain threshold. Use moderate finger pressure sufficient to blanch your fingernail bed (Fig. 3–51A, B). Beginning at the wrist, apply thumb pressure to the forearm extensor surface at two or three points distal to the elbow

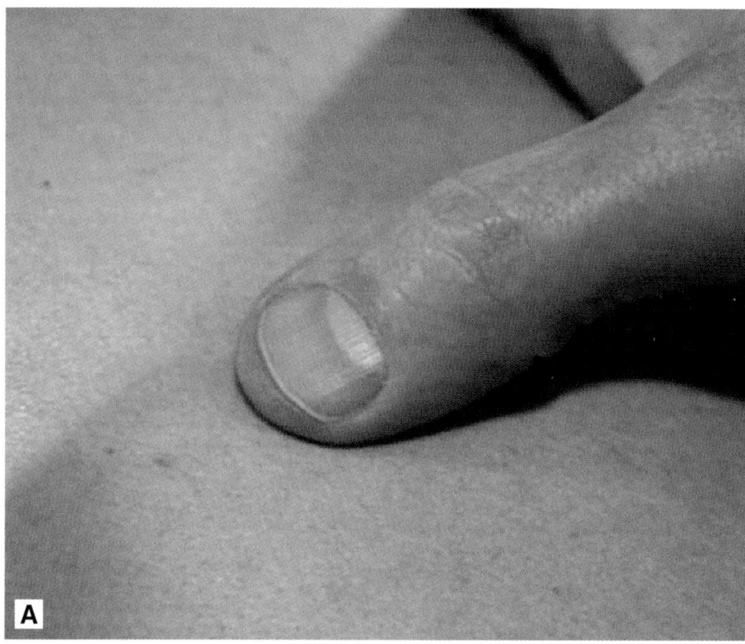

Fig. 3–51

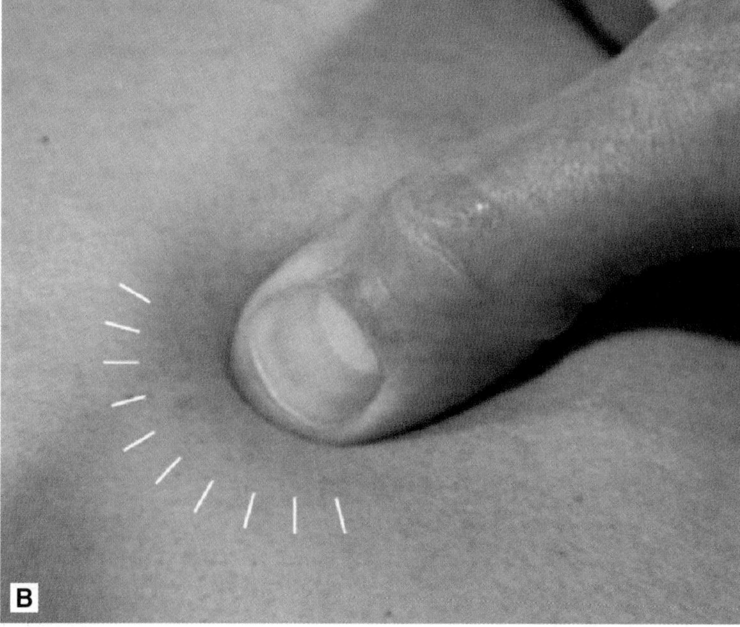

Fig. 3–51

(Fig. 3–52A). While palpating for tenderness, ask the patient: "Does this feel like pressure or pain?" Most patients with fibromyalgia experience pressure more distally but have significant pain and tenderness at the tender point of the forearm extensor muscles, just distal to the lateral epicondyle (Fig. 3–52B). Next, assess for tenderness at the manubriosternal joint. Apply moderate pressure centrally in

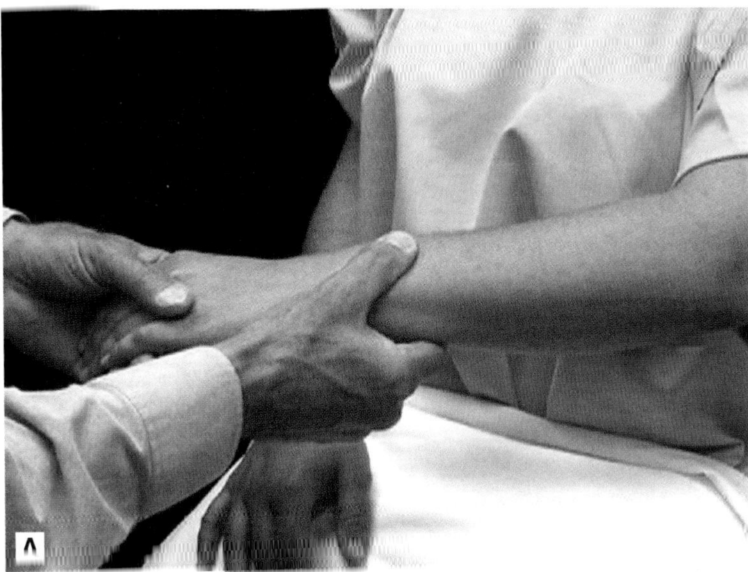

Fig. 3–52

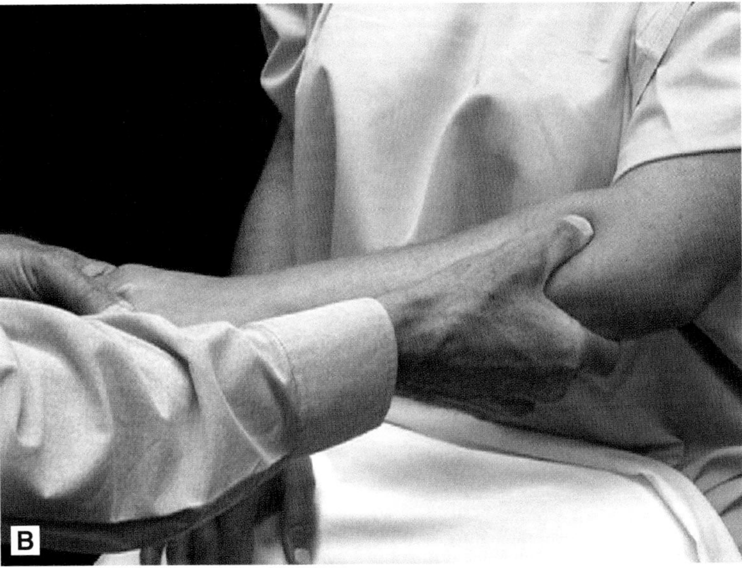

Fig. 3–52

the midline (Fig. 3–53A), often appreciated by the patient only as pressure, then move laterally to assess the second costosternal articulations, frequently associated with wincing and withdrawal of the chest from beneath the examiner's fingers in patients with fibromyalgia (Fig. 3–53B). Next, palpate the suboccipital muscle insertions, posteromedial to the mastoids on each side (Fig. 3–54). Note any tenderness.

Move your fingers to the midpoint of the upper trapezius and assess for local tenderness on each side (Fig. 3–55). Next, move your fingers slightly laterally and inferiorly to the origin of the supraspinatus,

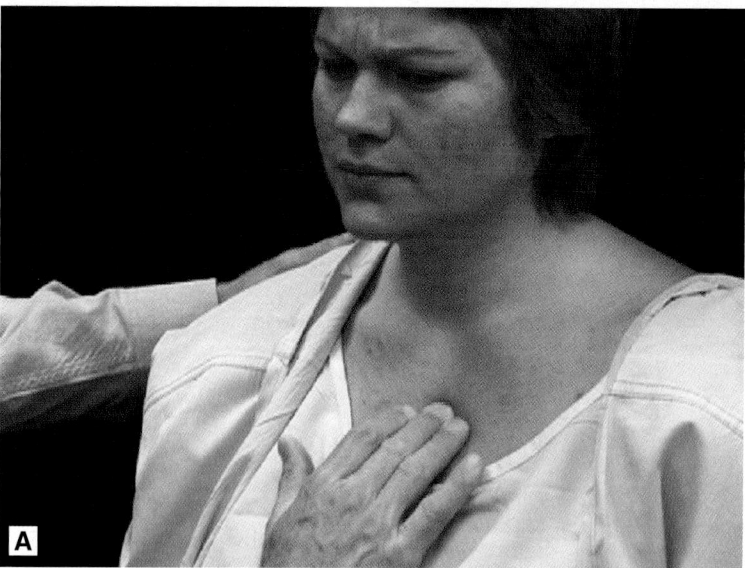

Fig. 3–53

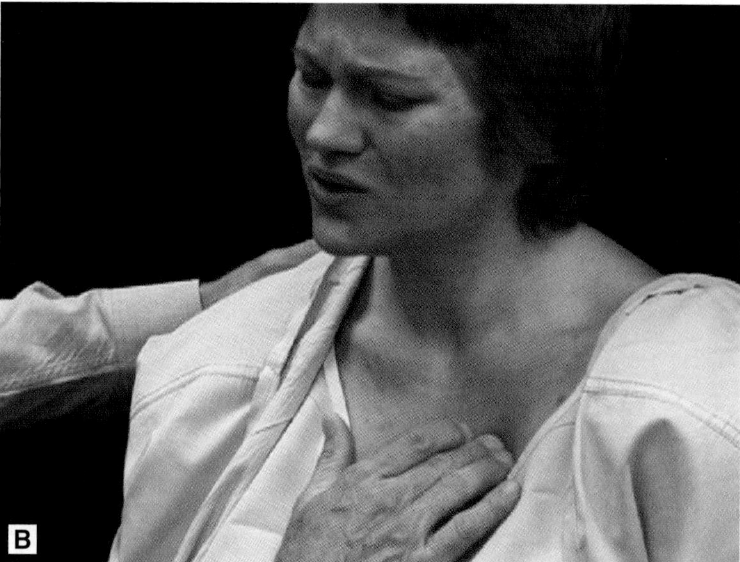

Fig. 3–53

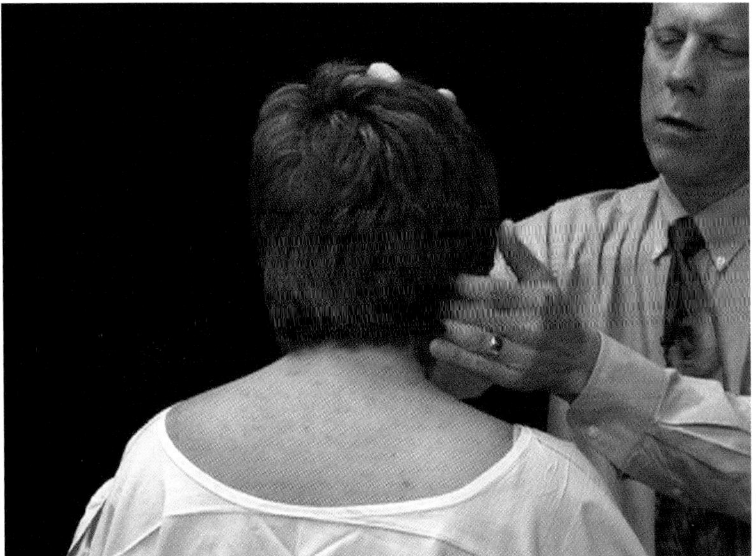

Fig. 3–54

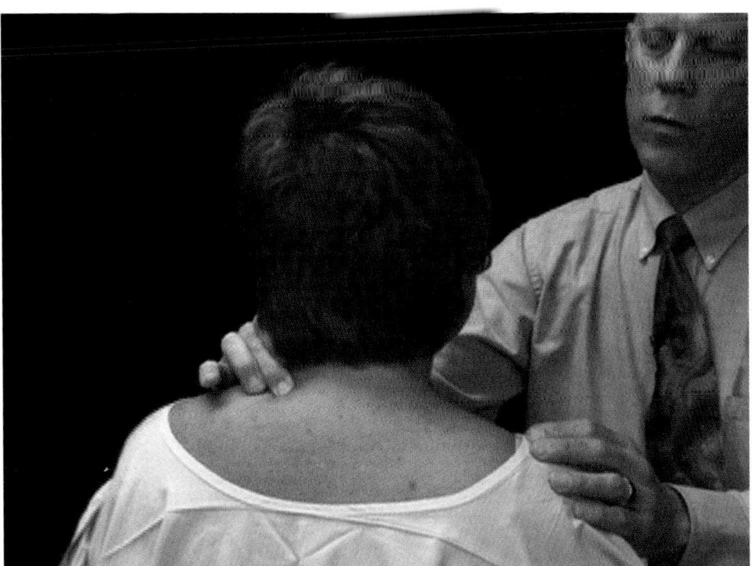

Fig. 3–55

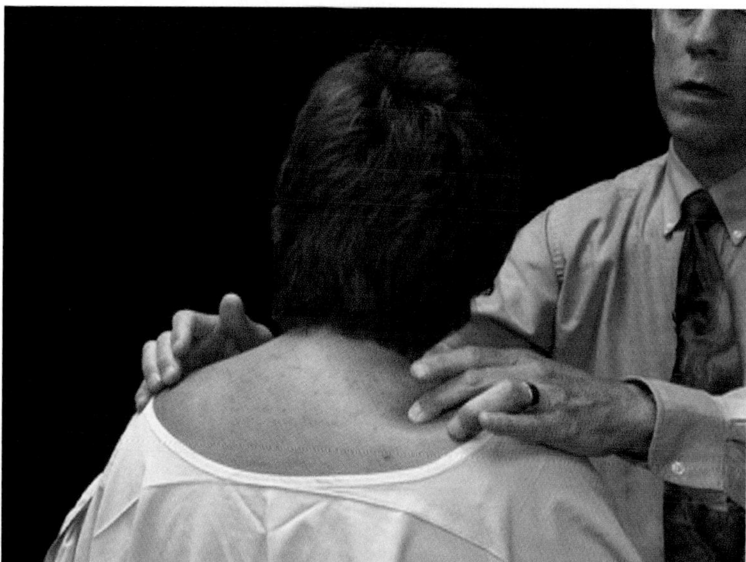

Fig. 3–56

just above the spine of the scapula (Fig. 3–56). Note any tenderness. Move your fingers inferiorly to the medial border of the scapula and assess tenderness in this location on each side (Fig. 3–57). (*Author's note: I use this site as an alternative to the low anterior cervical tender point because many normal patients find pressure over the carotid and root of the neck distinctly uncomfortable.*) Next, check tenderness at the lumbosacral junction in the midline between the sacral dimples, often appreciated by the patient only as

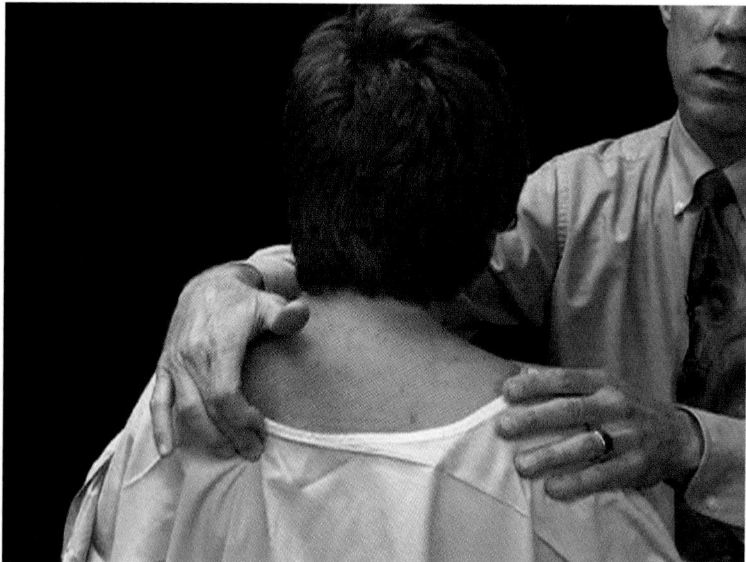

Fig. 3–57

pressure (Fig. 3–58A), then move your fingers laterally and apply pressure in the region of the sacral dimples (Fig. 3–58B). Note any tenderness. Next, assess for tenderness at the greater trochanters on each side (Fig. 3–59). Note any tenderness. Finally, apply pressure to the medial knees, just proximal to the joint line (Fig. 3–60). Assess for tenderness. This completes the tender point assessment.

Finally, if appropriate, conclude the GMSE with a **neurovascular** assessment.

Palpate the peripheral pulses and assess adequacy of distal perfusion.

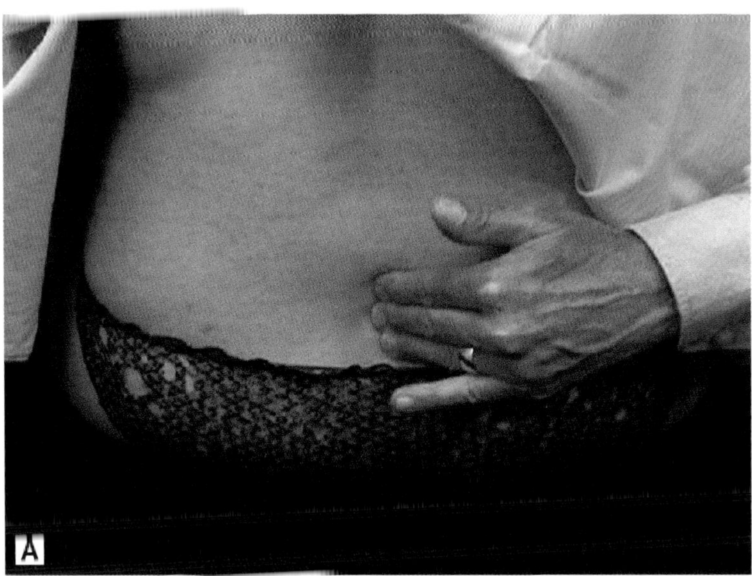

Fig. 3–58

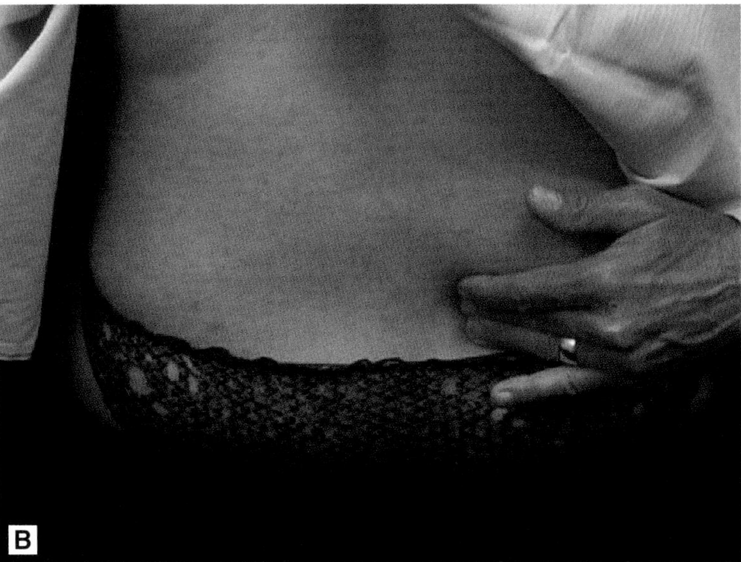

Fig. 3–58

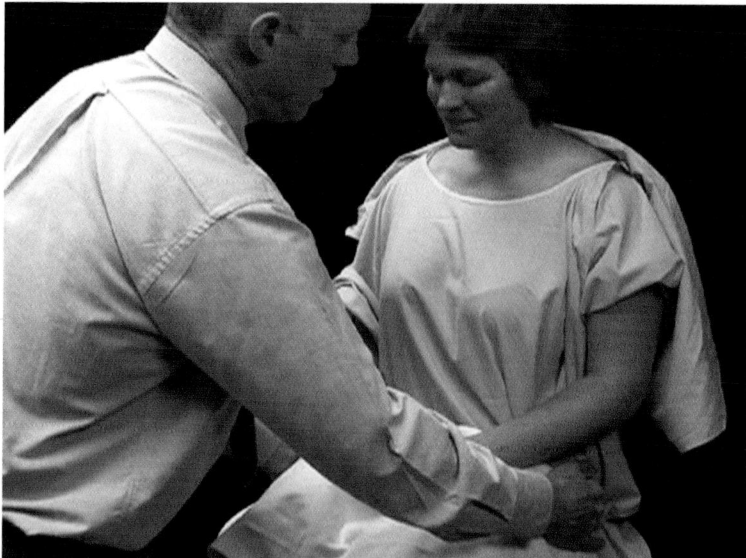

Fig. 3–59

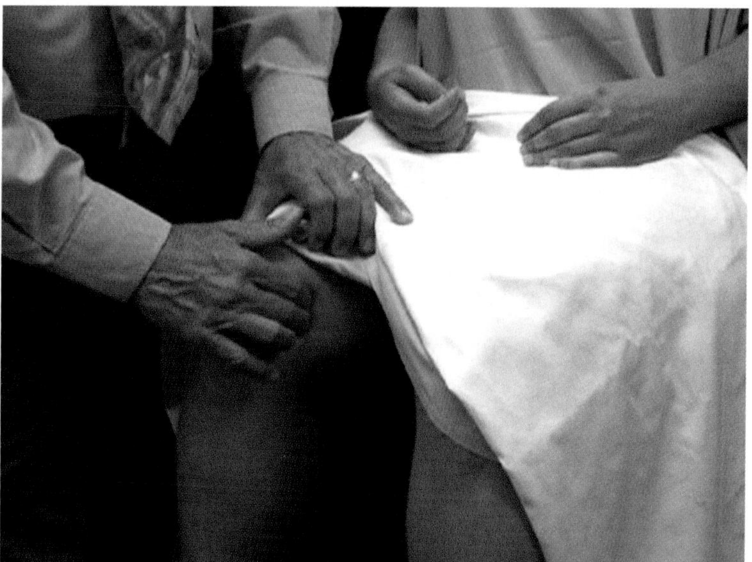

Fig. 3–60

Assess proximal and distal strength by assessing grip (distal), resisted neck flexion, shoulder abduction, and thigh flexion (proximal) and heel and toe walking (distal).

Assess the biceps, brachioradialis, triceps, knee, ankle, and plantar reflexes bilaterally.

Check sensation in the upper and lower extremities.

(Note: In the setting of ***acute trauma,*** *the* ***neurovascular examination*** *is performed* ***prior*** *to and* ***repeated after*** *the other components of the musculoskeletal examination to ensure that no injury to neurovascular structures has occurred during manipulation itself.)*

GENERAL MUSCULOSKELETAL EXAMINATION

Practice Checklist

Patient seated

______Inspect dorsal and palmar surface of hands
______Spread fingers/make fists
______Inspect [illegible]/supinate and pronate forearms
______Palpate DIP joints 5 through 2
______Palpate PIP joints 5 through 2
______Palpate MCP joints 5 through 2
______Palpate thumb, IP, MCP, and first CMC joints
______Inspect wrists
______Palpate wrists (dorsal surface)
______Wrist extension
______Wrist flexion
______Inspect elbows
______Palpate olecranon
______Palpate elbow joint
______Elbow flexion
______Elbow extension
______Inspect and palpate SC joints
______Inspect and palpate AC joints
______Inspect deltoid muscles and deltopectoral grove
______Shoulder flexion
______Shoulder internal rotation
______Shoulder external rotation

Patient lying down

______Palpate greater trochanters
______Hip flexion
______Hip external rotation
______Hip internal rotation
______Inspect quadriceps muscles
______Inspect knees
______Check for bulge sign (or ballotable patella or gross distention)
______Compress patella (assess patellofemoral joint)
______Knee flexion
______Knee extension
______Inspect ankles
______Ankle dorsiflexion
______Ankle plantar flexion
______Subtalar joint motion
______Palpate posterior calcaneus (insertion of Achilles)

______Palpate plantar calcaneus (insertion of plantar fascia)
______Inspect midfoot
______Inspect forefoot and toes
______Palpate MTPs 5 through 2
______Palpate first toe IP and MTP joints
______Inspect PIP and DIP joints of toes
______Inspect sole of feet

Patient standing

______Inspect knee alignment, calf muscle bulk, and alignment of heels and feet (from behind)
______C spine flexion
______C spine extension
______C spine rotation, R and L
______C spine lateral flexion (side bending), R and L
______Inspect thoracolumbar spine and lumbar lordosis
______LS spine flexion
______LS spine extension
______LS spine lateral flexion (side bending), R and L
______Observe gait (swing and stance phases)

Fibromyalgia tender points*

______Proximal forearms
______Second costosternal junctions
______Suboccipital muscle insertions
______Trapezius muscles
______Supraspinatus muscles
______Medial scapular border
______Lumbosacral junction, sacral dimples
______Greater trochanters
______Medial knees (proximal to the joint line)

Neurovascular assessment*

______Check pulses/perfusion
______Check proximal and distal strength, reflexes, and sensation

*If indicated

RECORDING MUSCULOSKELETAL EXAMINATION FINDINGS

A rapid and simple format for recording your MS examination is to divide the examination into its four major components: UE (upper extremities), LE (lower extremities), spine, and gait.

UE: fingers, wrists, elbows, and shoulders

LE: hips, knees, ankles, and feet

Spine: cervical, thoracic, lumbosacral, and SI joints

Gait: observe gait

If your examination is normal, you can record these findings as follows:

MS examination: no synovitis or deformity; full ROM; spine and gait normal

If your examination reveals abnormalities, note any deformity, muscle atrophy, joint tenderness, and/or swelling and altered ROM as follows* (sample patient with active rheumatoid arthritis and multiple findings):

UE: mildly tender, mod cool swelling R and L 2,3,4 PIPs and R 1,2,3,5 and L 2,3 MCPs; warm mild swelling R wrist; mod painful swelling L elbow with 20° FC; mildly painful but full active shoulder ROM; mild atrophy of supra- and infraspinatus

LE: R hip 90° flex, 40° ER, 10° IR with groin pain at end flex and IR; L hip 120° flex, 60° ER and 40° IR; R knee cool fluid wave; L knee mod effusion/ballotable patella with 20° FC; bilat warm, mod swelling at ankles with ↓ subtalar motion; tender swelling R and L 2,3 MTPs

Spine: full, painless ROM

Gait: antalgic due to knee and ankle pain

SKILL BUILDING

The GMSE is designed to build directly upon the techniques and sequence of the SMSE. While the skills involved are more complex than those of the screening examination, the proper techniques of joint palpation can be mastered on normal individuals. Acquiring confidence in these techniques and developing a smoothly integrated examination will require practice. Set aside some blocks of time to practice the examination with a friend, roommate, or your spouse. Using the checklist may make it easier for you to review the order and content of the examination.

Once you are more confident of your technique, you should periodically perform segments of the GMSE while examining patients presenting with other problems. This will allow you to continue to practice in the context of your day-to-day patient care without losing the important musculoskeletal skills you are now developing. The time you invest will pay rich rewards through the development of excellence in your skills of physical examination.

---

*bilat = bilateral; ER = external rotation; ext = extension; FC = flexion contracture; flex = flexion; IR = internal rotation; lat = lateral.

CONCLUSION

A rapid, yet thorough musculoskeletal examination, performed in an organized, sequential fashion is essential for accurate diagnosis of musculoskeletal problems. The GMSE is designed as an efficient, yet comprehensive assessment for the presence of arthritis and provides the foundation for learning more detailed RMSEs at a later point in your training.

4

The Regional Musculoskeletal Examination of the Shoulder

INTRODUCTION

The *regional musculoskeletal examination* (RMSE) of the **shoulder** is designed to build on the sequences and techniques taught in the SMSE and GMSE. It is intended to provide a comprehensive assessment of structure and function combined with special testing to permit you to evaluate common, important musculoskeletal problems of the shoulder seen in an ambulatory setting. The skills involved require practice and careful attention to technique. However, they can be learned and mastered on normal individuals.

CLINICAL UTILITY

The RMSE of the shoulder is clinically useful as the initial examination in individuals whose history clearly suggests an isolated shoulder problem. In individuals whose history is less straightforward (a seemingly local shoulder problem with additional musculoskeletal complaints of unclear relevance), a rapid SMSE may be the most appropriate first step in physical assessment. If significant, possibly related, abnormalities are found (and the patient's presenting shoulder complaint appears to be part of a more generalized musculoskeletal process), then performing a GMSE would be most appropriate.

With practice, a systematic, efficient RMSE of the shoulder can be performed in ~3 to 4 minutes.

Furthermore, the RMSE of the shoulder provides the foundation for learning additional, more refined diagnostic techniques through your later exposure to orthopedic surgeons, rheumatologists, physiatrists, physical therapists, and others specifically involved in the diagnosis and treatment of shoulder problems.

OBJECTIVES

This instructional program will enable you to identify important anatomic, functional, and pathologic relationships at the shoulder, including:

- Cervical spine ROM
- Sternoclavicular (SC) joint
- Acromioclavicular (AC) joint
- Subacromial bursa, rotator cuff, and biceps tendons
- Impingement testing
- Glenohumeral (GH) joint ROM

Most importantly, it will prepare you to perform an organized, integrated, and clinically useful regional examination of the shoulder.

ESSENTIAL CONCEPTS

Structural and Functional Anatomy The **scapula** is a thin, flat bone that serves as the attachment for muscles of the shoulder (rotator cuff, deltoid, and others), articulates with the chest wall at the **scapulothoracic joint** and the clavicle at the **AC joint**, and provides the shallow socket for the humeral head, the **glenoid fossa** (Fig. 4–1).

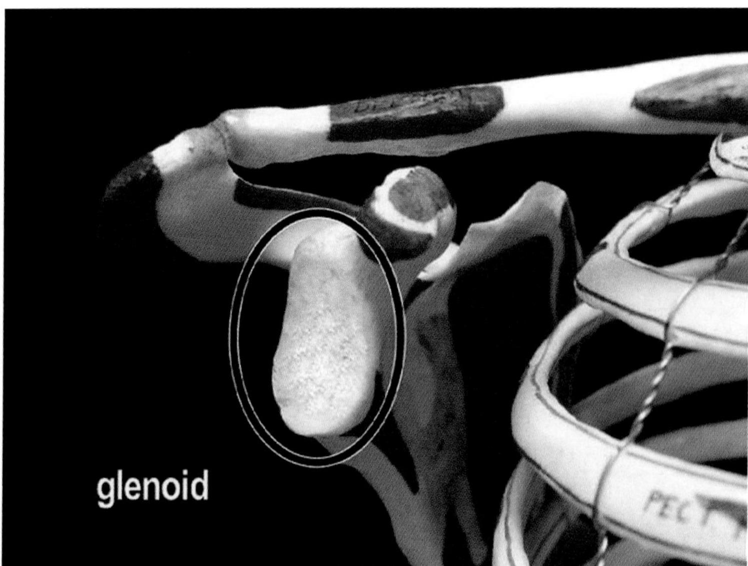

Fig. 4–1

In addition, the scapula provides the superior, protective bony "roof" of the shoulder joint, the **acromion** (Fig. 4–2) and an anterior hook-like projection for the attachment of tendons and ligaments, the **coracoid** (Fig. 4–3).

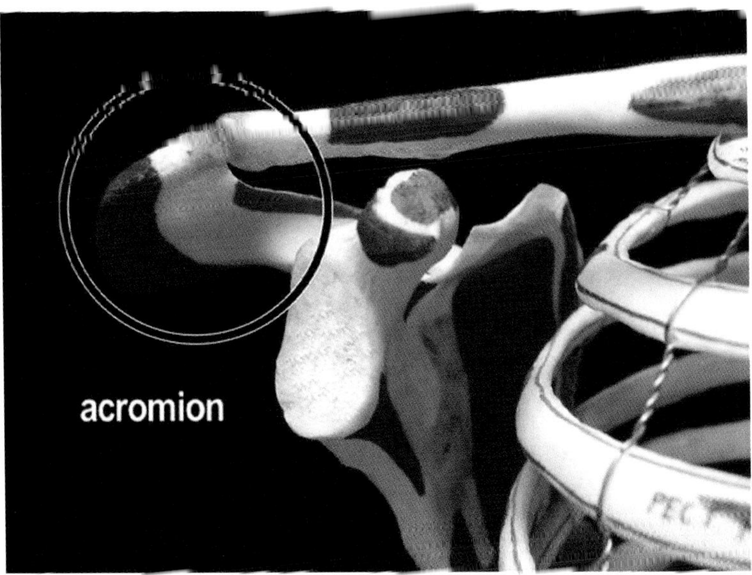

Fig. 4–2

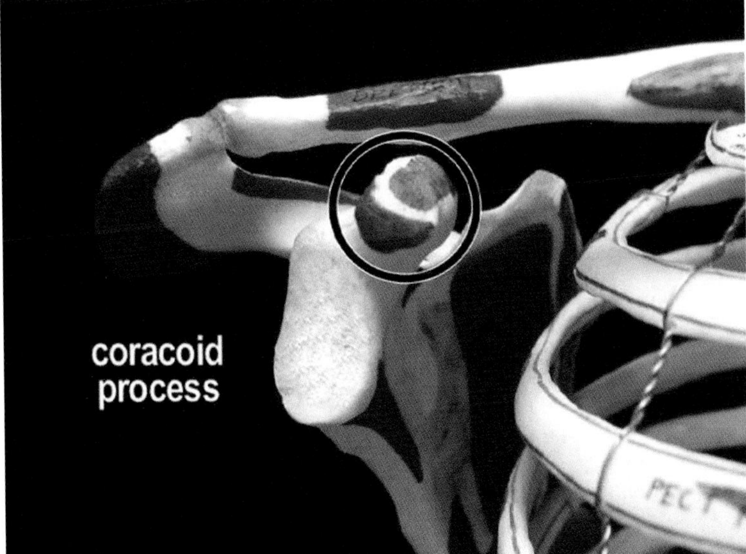

Fig. 4–3

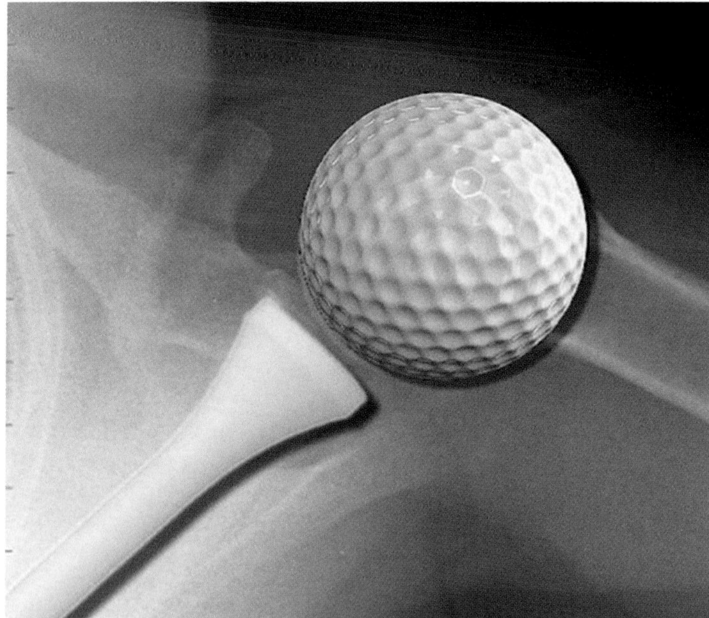

Fig. 4–4

The **GH joint**, rather than a ball and socket like the hip, can better be likened to a "golf ball" (humeral head) on a "golf tee" (glenoid) (Fig. 4–4). This shallow socket permits a significant range of motion at the expense of stability. A ring of fibrocartilage (glenoid labrum) surrounds the glenoid fossa, deepening the surface of the glenoid (Fig. 4–5). The proximal end of the clavicle attaches to the chest wall at the **SC joint** and the distal end of the clavicle attaches to the scapula at the **AC joint**.

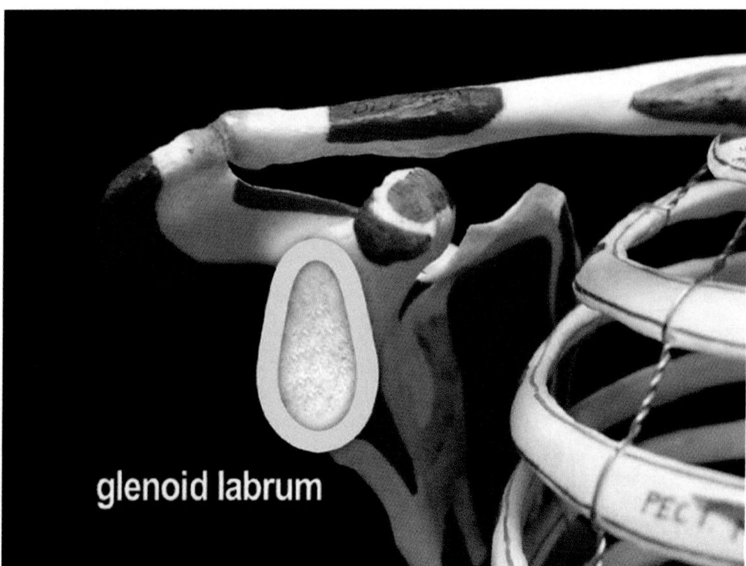

Fig. 4–5

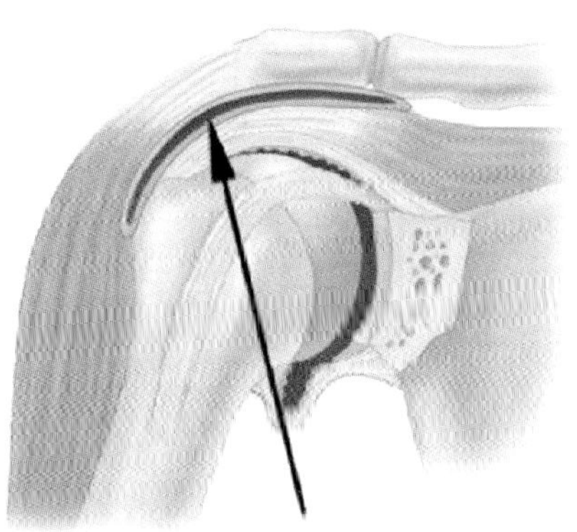

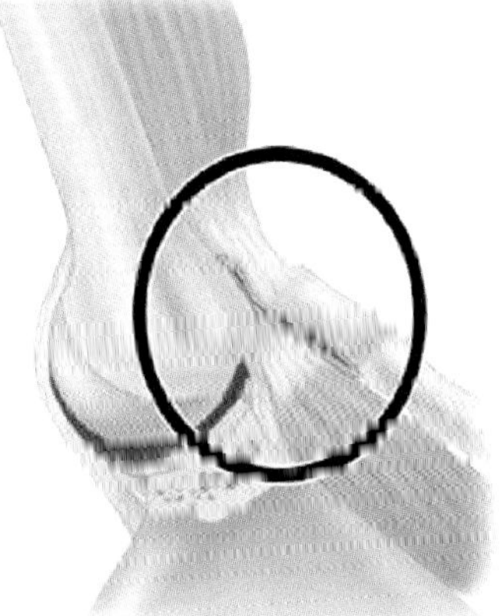

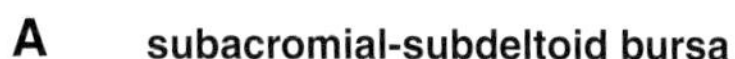

Fig. 4–6. (Modified with permission from Fam AG, Lawry GV, Kreder HJ. Musculoskeletal Examination and Joint Techniques, 1st ed. Mosby/Elsevier 2006, p. 8.)

The **subacromial-subdeltoid bursa**, a thin synovially lined cushion, lies beneath the acromion and proximal deltoid muscle (Fig. 4–6A). It functions to reduce compressive forces between the humeral head and acromion during shoulder elevation (flexion and abduction) beyond 90° (Fig. 4–6B).

The **rotator cuff** is a group of four muscles whose tendons blend together forming a tendinous cup surrounding the humeral head (Fig. 4–7).

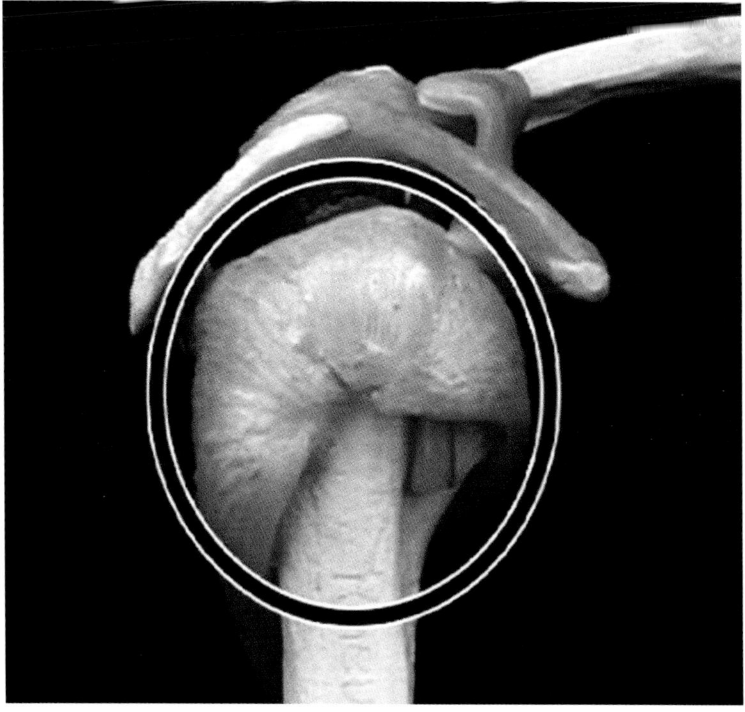

Fig. 4–7

It functions to stabilize the humeral head in the glenoid and rotate the humerus (hence the name "rotator cuff"). A prominence (tuberosity) on the lateral humeral head provides the bony attachment site for the rotator cuff tendons (Fig. 4–8A). It has a channel (bicipital groove; Fig.4–8B) which divides the tuberosity into and anterior one-third (lesser tuberosity) and posterior two-thirds (greater tuberosity) (Fig. 4–8C).

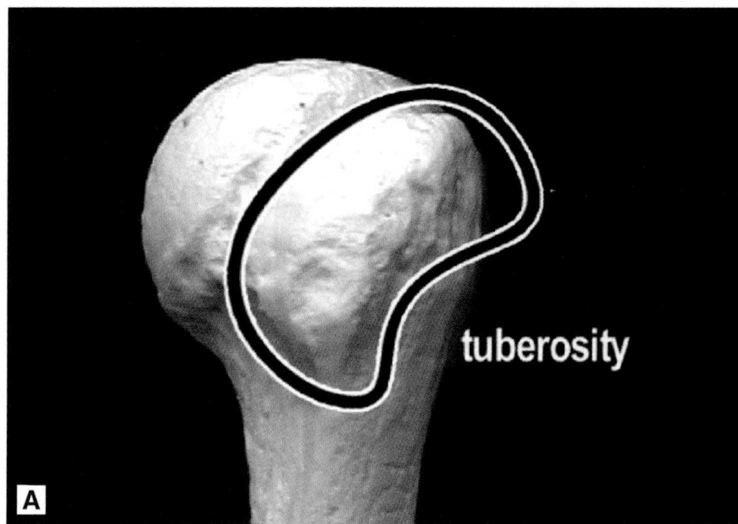

Fig. 4–8

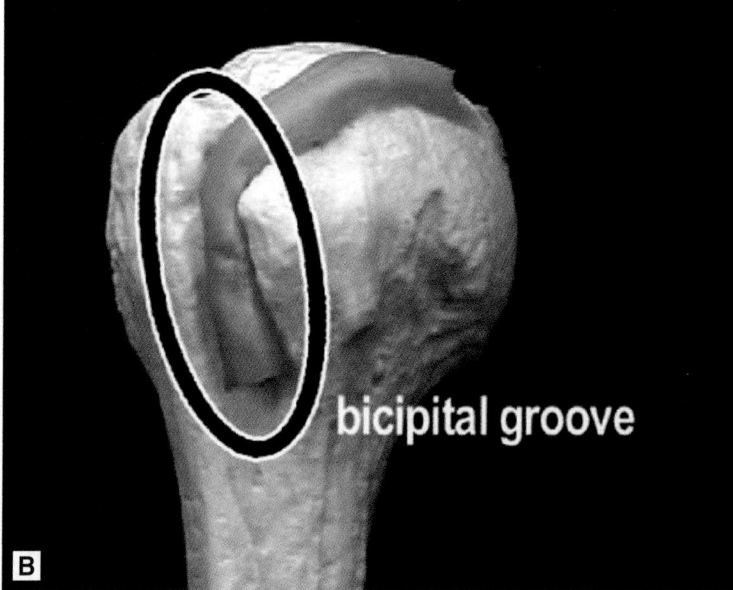

Fig. 4–8

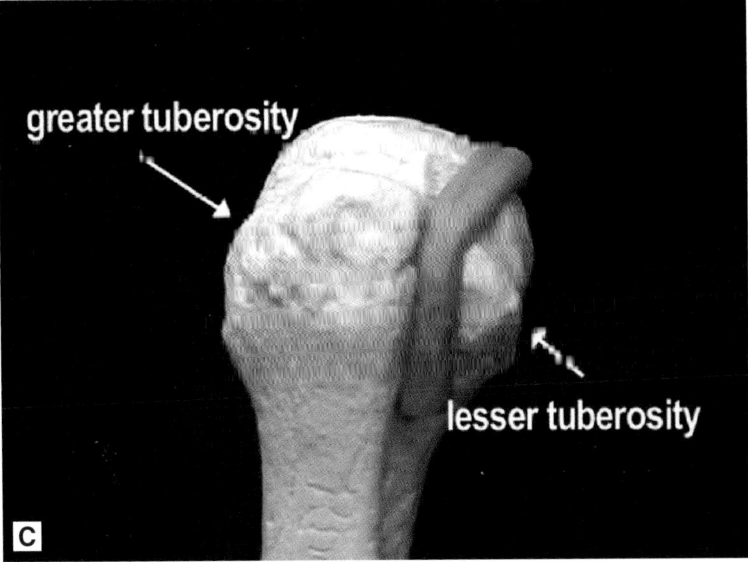

Fig. 4–8

The bony channel between these tuberosities provides a pulley for the long head of the biceps tendon. The **supraspinatus muscle** originates in the supraspinatus fossa (above the spine of the scapula, Fig. 4–9A) and inserts on the superior greater tuberosity, functioning as an abductor of the shoulder (Fig. 4–9B).

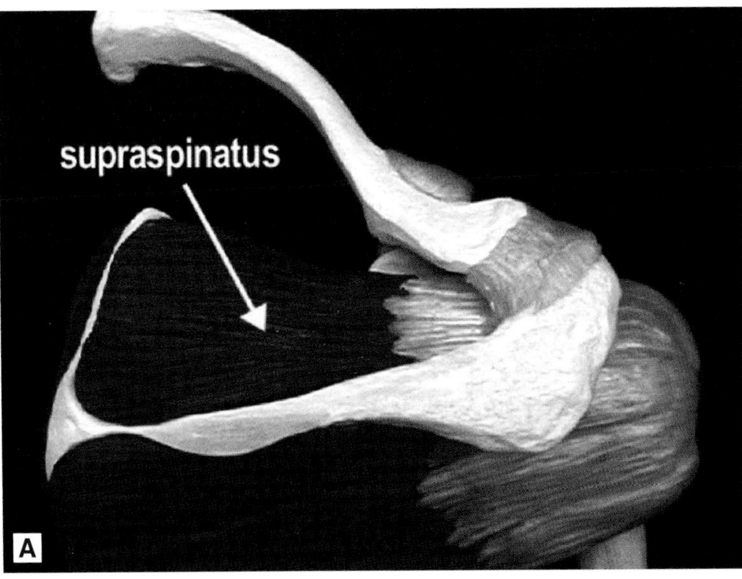

Fig. 4–9

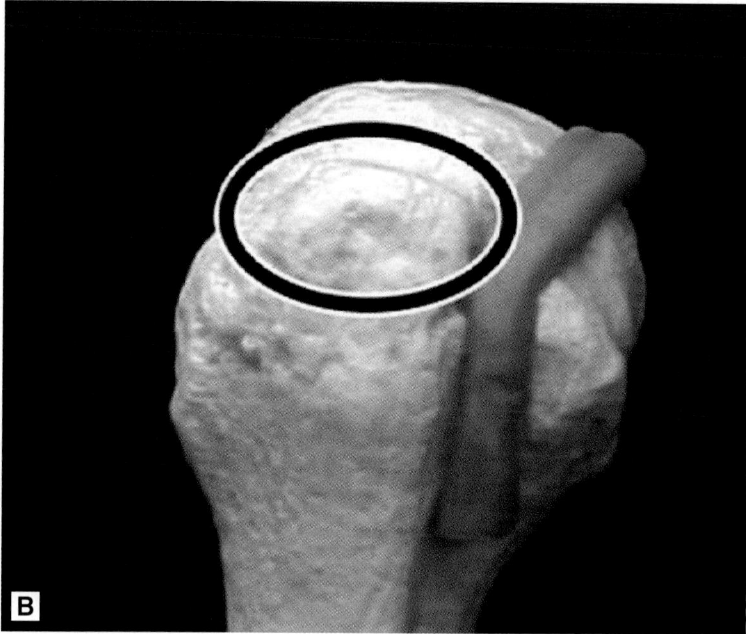

Fig. 4–9

The **infraspinatus muscle** originates in the infraspinatus fossa (below the spine of the scapula, Fig. 4–10A) and attaches to the posterior greater tuberosity and is an external rotator of the shoulder (Fig. 4–10B).

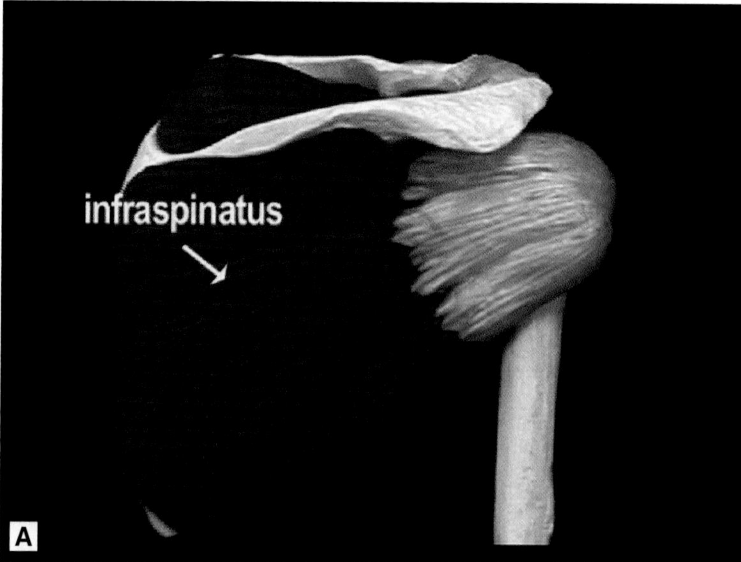

Fig. 4–10

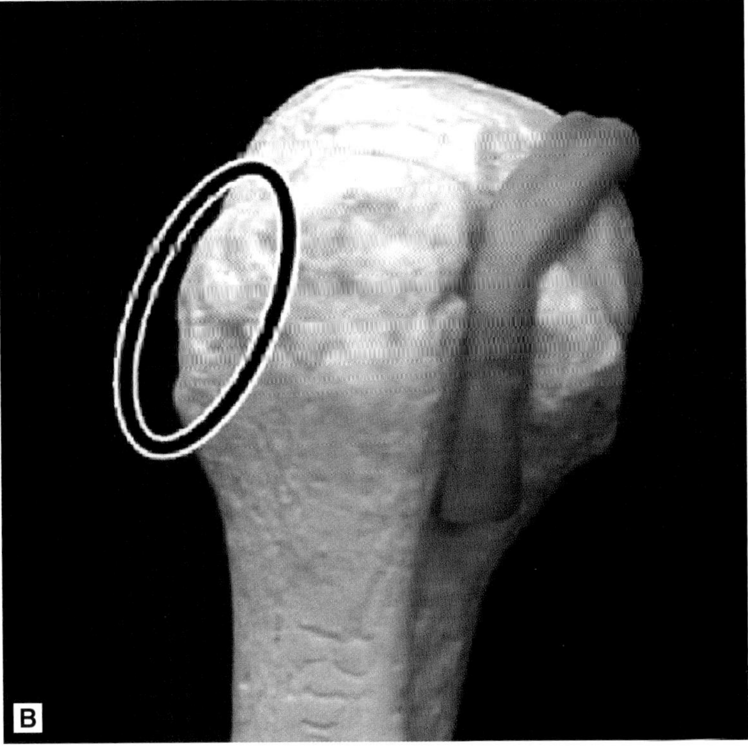

Fig. 4–10

The **teres minor muscle** originates below the infraspinatus muscle and also attaches to the posterior greater tuberosity and is an external rotator of the shoulder (Fig. 4–11A, B).

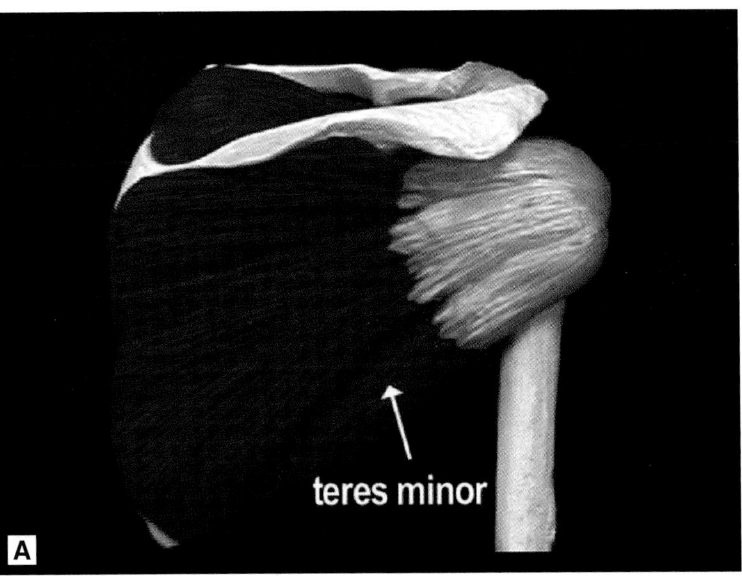

Fig. 4–11

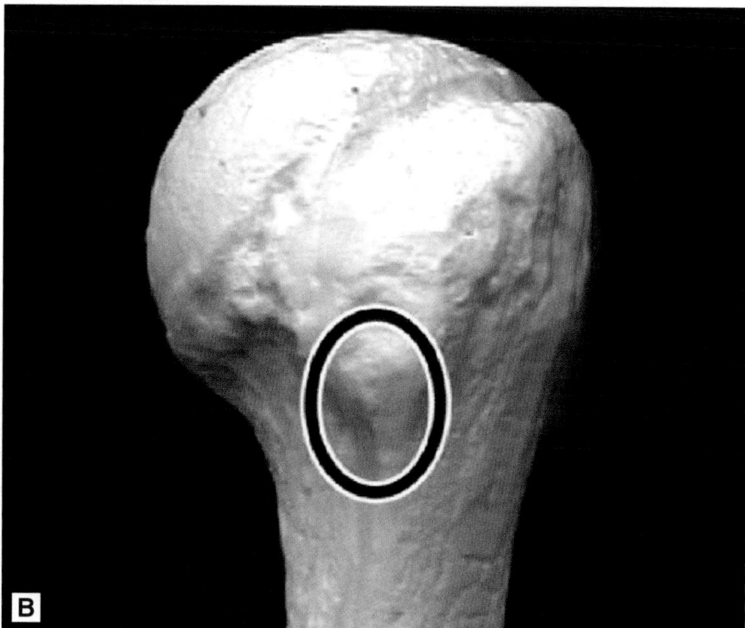

Fig. 4–11

The **subscapularis muscle** originates from the underside of the scapula and runs anterior to the humeral head, attaching on the anterior humerus at the lesser tuberosity, functioning as an internal rotator of the shoulder (Fig. 4–12A, B).

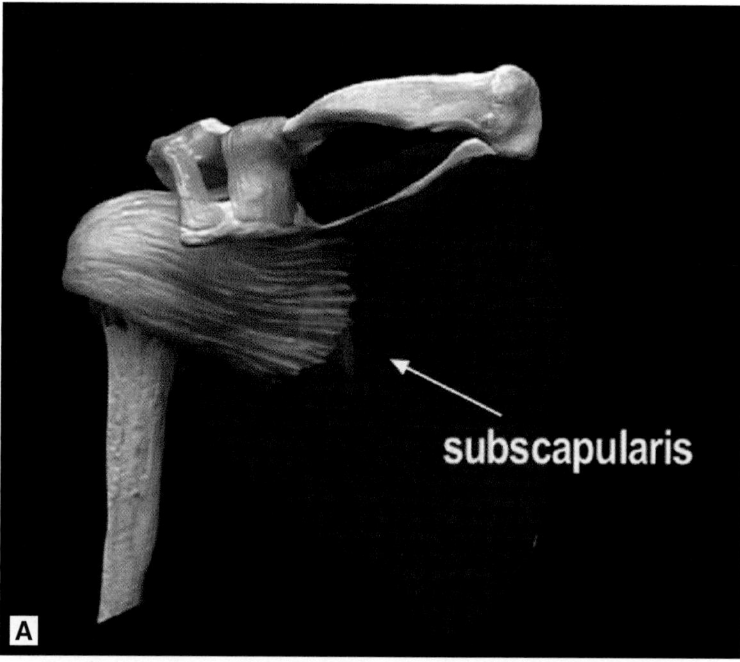

Fig. 4–12

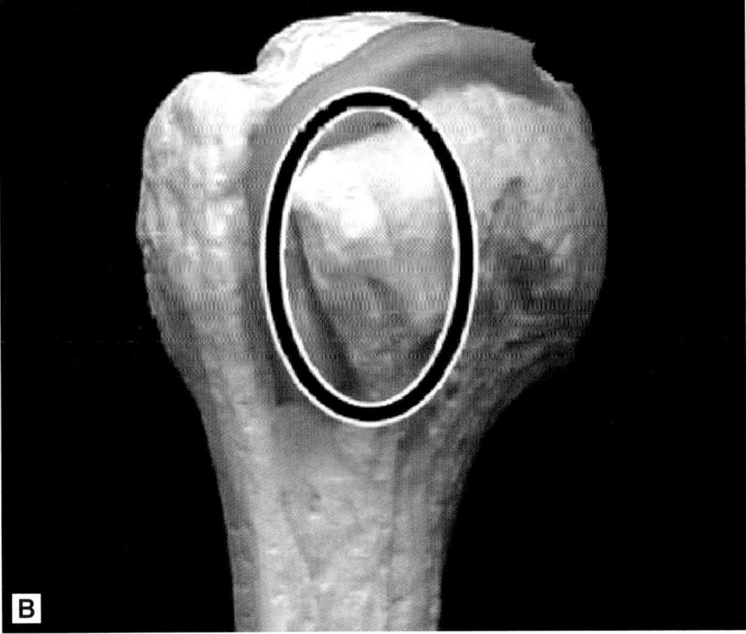

Fig. 4–12

The rotator cuff's most important function is stabilizing the shoulder joint by holding the humeral head in the glenoid during shoulder motion (Fig.4–13). The powerful pectoralis, latissimus dorsi, and deltoid muscles provide additional strength and stability.

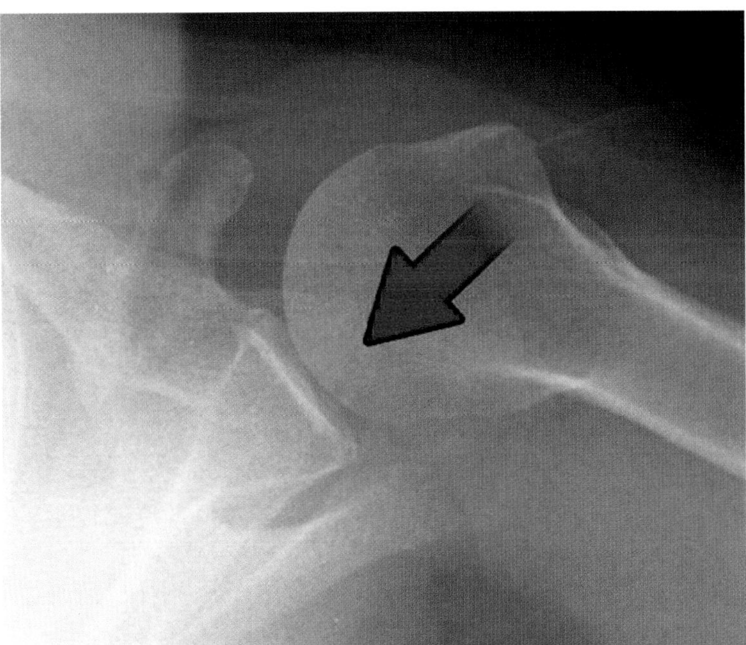

Fig. 4–13

The **biceps muscle** is composed of two (bi) heads (ceps) which flex the elbow and supinate the forearm. The short (medial) head runs between the proximal radius and the coracoid (Fig. 4–14A, B), and the long (lateral) head runs between the proximal radius and a tubercle on the superior rim of the glenoid (Fig. 4–15A, B).

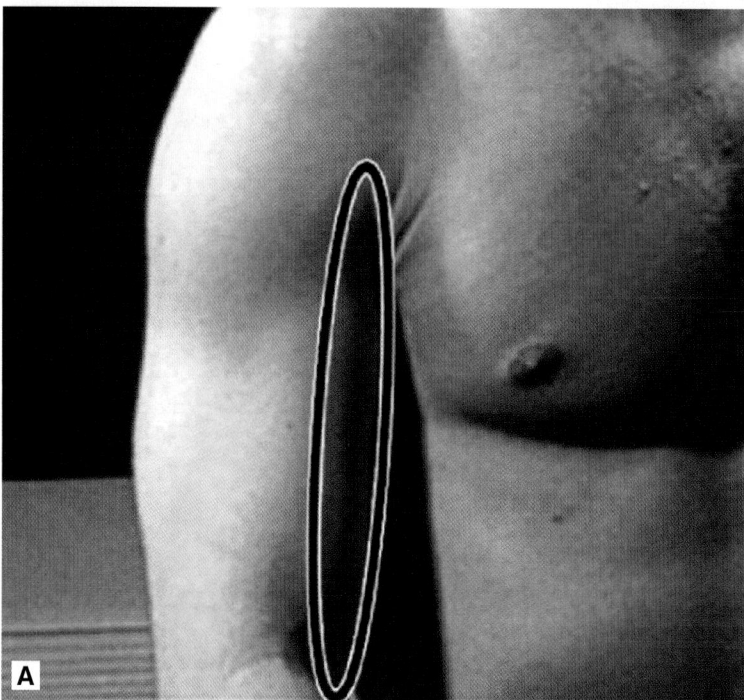

Fig. 4–14

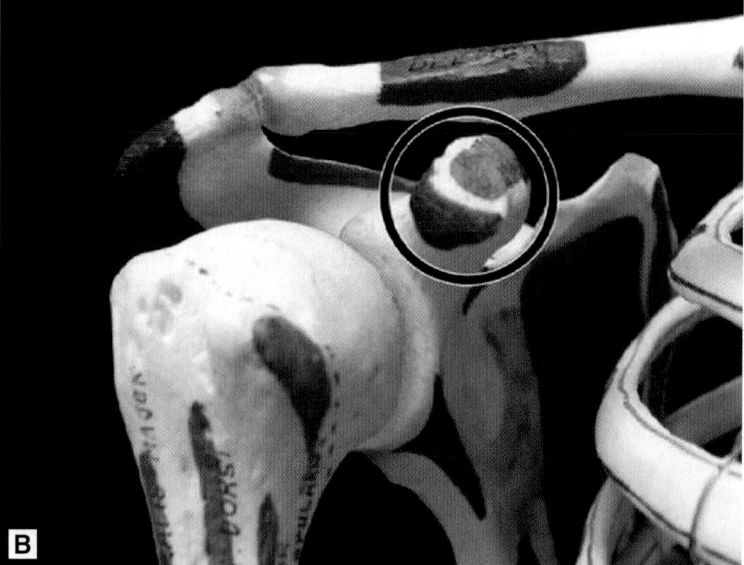

Fig. 4–14

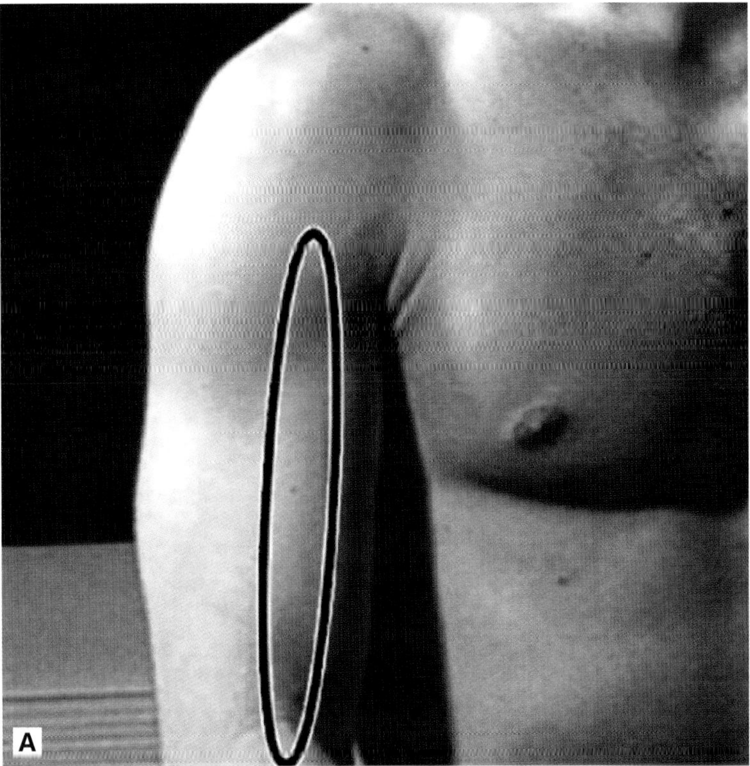

Fig. 4–15

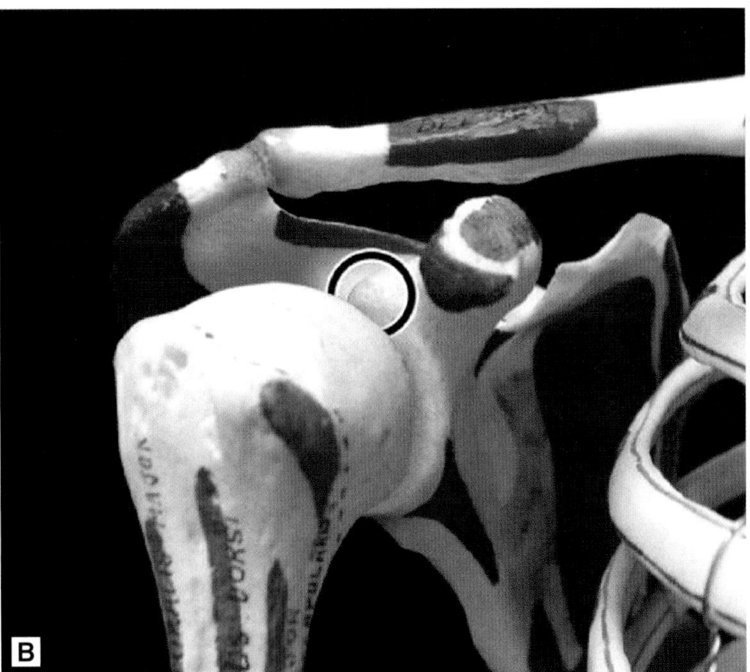

Fig. 4–15

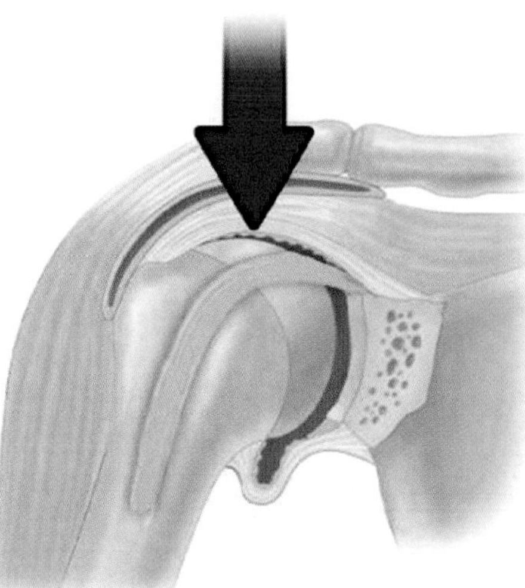

Fig. 4–16. (Modified with permission from Fam AG, Lawry GV, Kreder HJ. Musculoskeletal Examination and Joint Techniques, 1st ed. Mosby/Elsevier 2006, p. 8.)

Hence, the **tendon of the long head of the biceps** enters the shoulder capsule itself anteriorly, proceeds over the humeral head, and attaches into the superior labrum of the glenoid, within the shoulder joint. It functions as a powerful supinator of the forearm and also provides downward force on the humerus, helping the humeral head stay seated in the glenoid during lifting (Fig. 4–16).

Three important soft tissue structures of the shoulder live in a "bone sandwich" (Fig. 4–17) between the acromion superiorly and the humeral head inferiorly: the subacromial bursa, the supraspinatus tendon, and biceps tendon (Fig. 4–18A, B, C). In this location, they are subjected to pinch between the

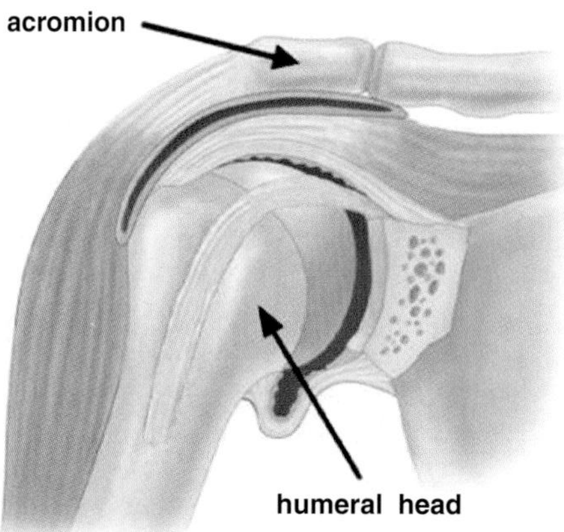

Fig. 4–17. (Modified with permission from Fam AG, Lawry GV, Kreder HJ. Musculoskeletal Examination and Joint Techniques, 1st ed. Mosby/Elsevier 2006, p. 8.)

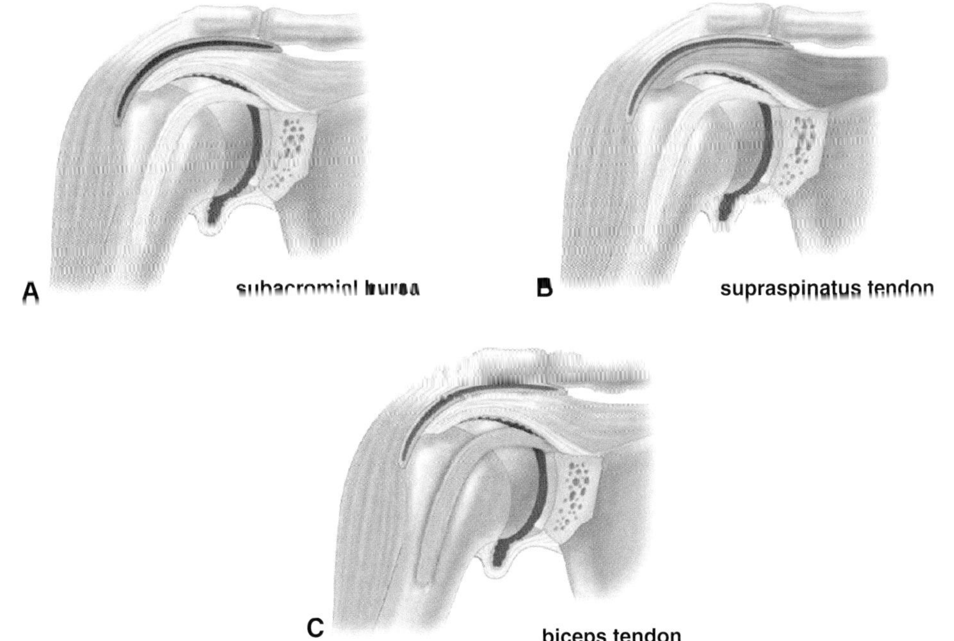

Fig. 4–18. (Modified with permission from Fam AG, Lawry GV, Kreder HJ. Musculoskeletal Examination and Joint Techniques, 1st ed. Mosby/Elsevier 2006, p. 8.)

acromion and humeral head whenever the arm is elevated beyond 90° (Fig. 4–19). Repetitive overhead activities and athletics, especially swimming, throwing, and racquet sports are common causes of a painful *impingement syndrome*. Given this anatomy and physiology, you can predict the three most common causes of shoulder pain in ambulatory adults: subacromial bursitis, supraspinatus tendonitis, and biceps tendonitis.

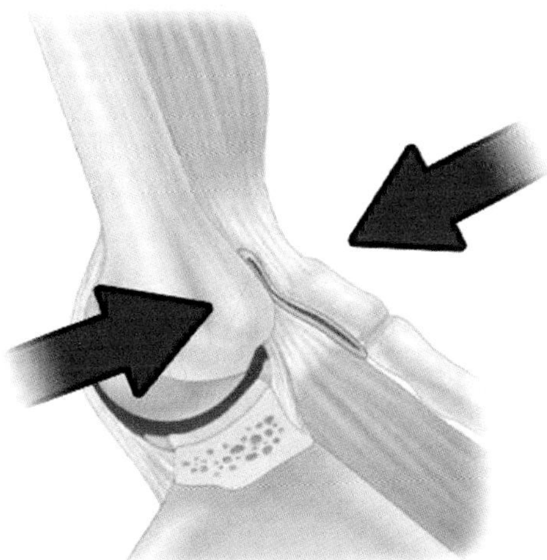

Fig. 4–19. (Modified with permission from Fam AG, Lawry GV, Kreder HJ. Musculoskeletal Examination and Joint Techniques, 1st ed. Mosby/Elsevier 2006, p. 8.)

Clinical History The patient's history is the essential first step in all musculoskeletal diagnosis and directs the focus of an appropriate physical examination. The musculoskeletal physical examination confirms or refutes diagnostic hypotheses generated by a thoughtful history.

An initial pain assessment can be well delineated with the use of the mnemonic **OPQRST**: **O** = Onset, **P** = Precipitating (and ameliorating) factors, **Q** = Quality, **R** = Radiation, **S** = Severity, **T** = Timing. This information can be quite helpful in narrowing the primary differential diagnosis of shoulder problems. Additional, particularly useful information in evaluating shoulder pain includes age and handedness; occupation or recreational activities and repetitive overhead movements; and a history of instability, prior injury, or any prior shoulder problems.

THE EXAMINATION, OVERVIEW

With the patient seated or standing, observe the shoulders from behind. Inspect the supraspinatus, infraspinatus, and deltoid muscles. Observe arm elevation and scapular motion. Next, observe the shoulders anteriorly. Inspect the deltoid and pectoralis muscles. Observe the deltopectoral groove.

Inspect the cervical spine. Assess neck flexion by instructing the patient to place his chin on the chest. Assess neck extension by asking the patient to look up at the ceiling. Observe right and left rotation by asking the patient to place his chin on each shoulder. Assess lateral flexion by asking the patient to incline his ear toward each shoulder.

Now, inspect and palpate the SC joints. Inspect and palpate the AC joints.

Next, palpate the lateral subdeltoid region of the subacromial bursa, then palpate the anterior subacromial region. Assess the resisted shoulder abduction with the "supraspinatus test." Next, assess rotator cuff integrity by checking resisted shoulder external rotation. Inspect and palpate the biceps tendon. Assess resisted supination of the forearm.

Next, check for signs of impingement. Assess for the Neer impingement sign by passively moving the shoulder into flexion while stabilizing the scapula with one hand. Assess for Hawkins sign by combining shoulder flexion, adduction, and forced internal rotation.

Next, complete your assessment of GH motion with passive shoulder abduction, internal rotation, and external rotation. If your assessment up to this point has been painful or guarded, ask the patient to *lie supine* while you complete the examination of GH internal and external rotation. Note any patient hesitation to passive external rotation in the abducted position.

THE EXAMINATION, COMPONENT PARTS

Inspection With the patient seated or standing, observe the shoulders from behind. Note any rashes or other cutaneous abnormalities. Check for deformity or resting asymmetry. Check for atrophy of the supraspinatus or infraspinatus muscles, frequently associated with rotator cuff pathology or GH arthritis (Fig. 4–20).

Next, ask the patient to raise the arms overhead slowly while you inspect the rhythm, timing, and symmetry of shoulder motion. Shoulder elevation (flexion and abduction) results from movement at the GH joint in combination with scapular movement on the chest wall, normally in a 2:1 ratio. Note any asymmetry or restricted range of motion (Fig. 4–21).

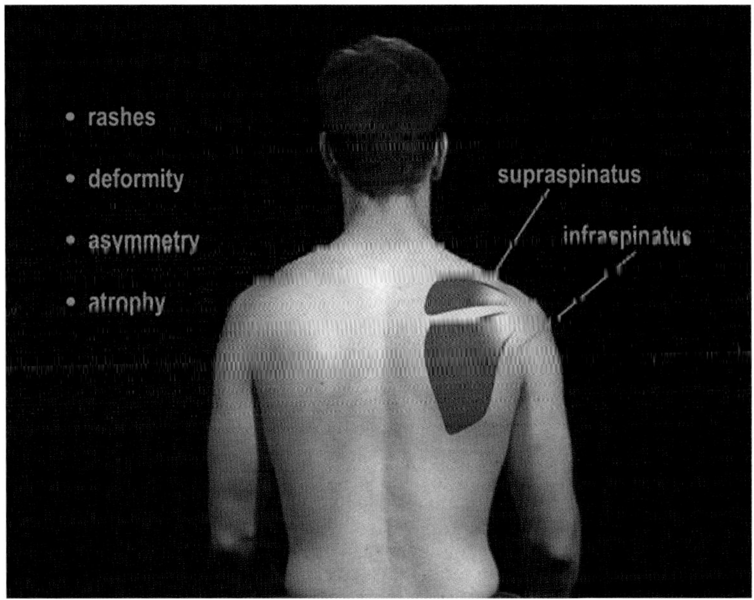

Fig. 4–20

Next, observe the shoulders anteriorly, again noting any cutaneous abnormalities, deformity, or resting asymmetry. Check for atrophy of the deltoid or pectoralis muscles. Inspect and compare each deltopectoral groove to assess for a possible shoulder effusion (Fig. 4–22). (A GH effusion may result in effacement of the normal sulcus between the deltoid and pectoral muscles.)

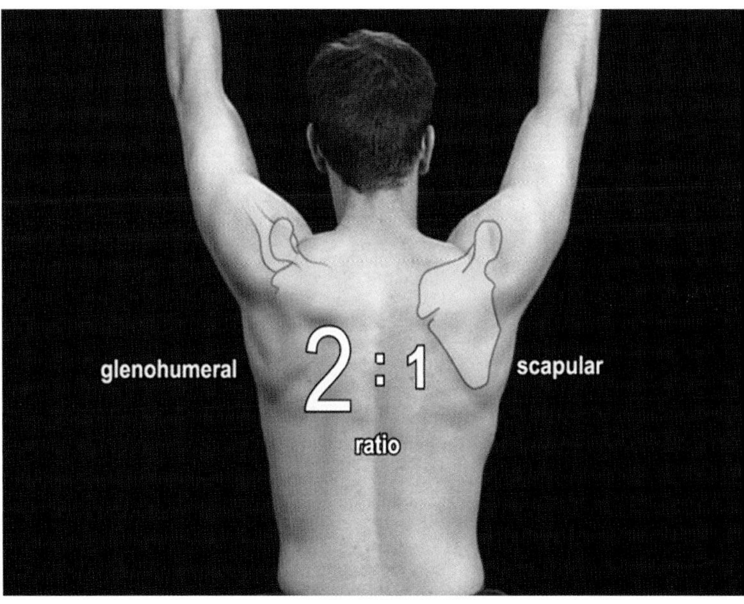

Fig. 4–21

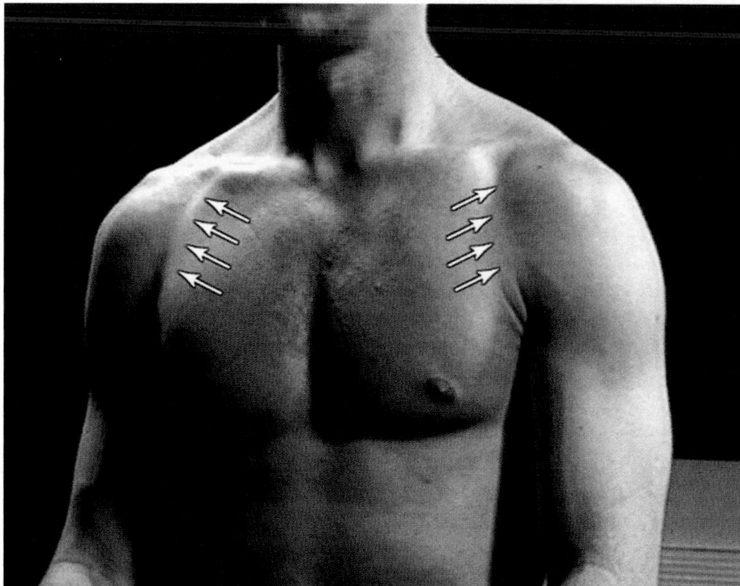

Fig. 4–22

Cervical Spine Next, check cervical spine range of motion to determine if the patient's shoulder symptoms may be originating from the cervical spine, with referred pain to the shoulder region. Assess neck flexion by asking the patient to touch his chin to the chest (Fig. 4–23A). Assess neck extension by asking the patient to look up at the ceiling (Fig. 4–23B). Observe right and left rotation by asking the patient

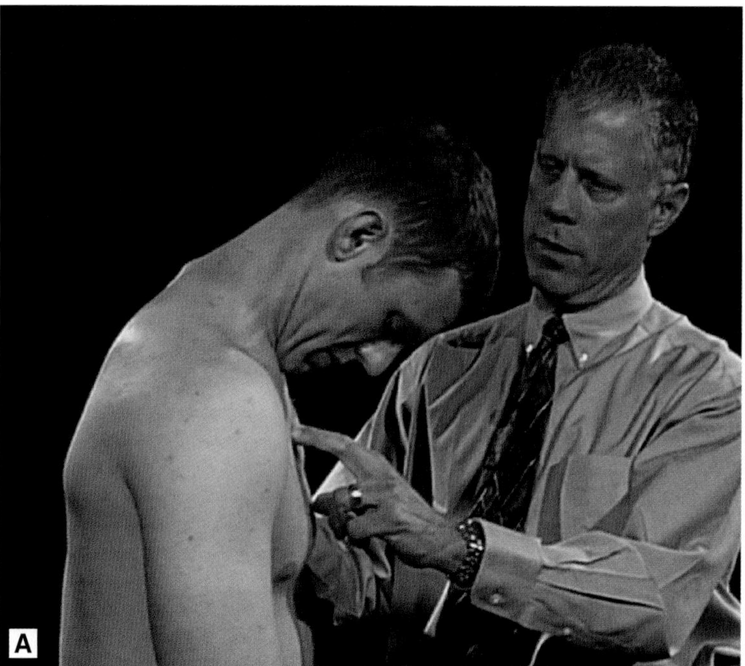

Fig. 4–23

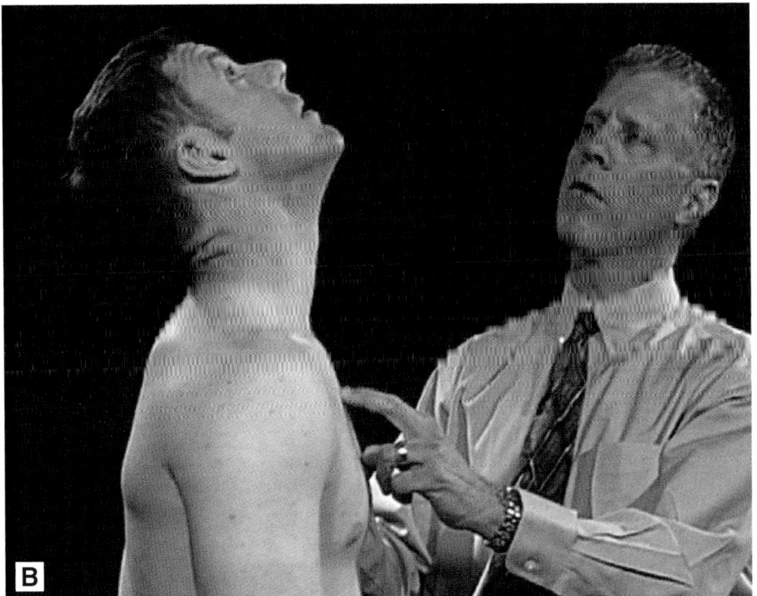

Fig. 4–23

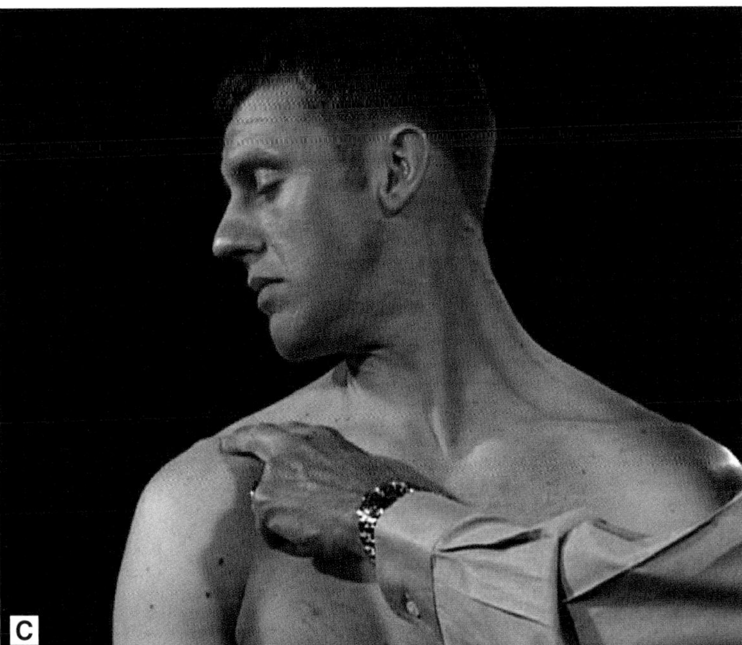

Fig. 4–23

to place his chin on each shoulder (Fig. 4–23C). Assess lateral flexion (or lateral bending) by asking the patient to incline his ear toward each shoulder (Fig. 4–23D).

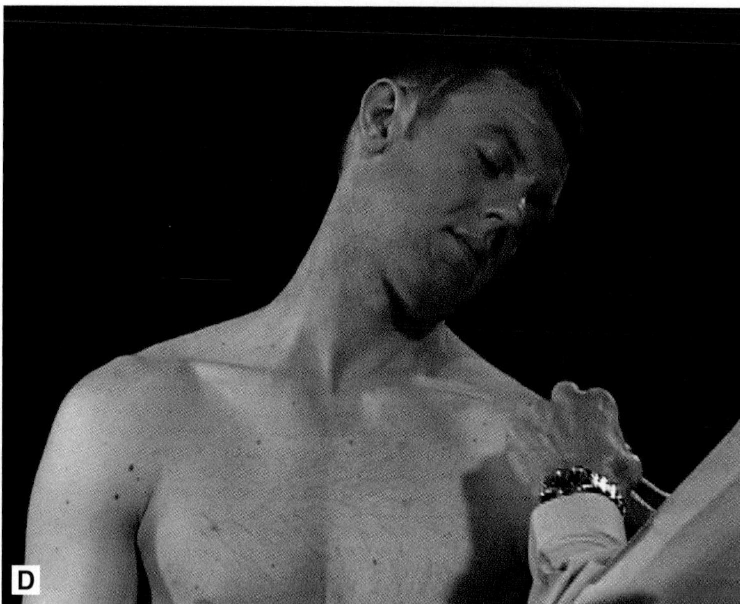

Fig. 4–23

Sternoclavicular Joints Next, observe the shoulders anteriorly. Now, inspect the sternoclavicular (SC) joints for visible swelling or asymmetry. Palpate the jugular notch with your index or middle finger, then slide slightly laterally (<1 cm) to feel the SC joint line (Fig. 4–24). The joint is subcutaneous and the bony margins of the proximal end of the clavicle and superolateral manubrium are normally easily palpable.

Note any tenderness or swelling.

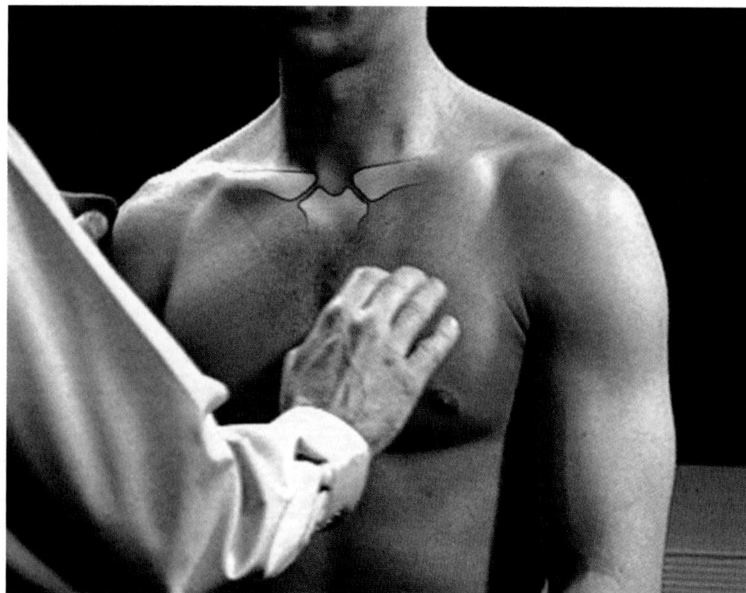

Fig. 4–24

Acromioclavicular Joints Next, inspect the acromioclavicular (AC) joints for asymmetry or visible swelling. Find the posterior angle of the acromion at the posterolateral edge of the shoulder (Fig. 4–25A). This bony "corner" is nearly always palpable, regardless of body weight or muscularity. Once you have identified the angle of the acromion, move your palpating fingers anteriorly to feel the lateral edge of the acromion (Fig. 4–25B). Now, palpate the AC joint by applying pressure with your index and middle fingers to the top of the shoulder, ~2 cm medial to the lateral edge of the acromion.

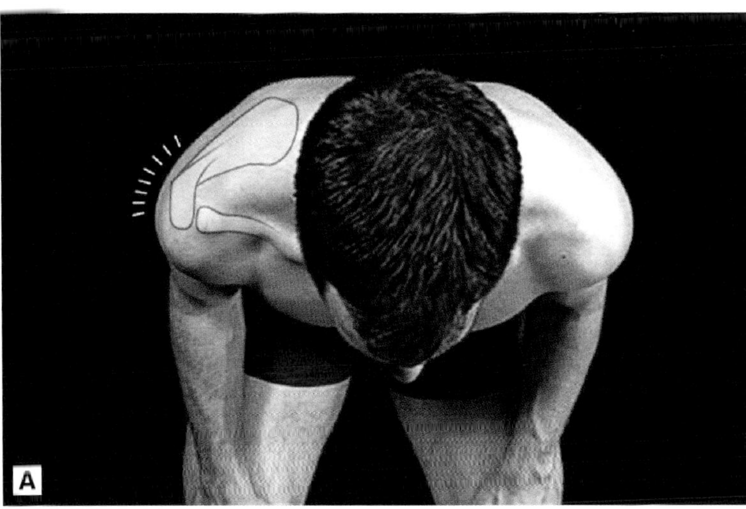

Fig. 4–25

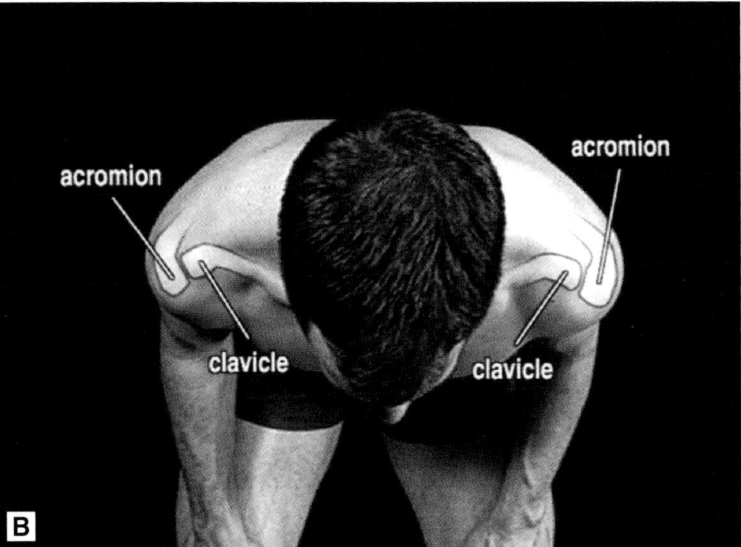

Fig. 4–25

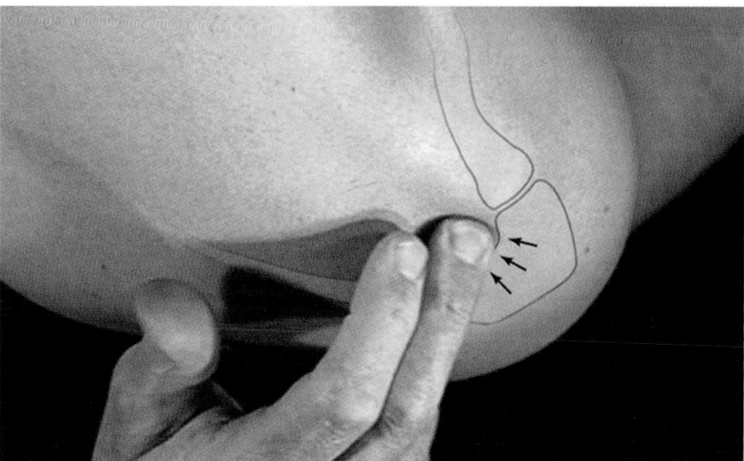

Fig. 4–26

More precise localization of the AC joint may be obtained by one of two techniques: Identify the spine of the scapula. Locate the supraspinatus fossa and palpate along the superior edge of the spine of the scapula until you feel the acromion laterally. Your finger is now touching the posterior AC joint line. Continue to palpate anteriorly and your fingers lie directly on top of the AC joint (Fig. 4–26).

Alternatively, palpate anteriorly along the distal clavicle and identify the small depression at the junction of the distal clavicle and the anterior surface of the acromion. Your finger is now touching the anterior AC joint line (Fig. 4–27A). Ask the patient to "place your hand on your hip and point your elbow behind you." This maneuver brings the shoulder into extension and causes the AC joint to open anteriorly, confirming the location of joint line (Fig. 4–27B). Continue to palpate superiorly and posteriorly and your finger will lie directly on top of the joint (Fig. 4–27C).

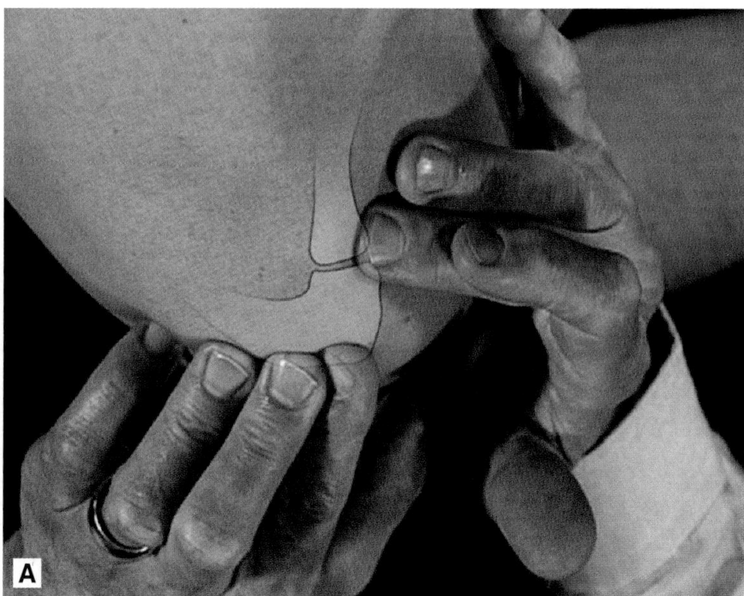

Fig. 4–27

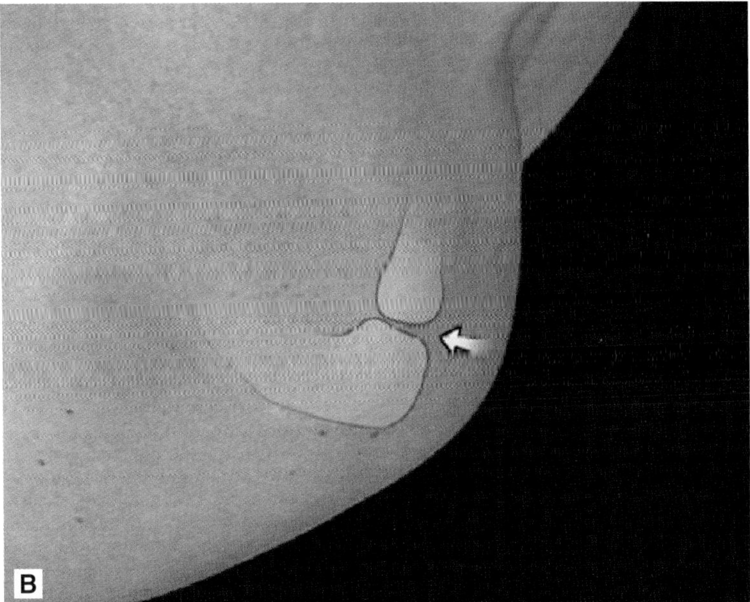

Fig. 4–27

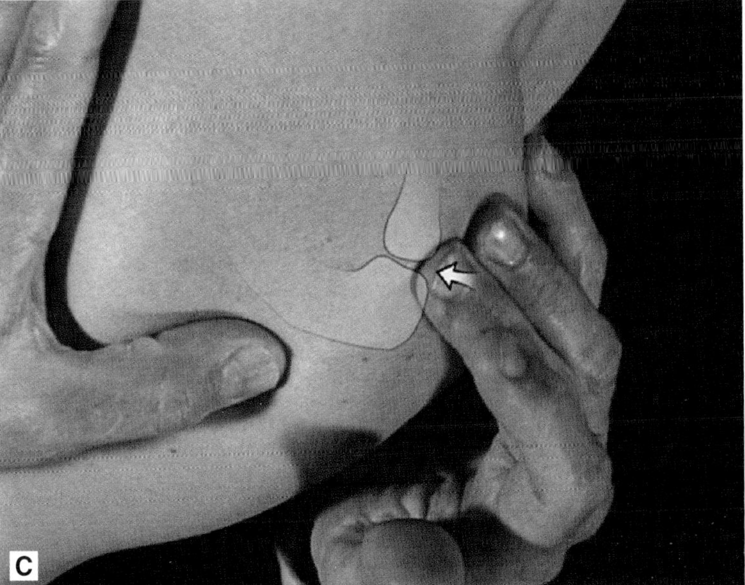

Fig. 4–27

Abnormalities of the AC joint are suspected from the history and local tenderness to direct palpation over the joint line. In addition, suspected AC joint pathology can be confirmed by passively adducting the arm across the chest, causing pain as the acromion is compressed against the distal clavicle. Pain originating from the AC joint is most often felt at the top of the shoulder, with little or no referral to other sites.

(Any visible or palpable bony prominence at the AC joint is almost always the distal clavicle itself or a distal clavicular osteophyte.)

Subdeltoid and Subacromial Bursa(e) With the patient's arms resting at the side, palpate just inferior to the lateral edge of the acromion to assess for subdeltoid tenderness. Tenderness in this area may indicate inflammation of the subdeltoid bursa (Fig. 4–28A). Next, ask the patient to "place your hands on your hips and point your elbows behind you." This maneuver brings the shoulder into extension and exposes the superior and anterior portion of the subacromial bursa (Fig. 4–28B).

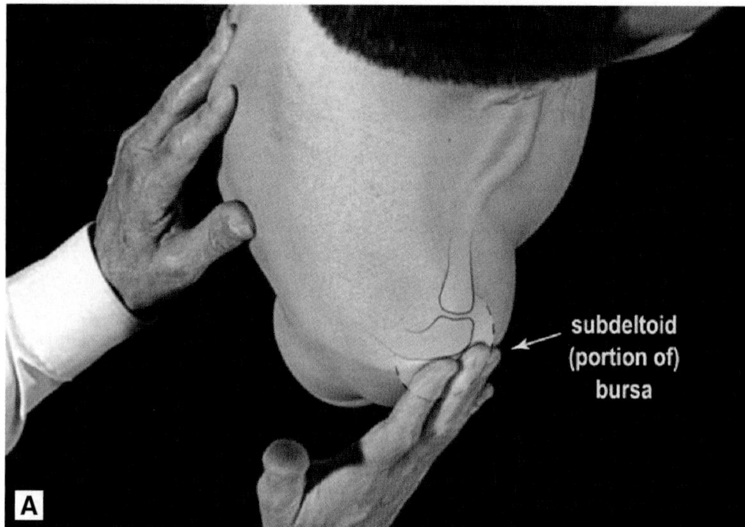

Fig. 4–28

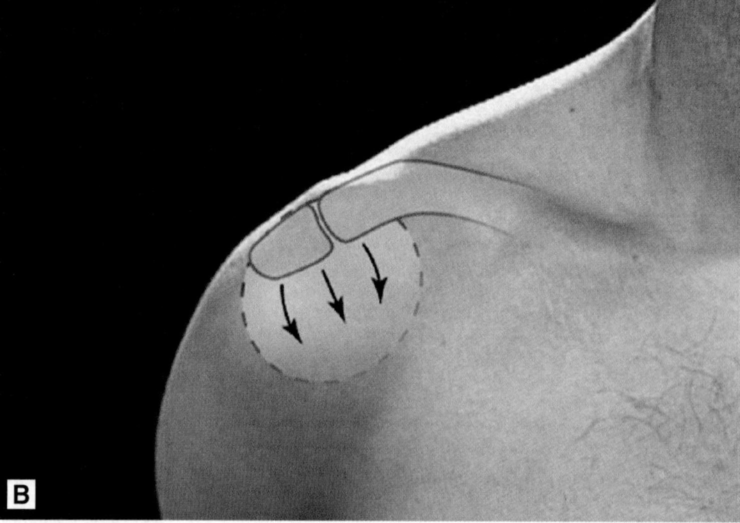

Fig. 4–28

You can now apply pressure to the subacromial bursa anteriorly, where it overlies the humeral head. Note any tenderness.

(Despite clinical features of bursitis, visible or palpable swelling of the subdeltoid and subacromial bursae is very uncommon.)

Supraspinatus and Infraspinatus Tendons Assess for pain or weakness in the rotator cuff by testing the supraspinatus and infraspinatus muscles.

Ask the patient to extend the elbows fully while you move their arms into a position of ~70° to 80° of abduction and 30° of forward flexion. The outstretched arms are now in the plane of the scapulae (Fig. 4–29A).

Next, ask the patient to turn the hands over so the thumbs are pointing at the floor (as though emptying cans or cups of water). Instruct the patient to hold the arms in this position while you supply downward force at the elbows, driving each arm down and in toward the body (Fig. 4–29B).

This maneuver stresses the supraspinatus tendon (the superior rotator cuff) and is referred to as the "supraspinatus test." Note any pain or weakness. Pain associated with supraspinatus tendonitis is often referred down the deltoid and anterolateral shoulder to the mid-humerus (Fig. 4–29C).

(Weakness of the supraspinatus may indicate a rotator cuff tear. Assessing supraspinatus strength may be difficult if resistance testing is painful, as guarding secondary to pain may inhibit maximal effort.)

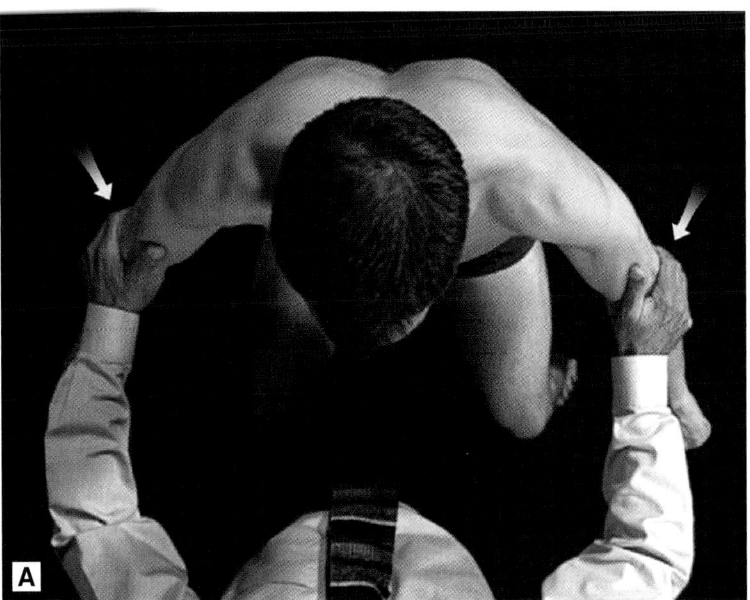

Fig. 4–29

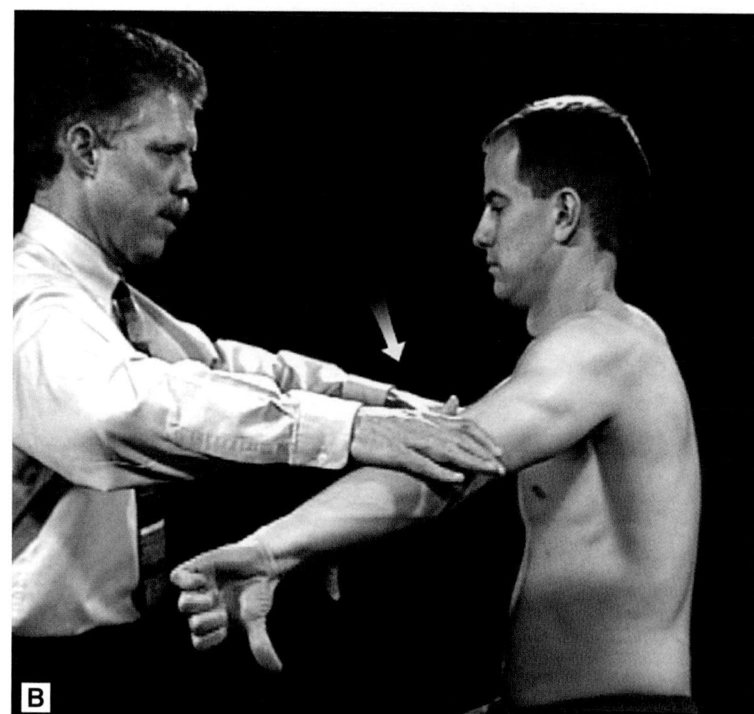

Fig. 4–29

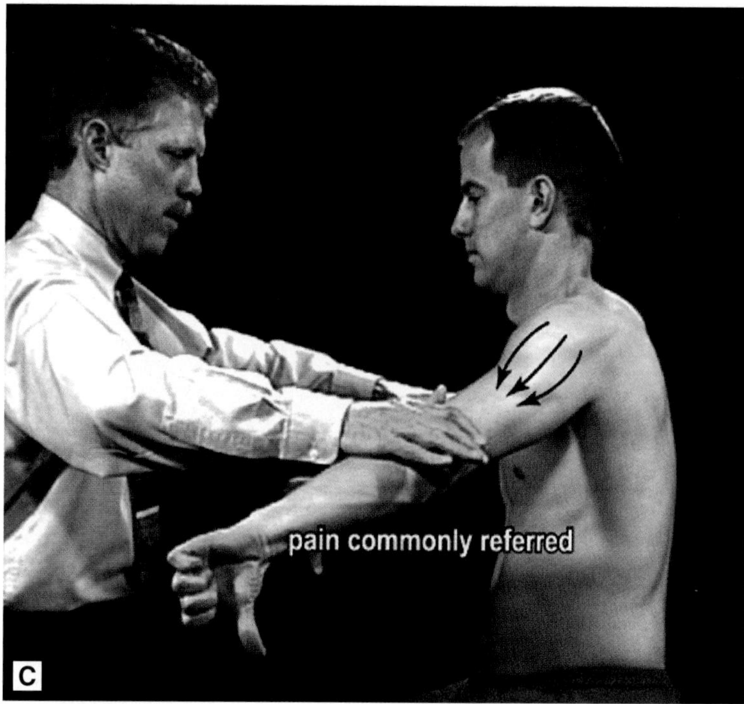

Fig. 4–29

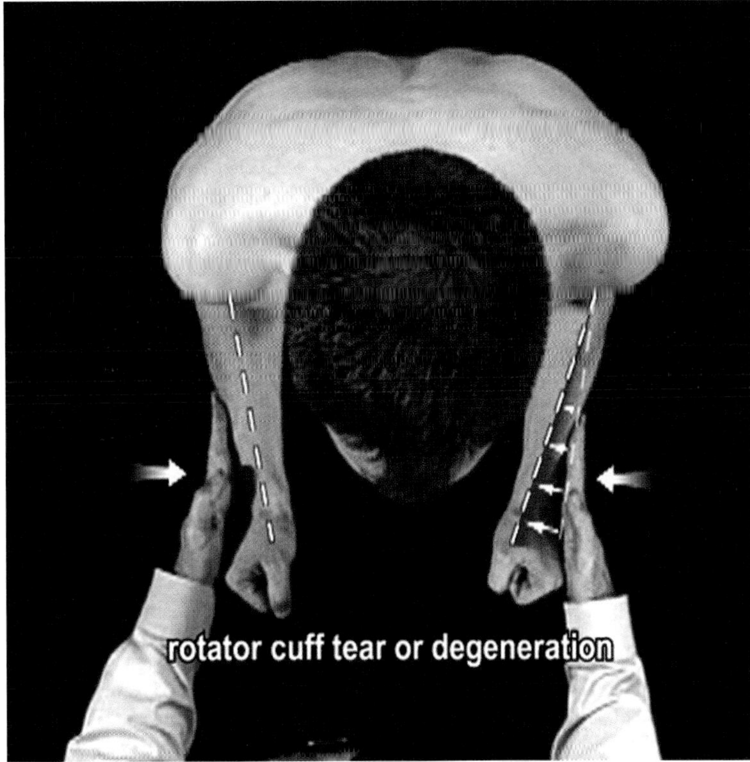

Fig. 4–30

Next, place the patient's arms at the side with the elbows flexed at 90° and the forearms directed anteriorly. Ask the patient to resist as you apply force to the distal forearm, pushing the hands medially. Weakness to resisted external rotation strongly suggests the possibility of a rotator cuff tear or degeneration (Fig. 4–30).

(While this maneuver, resisted external rotation, stresses the infraspinatus and teres minor tendons, it is helpful as a test of rotator cuff integrity. Significant rotator cuff tears most often involve the fibers of the supraspinatus and put the infraspinatus and teres minor at a mechanical disadvantage.)

Biceps Tendon Next, inspect and palpate the biceps tendon. The bicipital groove runs vertically between the greater and lesser tuberosities on the anterior surface of the humoral head, in a direct line with the forearm (Fig. 4–31A). Locate the biceps tendon by flexing the patient's elbow to 90° and running your fingers up the biceps muscle until you reach the humeral head. Next, identify the coracoid process (Fig. 4–31B). Palpating the humeral head anteriorly, at the level of the coracoid, place your examining fingers directly over the tendon in the bicipital groove (Fig. 4–31C). Many normal, noninflamed biceps tendons are tender when palpated in the bicipital groove. Be sure to compare one side with the other to assess for differential tenderness. Tenderness of the biceps tendon, suggesting tendonitis, needs to be confirmed with another maneuver to be certain that it is not simply an artifact of firm palpation.

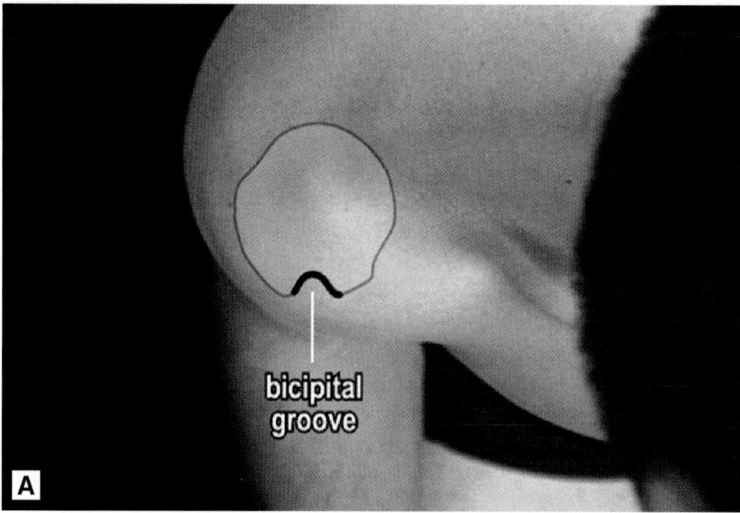

Fig. 4–31

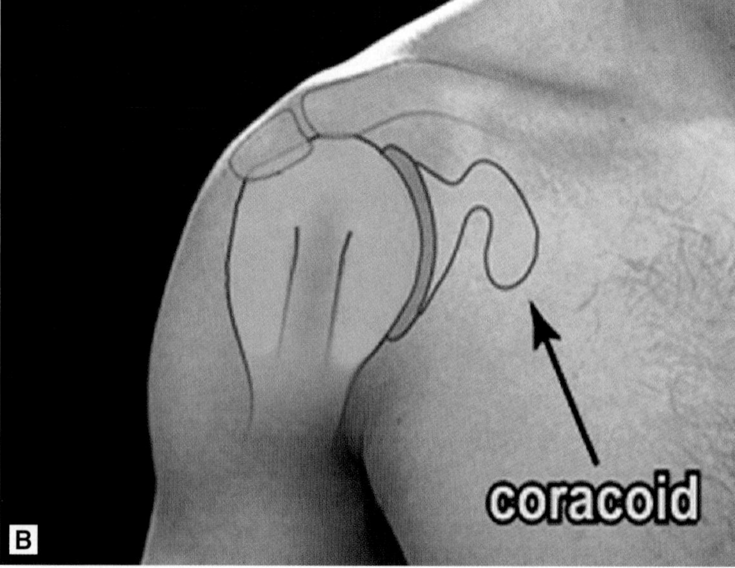

Fig. 4–31

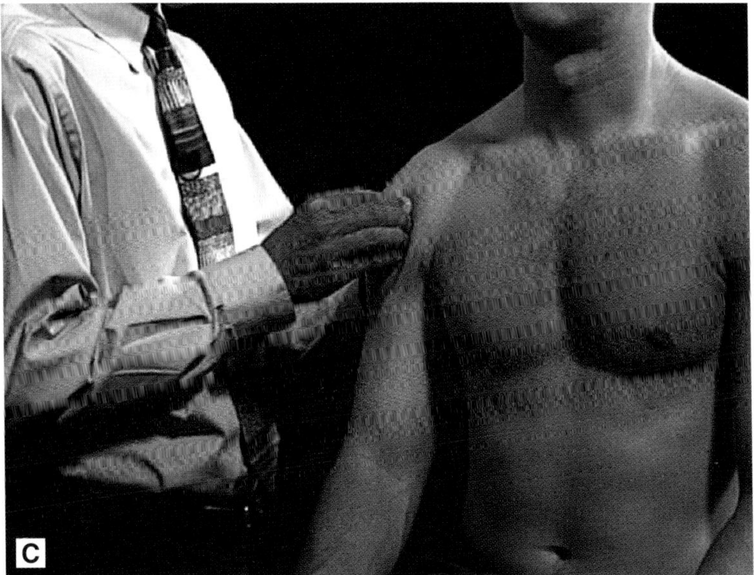
Fig. 4–31

Supination of the forearm against resistance applies considerable stress to the biceps tendon and provides an indirect means of assessing for tendonitis. Place the patient's hand with the palm facing up and grasp their hand in yours. Use your right hand with their right hand (and vice versa) and support the back of their hand and wrist with your other hand to avoid unnecessarily squeezing their fingers (Fig. 4–32A, B).

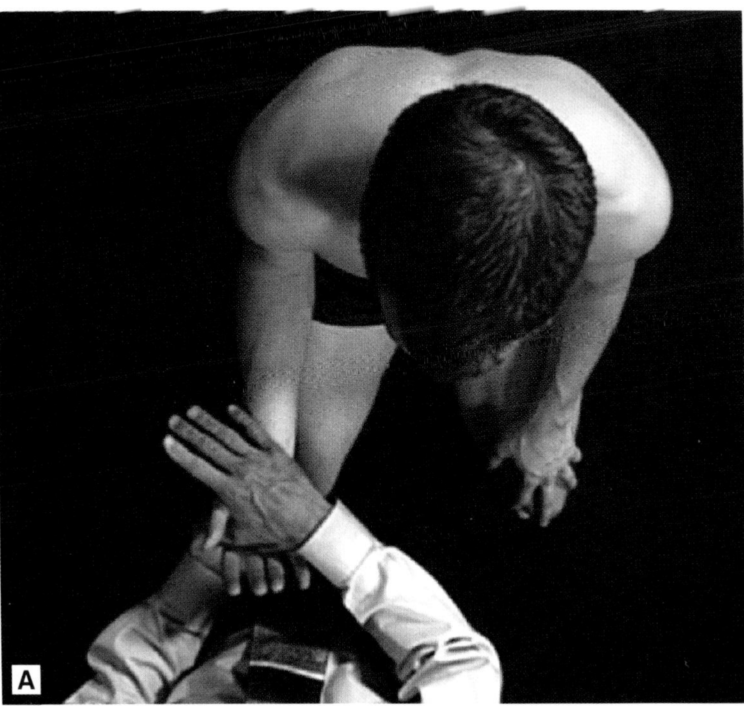
Fig. 4–32

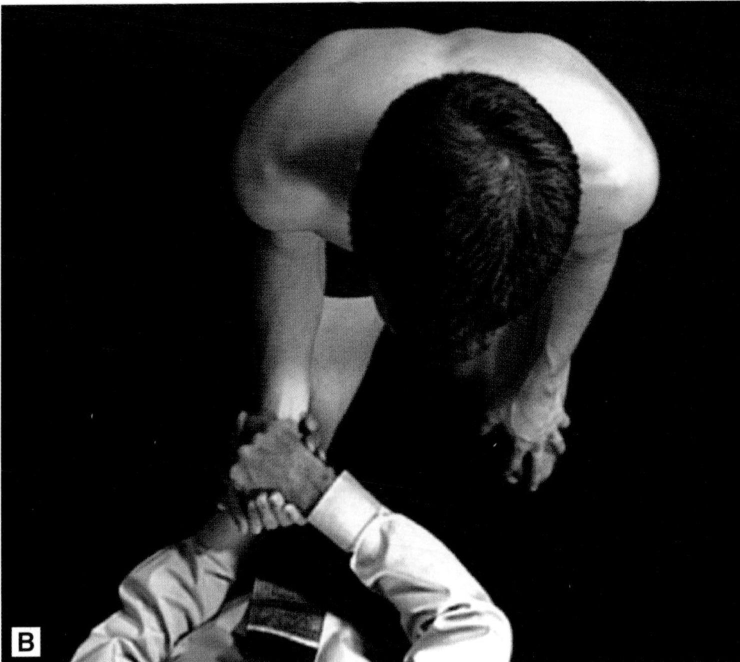

Fig. 4–32

Instruct the patient to "hold your hand flat and don't let me turn it over," as you attempt to pronate the patient's hand (turn their palm down) against their resistance (Fig. 4–33A, B).

This maneuver, called the Yerguson test, is frequently positive if the bicipital tendon is inflamed and should result in pain felt anteriorly, directly over the bicipital groove (Fig. 4–33C).

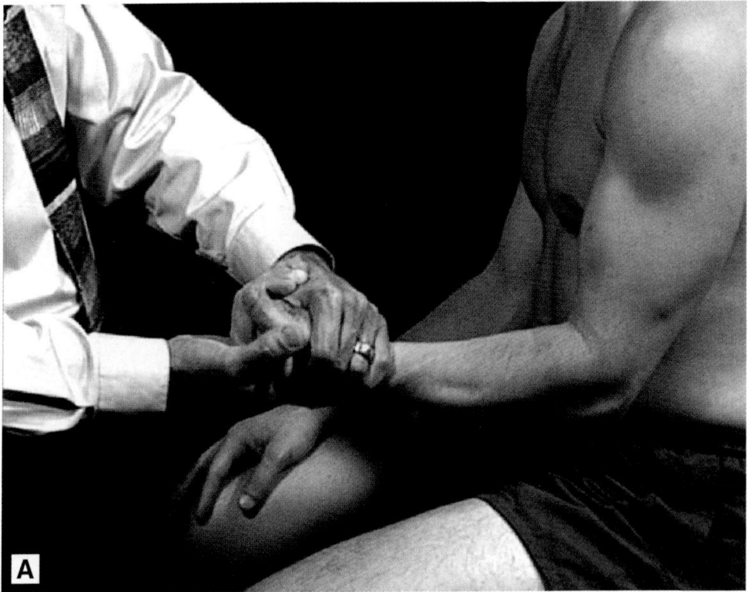

Fig. 4–33

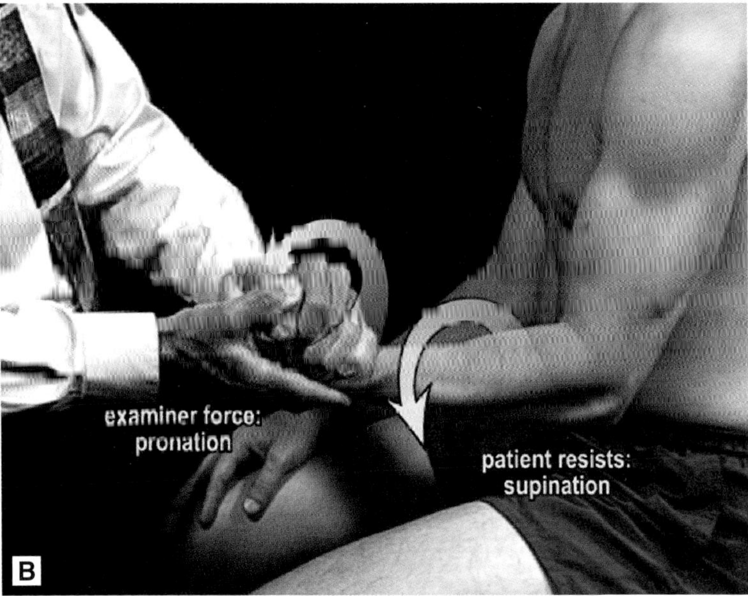

Fig. 4–33

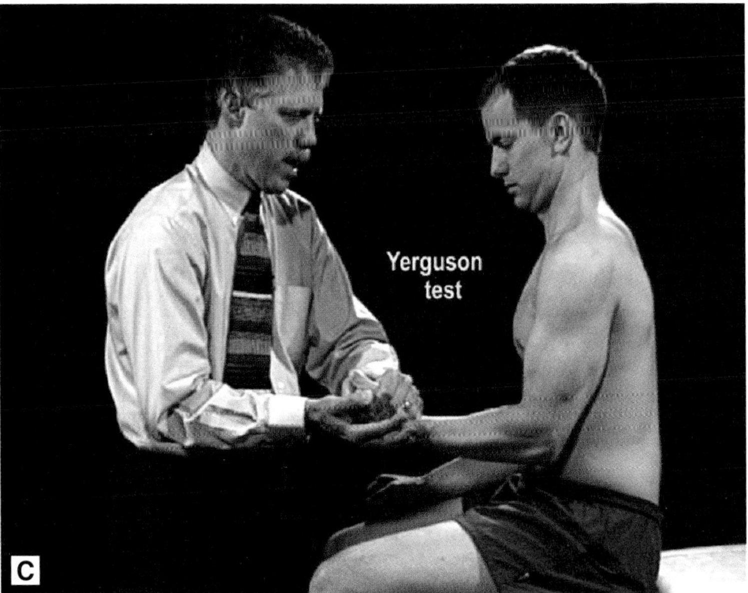

Fig. 4–33

Neer Impingement Sign Place one hand on top of the patient's acromion to stabilize the scapula while you grasp the forearm (Fig. 4–34A).

With the patient's arm relaxed and palm facing down, passively flex the shoulder anteriorly, raising the arm overhead (Fig. 4–34B). This maneuver compresses the greater tuberosity of the humerus against the anterior undersurface of the acromion, compressing the superior rotator cuff (supraspinatus tendon) near its insertion site (Fig. 4–34C). Note any pain or tenderness. Pain produced with this movement, often referred down the deltoid and anterolateral shoulder to the level of the mid-humerus, is considered a positive test and may indicate inflammation, an overuse injury, or tear of the rotator cuff (Fig. 4–35).

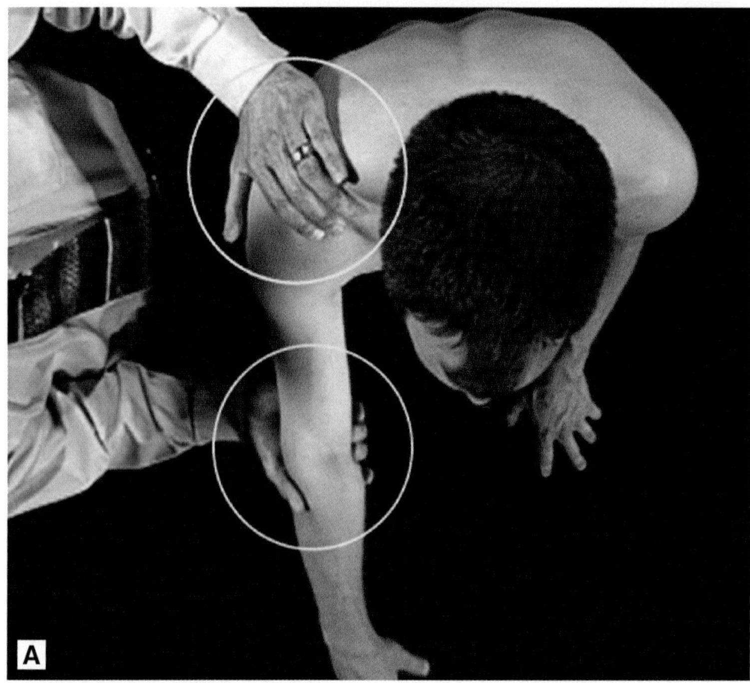

Fig. 4–34

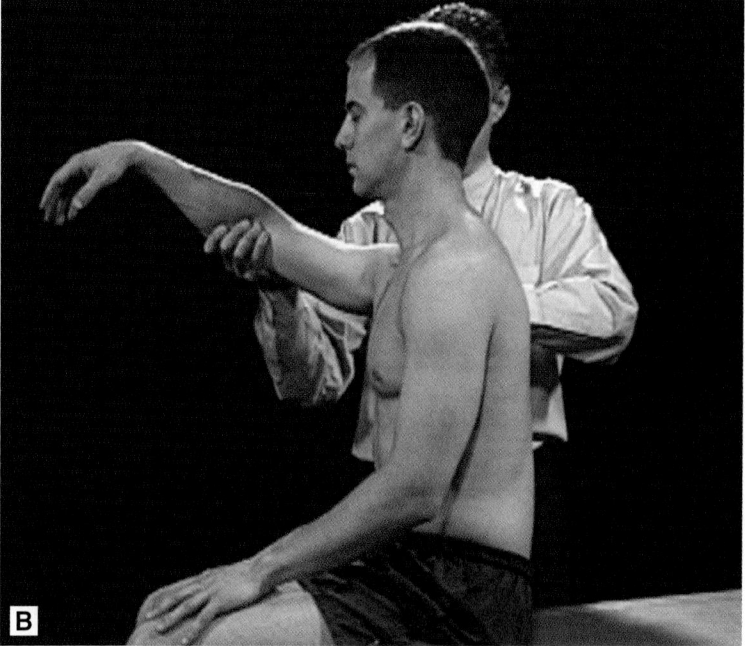

Fig. 4–34

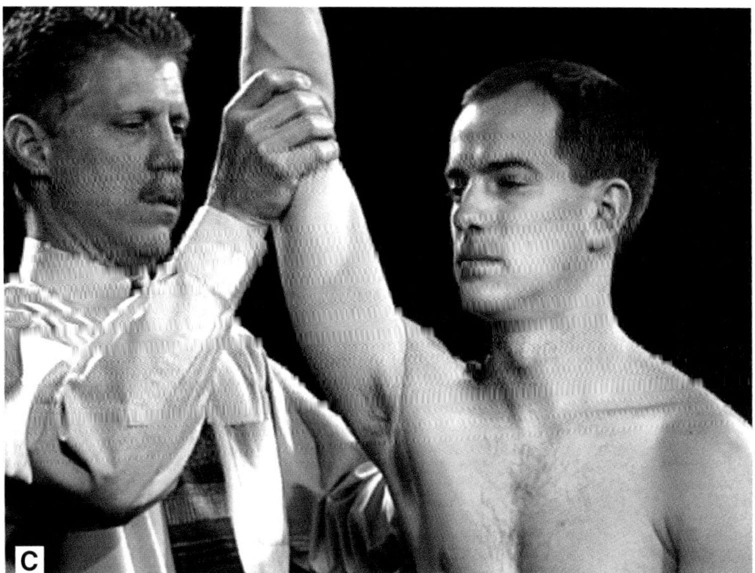

Fig. 4–34

(Patients with GH arthritis may experience pain [and restricted range of motion] during passive flexion of the shoulder. Therefore, final interpretation of the significance of a "positive" impingement sign needs to await your later, more complete assessment of GH joint range of motion.)

It is important that you maintain one hand on the patient's acromion to stabilize the scapula in order to recognize the end of GH motion (and the onset of scapulothoracic motion) during passive flexion (Fig. 4–34A). This is felt by your palpating hand as early movement of the scapula, prior to the ~120° of flexion contributed to by normal GH motion.

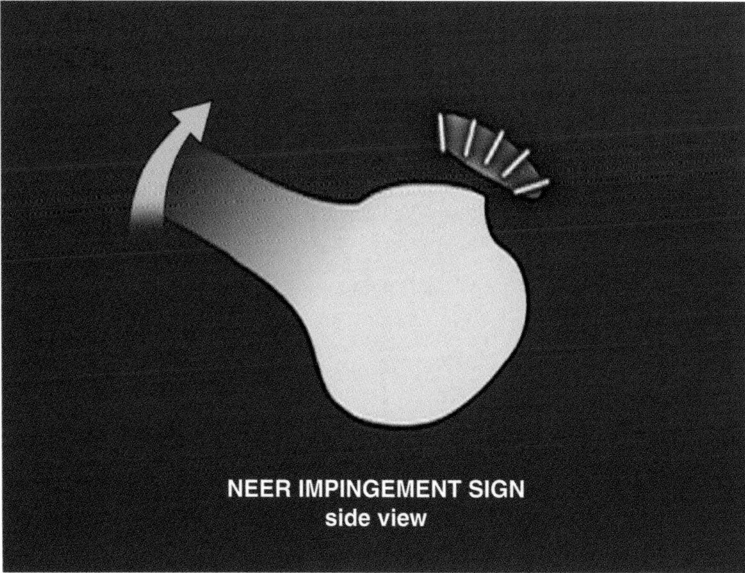

Fig. 4–35

Hawkins Impingement Sign Place one hand on top of the patient's acromion to stabilize the scapula. Passively flex the shoulder to 90° and bring the elbow into 90° of flexion with the forearm parallel to the floor (Fig. 4–36A).

Next, internally rotate the humerus by moving the hand toward the floor (Fig. 4–36B). This maneuver compresses the greater tuberosity against the anterior undersurface of the coracoacromial ligament,

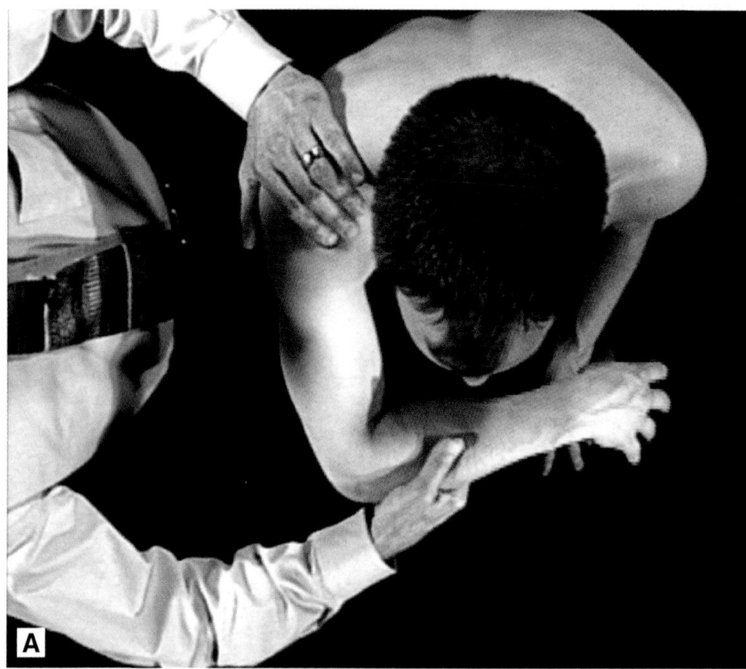

Fig. 4–36

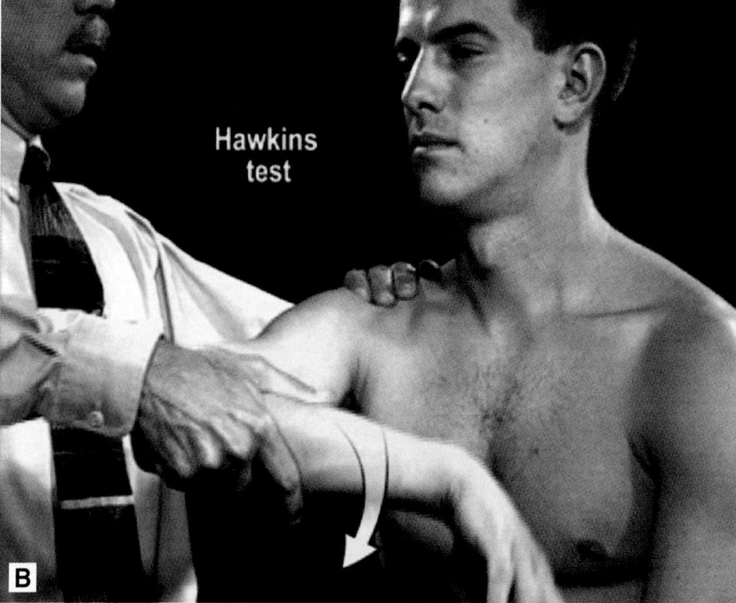

Fig. 4–36

compressing the superior rotator cuff (supraspinatus tendon) near its insertion site (Fig. 4–36C). Note any pain or tenderness.

Both the Neer and Hawkins tests are helpful in diagnosing impingement and are complementary, directing the compressive force at two different areas of the coracoacromial arch.

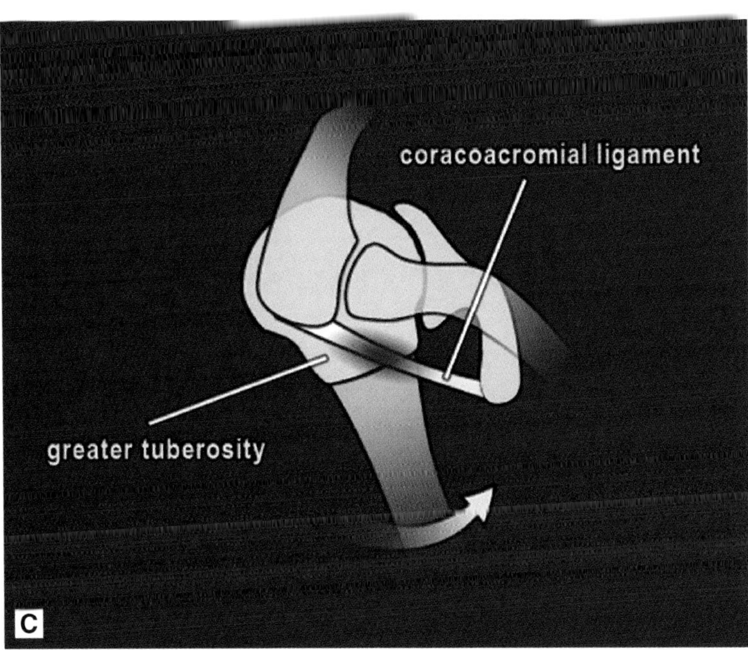

Fig. 4–36

Glenohumeral Joint Range of Motion: Seated

Flexion Passive shoulder flexion was previously assessed at the time of the Neer impingement test (and need not be repeated).

Abduction Place one hand on top of the patient's acromion to stabilize the scapula while you passively abduct the shoulder, raising the arm overhead (Fig. 4–37A).

You can facilitate relaxation of the arm by grasping the patient's forearm at or just distal to the elbow joint while gently shaking the hand and wrist during elevation. Note any pain and estimate the approximate degrees of motion (Fig. 4–37B). Pain on passive abduction is most commonly secondary to impingement of inflamed subacromial structures, movement of an abnormal GH joint (*arthritis*), or contracted shoulder joint capsule (*adhesive capsulitis*).

It is important that you maintain one hand on the patient's acromion to stabilize the scapula in order to recognize the end of GH motion (and the onset of scapulothoracic motion) during passive abduction (see Fig. 4–37A). This is felt by your palpating hand as early movement of the scapula, prior to the ~120° of abduction expected with normal GH motion.

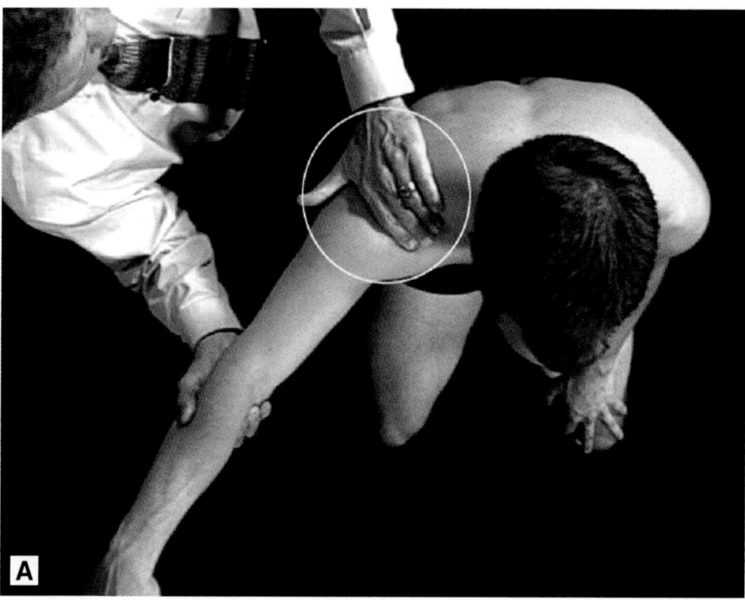

Fig. 4–37

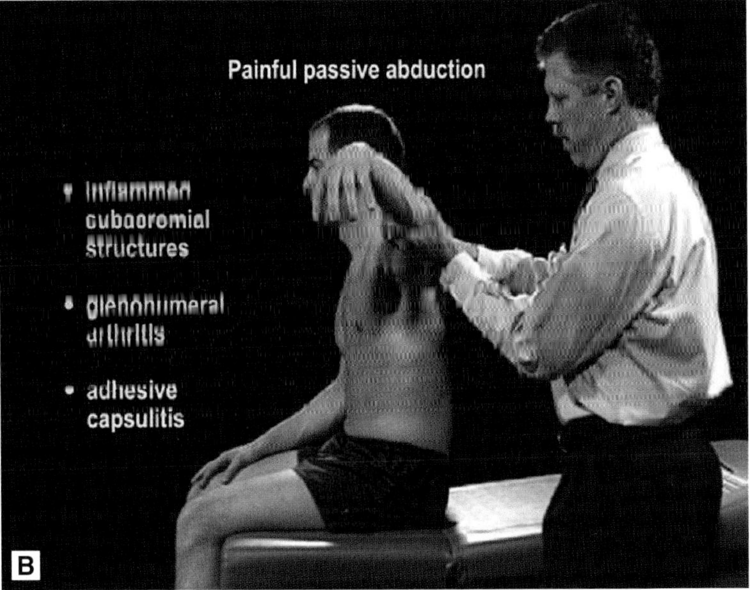

Fig. 4–37

Internal Rotation Abduct the arm to ~80° (just short of impingement) and flex the elbow to ~90°. Assess GH internal rotation by gently moving the forearm toward the patient's feet. Watch the acromion carefully to detect any early scapular motion, indicating reduced GH motion. Note any pain and the approximate degrees of total internal rotation. (In the abducted position, the normal total arc of internal rotation is ~80°.) (Fig. 4–38A, B.)

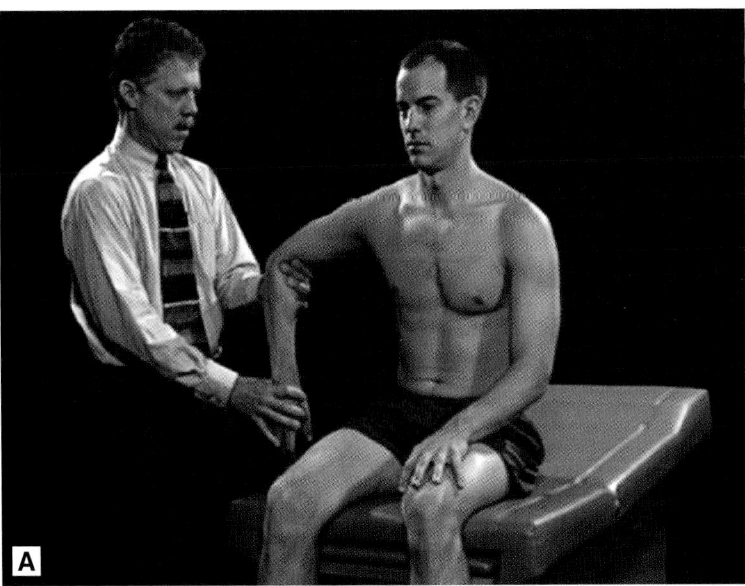

Fig. 4–38

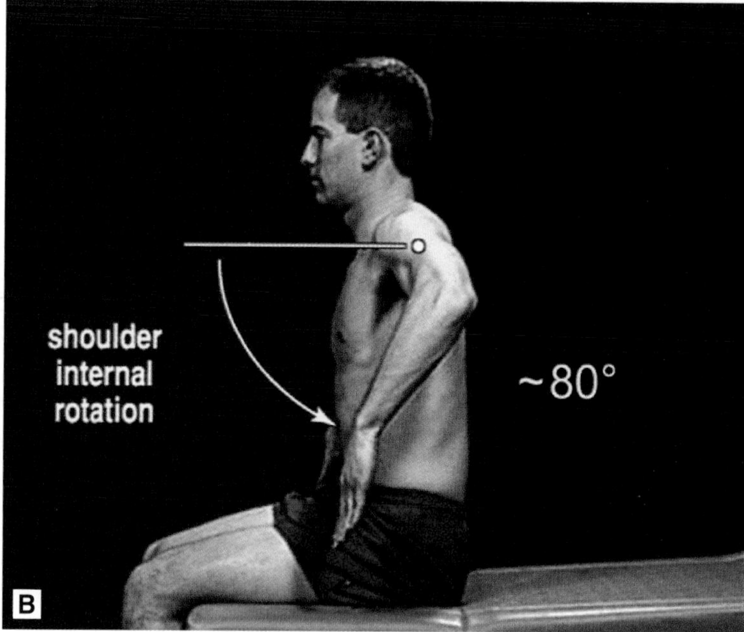

Fig. 4–38

External Rotation Return the shoulder to the abducted position with the forearm directed anteriorly. Assess GH external rotation by moving the forearm toward the patient's head gently and slowly. Again, watch the acromion carefully to detect any early scapular motion. Note any pain and the approximate degrees of total external rotation. In the abducted position, the normal total arc of external rotation is ~90° (Fig. 4–39A, B).

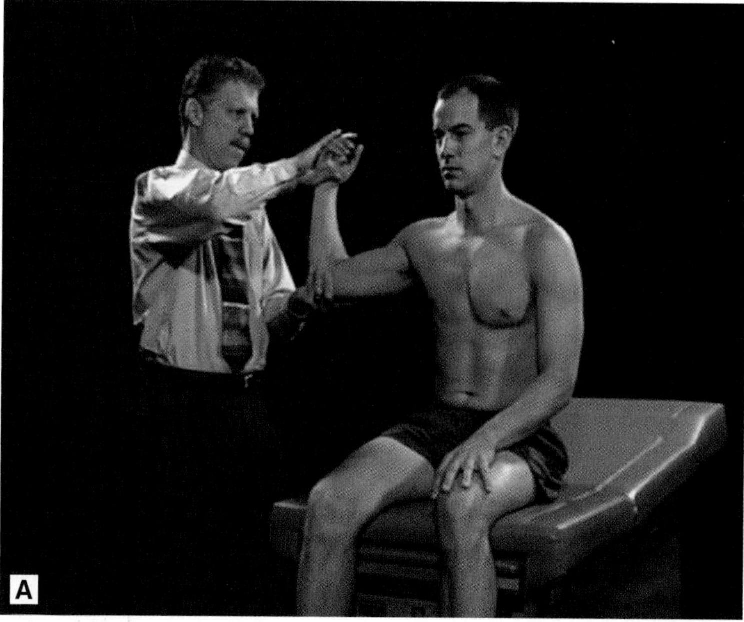

Fig. 4–39

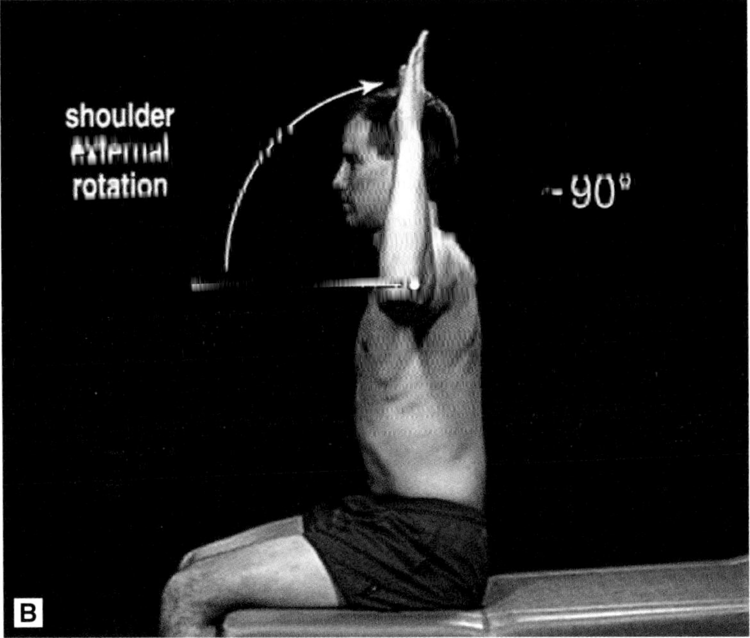

Fig. 4–39

Anterior Instability Testing In addition, while performing passive external rotation, you can assess for anterior instability of the shoulder. A patient with anterior instability or prior dislocations will often ask you to stop (or grab your hand) midway through passive ER because of apprehension generated by assuming this position (Fig. 4–40). This maneuver, called the "apprehension test," is a valuable sign suggesting anterior instability and can be performed in the seated or supine position.

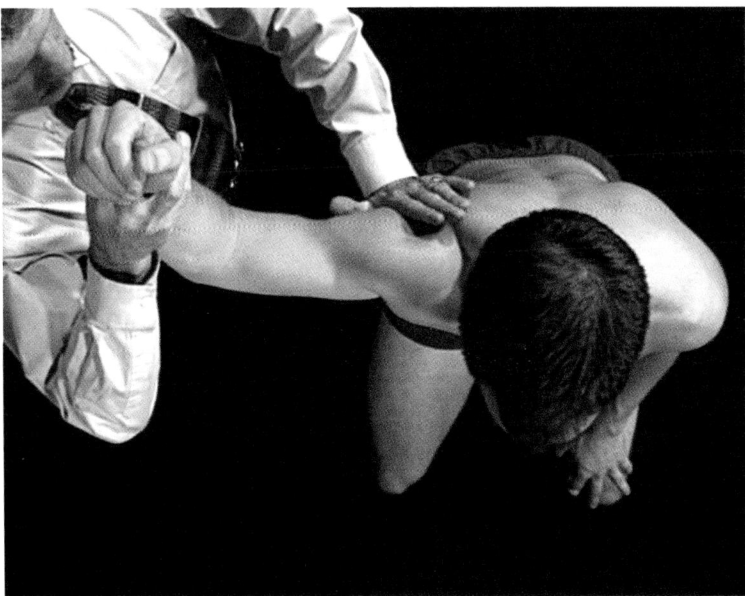

Fig. 4–40

Glenohumeral Joint Range of Motion: Supine If the patient has *any* pain or apprehension while attempting shoulder IR or ER in the seated position, ask the patient to lie supine to complete your assessment of GH joint motion (Fig. 3–41A).

The technique of assessing IR and ER is identical to that used in the seated position (Fig. 3–41B, C).

(In the supine position, the patient is more likely to relax. The scapula is stabilized against the examining table and the arcs of internal and external rotation are easy to visualize.)

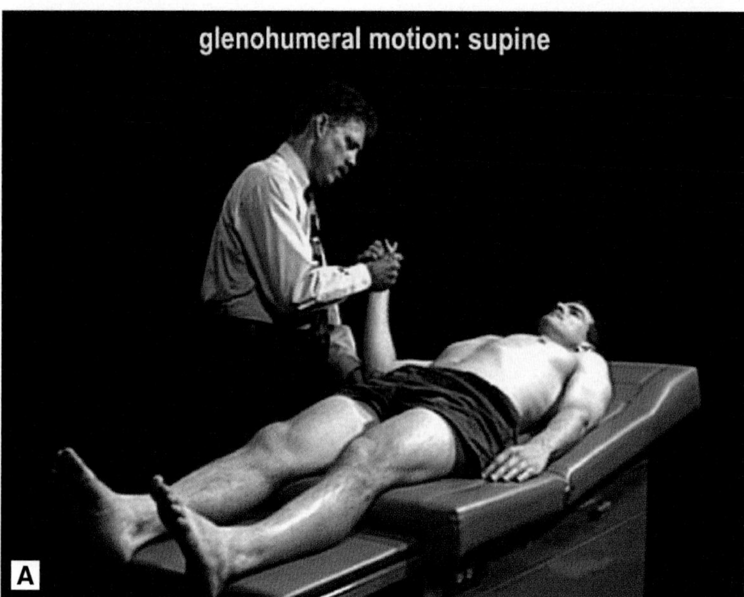

Fig. 4–41

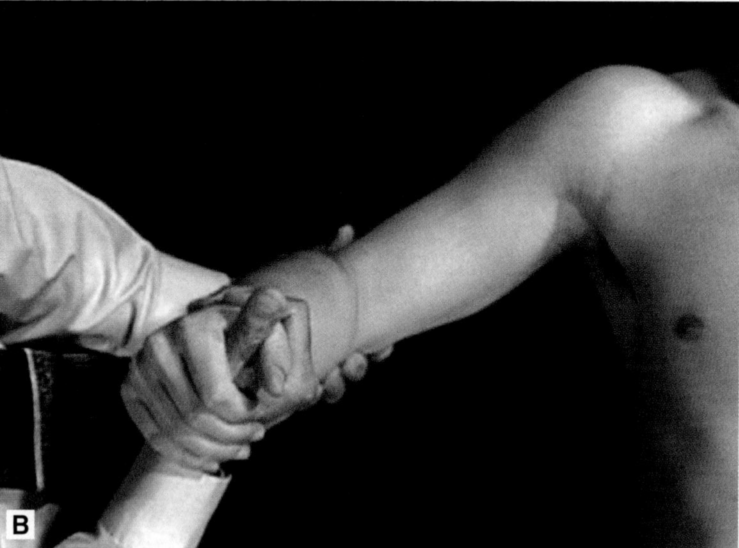

Fig. 4–41

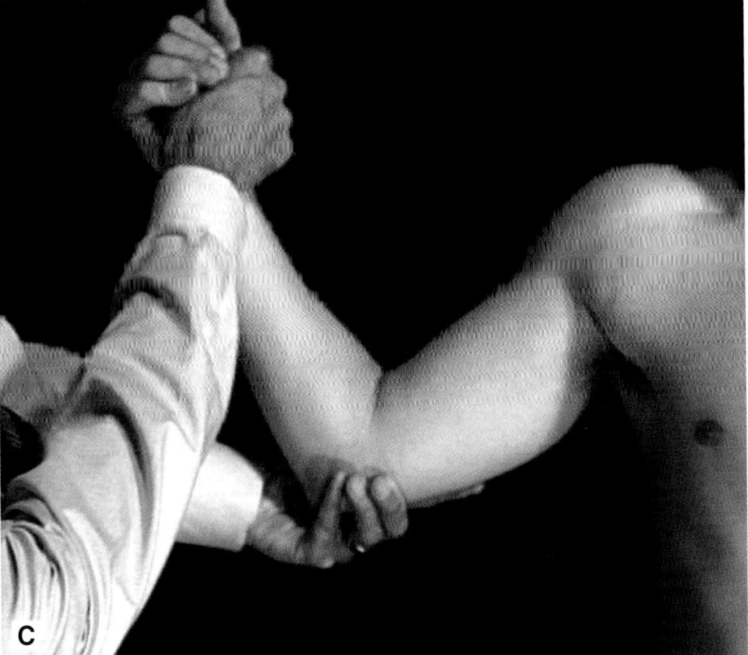

Fig. 4–41

In the absence of an apprehension sign, loss of GH motion (particularly external rotation) is a very helpful indicator of GH arthritis or adhesive capsulitis. Patients who demonstrate globally diminished range of GH motion (flexion, abduction, internal and external rotation) most commonly have either GH arthritis or adhesive capsulitis.

It is frequently not possible to differentiate between these two possibilities on the basis of your clinical examination alone. A plane x-ray of the shoulder (two views) may be required to finalize your diagnosis. Adhesive capsulitis is associated with a normal x-ray and GH arthritis may be associated with joint space loss, osteophytes, sclerosis, erosions, etc.

RMSE OF THE SHOULDER
Practice Checklist

Patient seated

Observe from behind

____Inspect supraspinatus, infraspinatus, and deltoid muscles

____Observe active arm elevation and scapular motion

Observe from the front

____Inspect deltoid and pectoralis muscles

____Observe deltopectoral groove

____Check C spine range of motion

____Inspect and palpate SC joints

____Inspect and palpate AC joints

____Palpate lateral subdeltoid region/bursa

____Palpate anterior subacromial region/bursa

____Resisted shoulder abduction: supraspinatus test ("empty cans")

____Resisted shoulder ER: rotator cuff integrity

____Inspect and palpate the biceps tendon

____Resisted supination of the forearm: Yerguson test

____Neer impingement sign: passive shoulder flexion

____Hawkins impingement sign: passive shoulder flexion, adduction, and forced IR

Patient seated or supine

____Shoulder flexion: *already performed with the Neer maneuver*

____Shoulder abduction

____Shoulder internal rotation*

____Shoulder external rotation (check apprehension sign)*

* If examination has been at all painful or guarded, ask the patient to lie *supine* to assess GH motion.

COMMON SHOULDER PROBLEMS

- Impingement
- Subacromial bursitis
- Supraspinatus/rotator cuff tendonitis and rotator cuff tear
- Biceps tendonitis
- Adhesive capsulitis (frozen shoulder)
- Glenohumeral arthritis
- Acromioclavicular arthritis
- Cervical spine referred pain
- Instability

Impingement Forward flexion and abduction of the arm beyond 90° (overhead activities, throwing, etc) will result in compression of the subacromial bursa, superior rotator cuff (supraspinatus tendon), and the tendon (long head) of the biceps. These three soft tissue structures "live" sandwiched between the head of the humerus (bone) and the acromion (bone), and coracoacromial arch (ligament) where they are subject to repetitive pinch, causing irritation and inflammation. This impingement results in the three most common ambulatory shoulder problems: subacromial bursitis, supraspinatus tendonitis, and biceps tendonitis.

Subacromial Bursitis Repetitive pinch of the subacromial bursa between the greater tuberosity of the humerus and the acromion can result in acute or chronic irritation and inflammation. Pain occurs during arm elevation beyond 90° (impingement position) and is frequently referred down the upper arm (deltoid region) to the mid humerus.

Supraspinatus Tendonitis/Rotator Cuff Tendnitis and Rotator Cuff Tears Sports or occupationally related repetitive activity and overuse injury may result in irritation, inflammation, and micro or macro tears of the rotator cuff. Because of its vascular supply and superior location (directly under the bony acromion), the supraspinatus tendon is the most frequent site of rotator cuff tendonitis. Pain occurs especially during active or resisted abduction and frequently radiates down the upper arm (deltoid region) to the mid-humerus.

Acute or chronic tears of the rotator cuff usually involve the supraspinatus (most common) and infraspinatus (less common) tendons.

Biceps Tendonitis Because of its intra-articular location (entering the shoulder joint capsule, passing through the bicipital groove, proceeding over the top of the humeral head, and attaching to the superior rim of the glenoid fossa), the biceps tendon (like the subacromial bursa and supraspinatus tendon) is subjected to subacromial impingement. Pain during forward flexion and forearm supination is usually felt anteriorly in the region of the bicipital groove.

(Because of its extra-articular location, the short head of the biceps is seldom a source of clinical symptoms.)

Adhesive Capsulitis (Frozen Shoulder) Adhesive capsulitis refers to the condition of progressive (painful or painless) globally decreased shoulder range of motion. This most commonly follows injury, shoulder bursitis or tendonitis, or stroke, and may occur in association with diabetes mellitus. Passive (examiner-initiated) movement is diminished in all planes and may be painful (early) or painless (late). Plain x-rays of the shoulder are normal.

Glenohumeral Arthritis Arthritis of the GH joint usually presents with diffuse, dull, aching discomfort and painful, restricted active and passive range of motion. GH joint swelling may sometimes cause loss of the normal deltopectoral groove anteriorly (uncommon). Advanced GH arthritis may be associated with palpable or audible crepitus on range of motion. Plain x-rays are abnormal with features of arthritis (joint space narrowing, sclerosis, osteophyte formation).

Acromioclavicular Joint Pain AC joint pain is most commonly felt directly over the joint, on the superior aspect of the shoulder. It can be reliably precipitated by direct palpation over the joint and passive (examiner-initiated) cross-chest adduction.

Cervical Spine Referred Pain The neck frequently refers pain to the shoulder. Nonradicular cervical pain frequently radiates along the trapezius muscles superolaterally and along the medial scapular border posteriorly, sometimes presenting as "shoulder" pain.

Instability Patients with shoulder instability may have recurrent episodes of subluxation and/or dislocation, with anterior instability being the most common. Patients may be aware of the arm slipping "out of joint," and have apprehension with certain movements (especially combined abduction and external rotation) and a prior history of trauma or generalized joint hypermobility. Shoulder instability may accompany joint laxity due to an associated tear of the glenoid labrum.

LESS COMMON SHOULDER PROBLEMS

- Sternoclavicular arthritis
- Visceral referred pain

Sternoclavicular Joint Pain SC joint pain is usually felt directly over the joint itself and (less commonly) radiates to the anterior chest on the same side. Visible and palpable swelling plus local tenderness suggest SC joint pathology. The SC joint may be the site of septic arthritis in injection drug users and inflammatory arthritis in patients with spondyloarthropathies.

Visceral Referred Pain The lungs, diaphragm, and heart can each refer pain to the shoulder. Referred visceral pain is first suspected from the clinical context and a careful history combined with a negative regional examination of the shoulder (despite shoulder pain complaints).

5

The Regional Musculoskeletal Examination of the Knee

INTRODUCTION

The *regional musculoskeletal examination* (RMSE) of the **knee** is designed to build on the sequences and techniques taught in the SMSE and GMSE. It is intended to provide a comprehensive assessment of structure and function combined with special testing to permit you to evaluate common, important musculoskeletal problems of the knee seen in an ambulatory setting. The skills involved require practice and careful attention to technique. However, they can be learned and mastered on normal individuals.

CLINICAL UTILITY

The RMSE of the knee is clinically useful as the initial examination in individuals whose history clearly suggests an acute knee injury or an isolated knee problem. In individuals whose history is less straightforward (a seemingly local, nontraumatic knee problem with additional musculoskeletal complaints of unclear relevance), a rapid SMSE may be the most appropriate first step in physical assessment. If significant, possibly related, abnormalities are found (and the patient's presenting knee complaint appears to be part of a more generalized musculoskeletal process), then performing a GMSE would be most appropriate.

With practice, a systematic, efficient RMSE of the knee can be performed in ~3 to 4 minutes.

Furthermore, the RMSE of the knee provides the foundation for learning additional, more refined diagnostic techniques through your later exposure to orthopedic surgeons, rheumatologists, physiatrists, physical therapists, and others specifically involved in the diagnosis and treatment of knee problems.

OBJECTIVES

This instructional program will enable you to identify important anatomical, functional, and pathologic relationships at the knee, including

- Important surface anatomy
- Presence of knee effusions
- Patellofemoral and tibiofemoral joints
- Anterior cruciate, medial and lateral collateral and posterior cruciate ligaments
- Meniscal cartilages
- Prepatellar and anserine bursae

Most importantly, this program will prepare you to perform an organized, integrated, and clinically useful examination of the knee.

ESSENTIAL CONCEPTS

Structural and Functional Anatomy The knee joint is made up of four bones: the distal **femur**, proximal **tibia**, **patella** (a large, sesamoid within the quadriceps tendon), and the proximal **fibula** (Fig. 5–1). These bones form three articulations: the **tibiofemoral joint** (hinge-like), the **patellofemoral joint** (gliding pulley), and the **tibiofibular joint** (small, lateral stabilizer) (Fig. 5–2).

Because the knee is an inherently unstable joint, it has two external (collateral) stabilizing ligaments: the long, broad **medial collateral ligament** (MCL) (between the medial femoral epicondyle and the medial tibia) and the smaller diameter **lateral collateral ligament** (LCL) (between the lateral femoral epicondyle and the head of the fibula) (Fig. 5–3A, B). The knee also has two internal (crossing or "cruciate") stabilizing ligaments which run centrally in the notch between the femoral condyles: the **anterior**

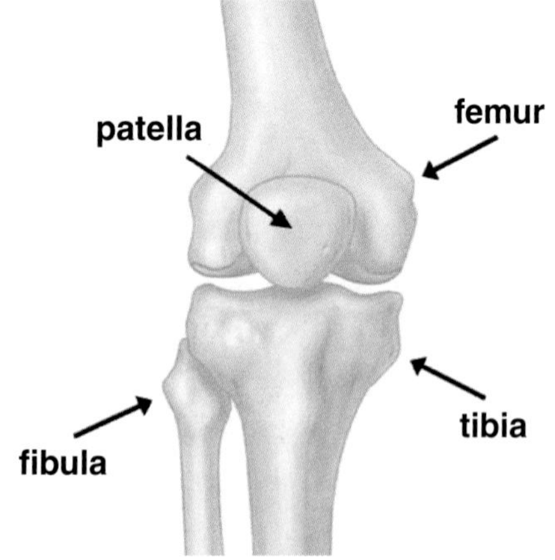

Fig. 5–1.

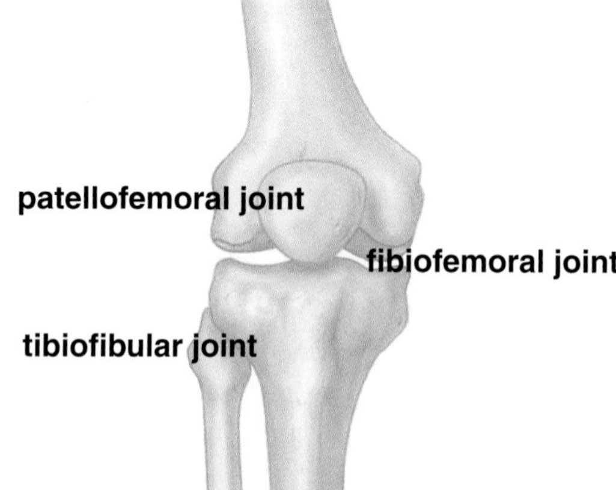

Fig. 5–2. (Modified with permission from Lawry GV, Kreder HJ, Hawker G, Jerome D. Fam's Musculoskeletal Examination and Joint Injection Techniques, 2nd ed. Mosby/Elsevier, 2010, p. 66.)

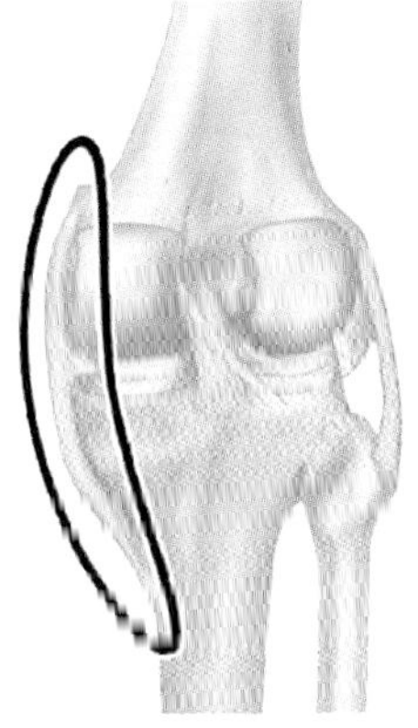

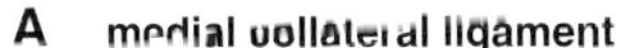

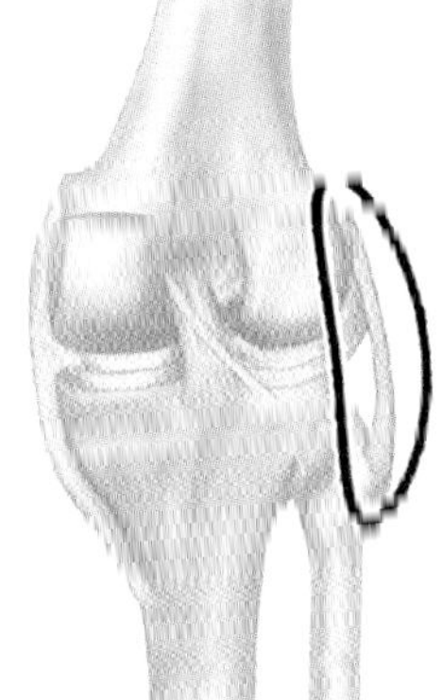

Fig. 5–3. (Modified with permission from Lawry GV, Kreder HJ, Hawker G, Jerome D. Fam's Musculoskeletal Examination and Joint Injection Techniques, 2nd ed. Mosby/Elsevier, 2010, p. 69.)

cruciate ligament (ACL) (Fig. 5–4A; between the posteromedial corner of the lateral femoral condyle and the anterior tibial plateau just medial to the midline) and the **posterior cruciate ligament** (PCL) (Fig. 5–4B; between the anterolateral corner of the medial femoral condyle and the posterior tibial plateau just lateral to the midline).

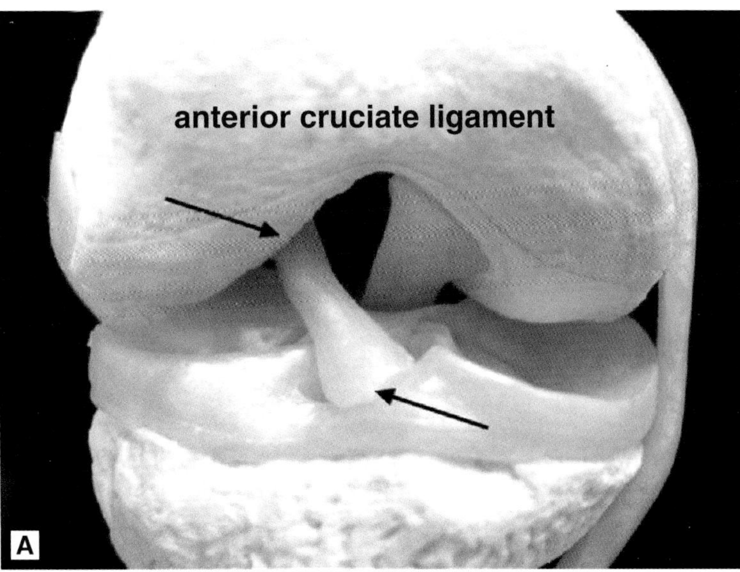

Fig. 5–4

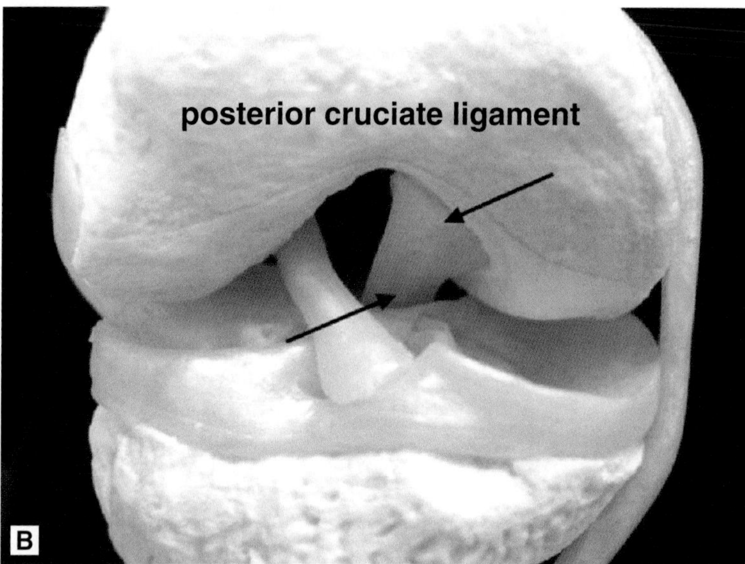

Fig. 5–4

To better visualize the relationship of these two ligaments to the femur and tibia, cross your fingers and place them next to the medial aspect of the corresponding knee (right hand to right knee or left hand to left knee; Fig. 5–5A). Now, uncross your fingers. Your middle finger corresponds to the orientation of the ACL (running from the posterior femur to the anterior tibia), and your index finger corresponds to the orientation of the PCL (running from the anterior femur to the posterior tibia; Fig. 5–5B). Understanding these relationships will become important when learning physical examination techniques to stress the ligaments.

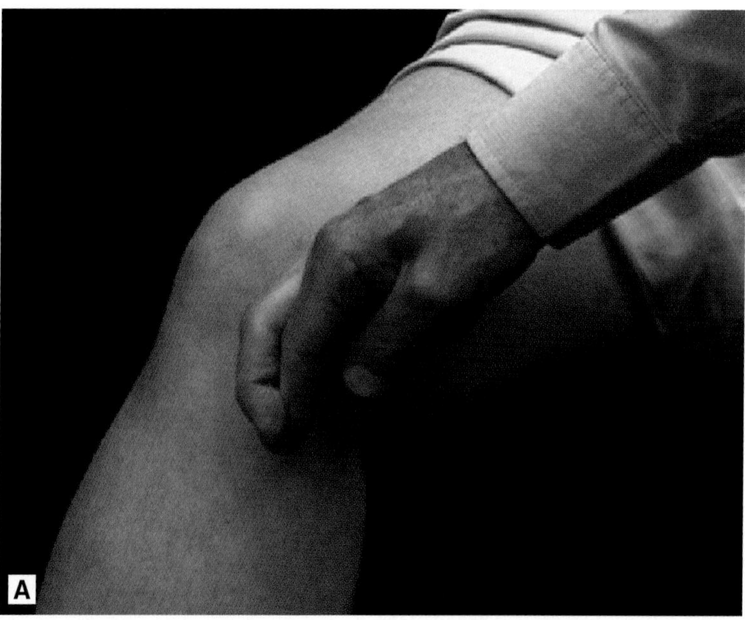

Fig. 5–5

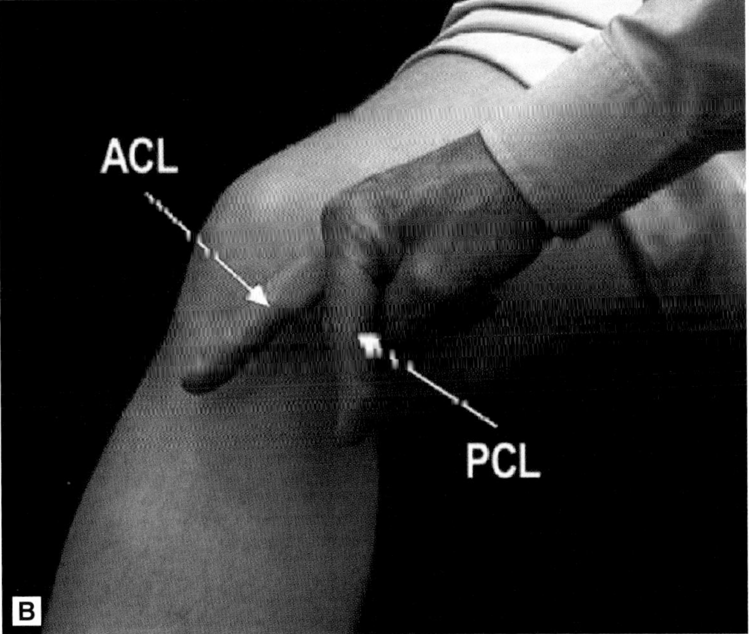

Fig. 5–5

In addition, each knee has two crescent-shaped fibrocartilages, the **medial** and **lateral menisci** (Fig. 5–6). These shock-absorbing cartilages are wedge-shaped in cross section and increase the contact surface area between each femoral condyle and the tibial plateau, thereby improving weight distribution and joint stability.

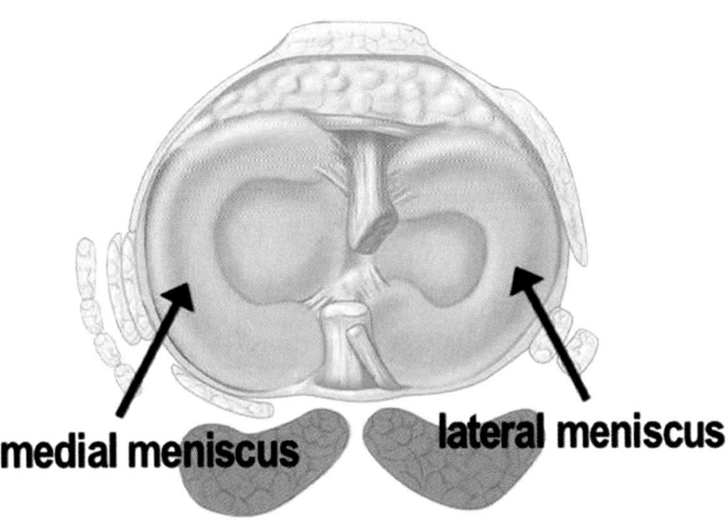

Fig. 5–6. (Modified with permission from Lawry GV, Kreder HJ, Hawker G, Jerome D. Fam's Musculoskeletal Examination and Joint Injection Techniques, 2nd ed. Mosby/Elsevier, 2010, p. 70.)

Subcutaneous and anterior to the patella lies the **prepatellar bursa** (Fig. 5–7A). Quite superficial and just beneath the insertion of the pes anserine tendons on the anteromedial flare of the proximal tibia lies the **anserine bursa** (Fig. 5–7B).

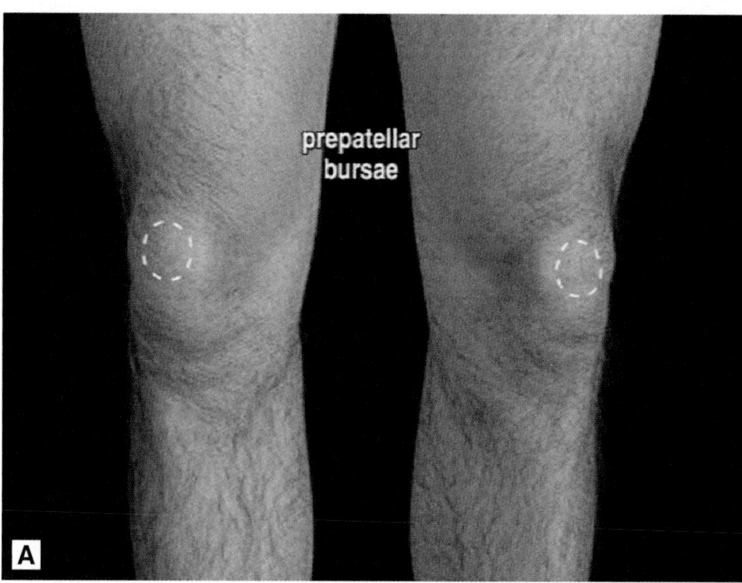

Fig. 5–7

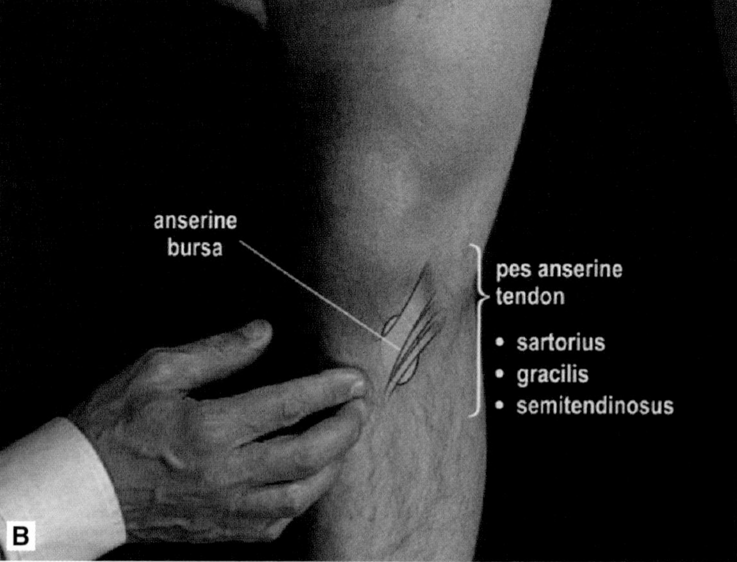

Fig. 5–7

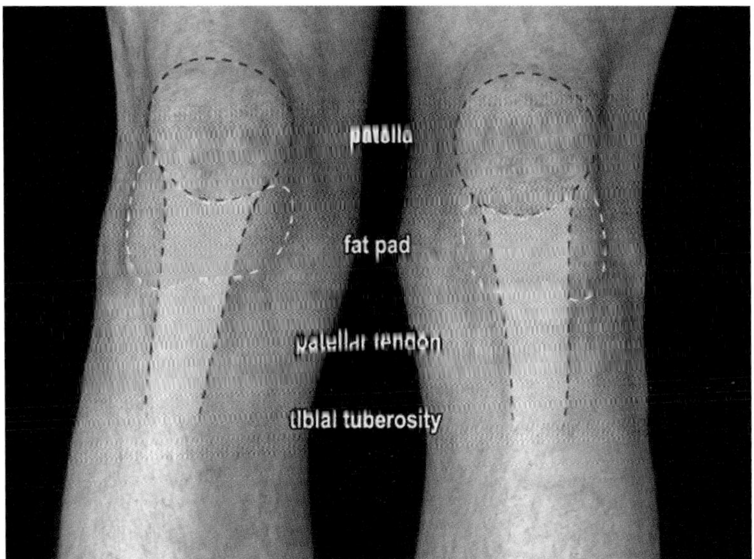

Fig. 5–8

Two additional structures are very important for clinicians and are essential to understanding the surface anatomy of the knee: the infrapatellar fat pad and the suprapatellar pouch of the knee joint cavity. The **infrapatellar fat pad** is a wide, fatty cushion which lies anteriorly below the patella (deep to the patellar tendon, between the joint capsule and synovial membrane; Fig. 5–8). Shaped like a bow tie or thyroid gland, it cushions the anterior joint line during kneeling. The infrapatellar fat pads are usually more prominent in women than men (Fig. 5–9A, B) and can vary in size from being barely

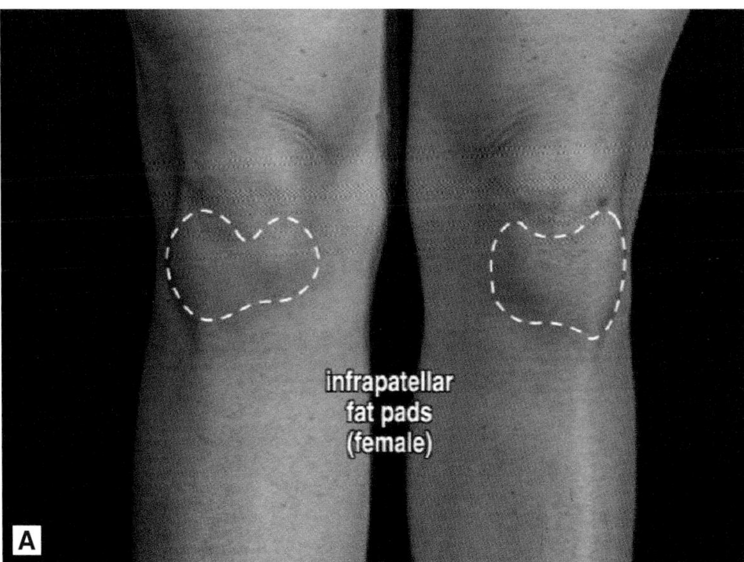

Fig. 5–9

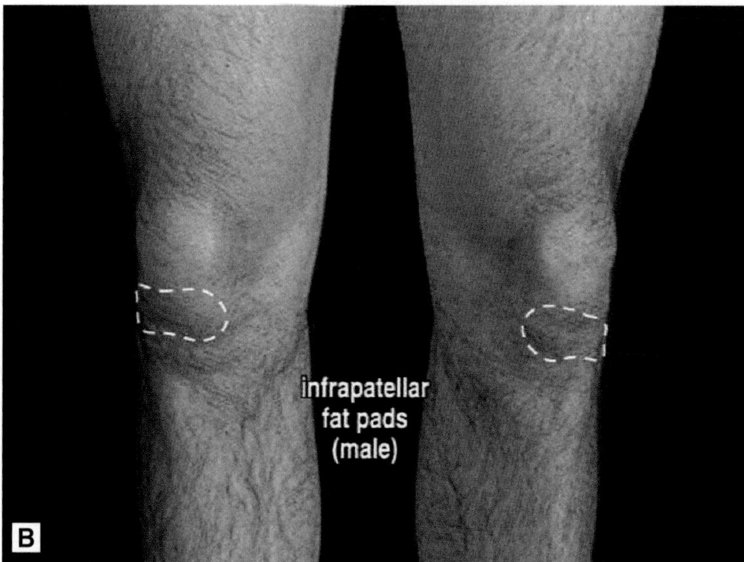

Fig. 5–9

visible to very large and prominent (sometimes easily confused with a "swollen knee"; Fig. 5–10A, B). The **suprapatellar pouch** is a large, superior reflection of the synovial cavity which extends ~6 cm above the patella (Fig. 5–11A).

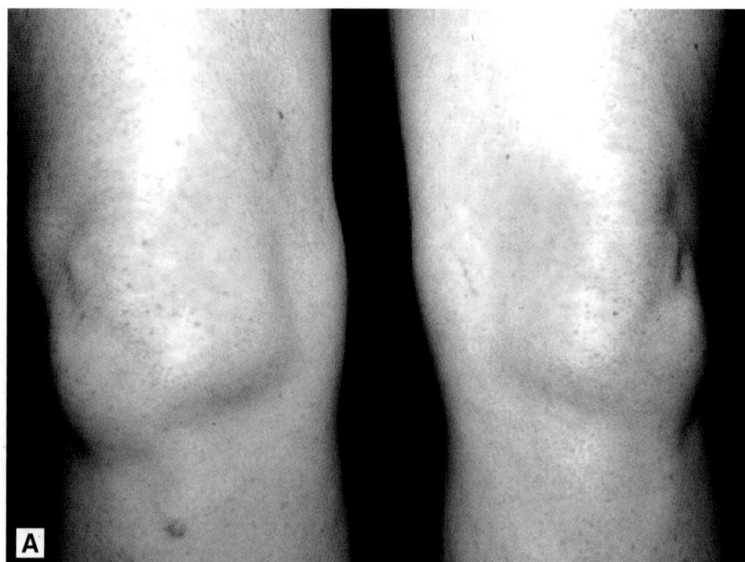

Fig. 5–10

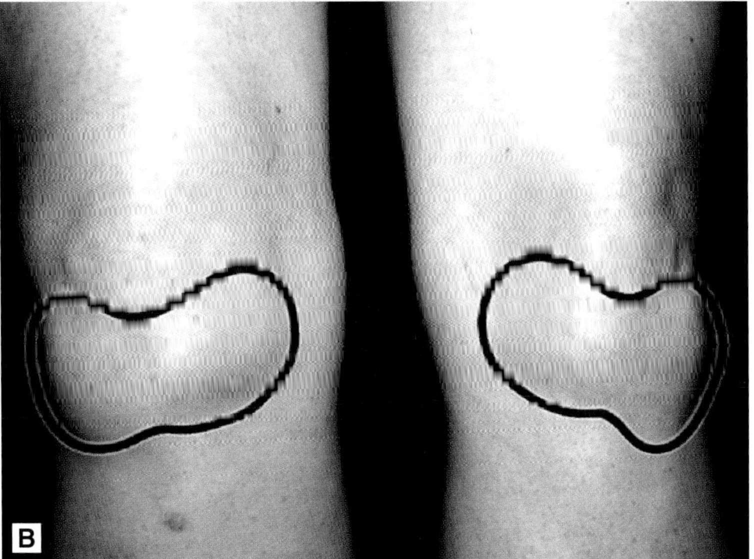

Fig. 5–10

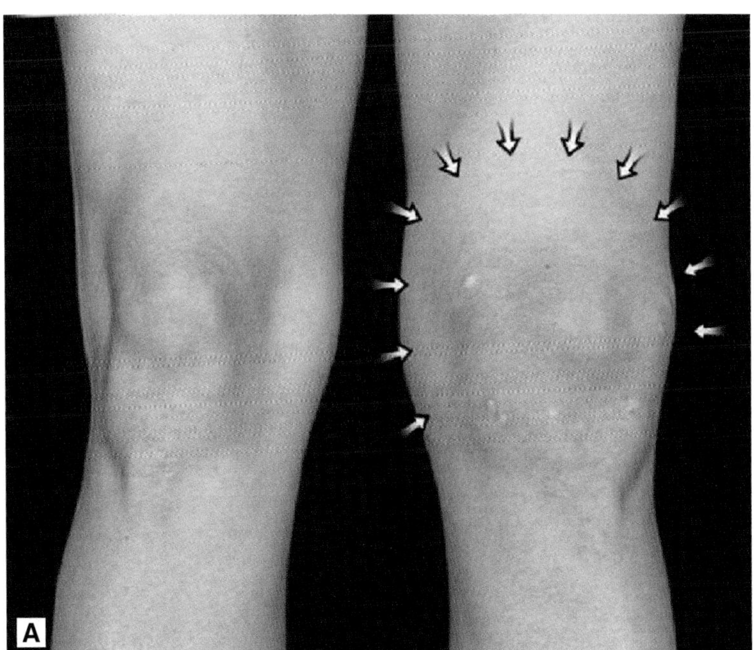

Fig. 5–11

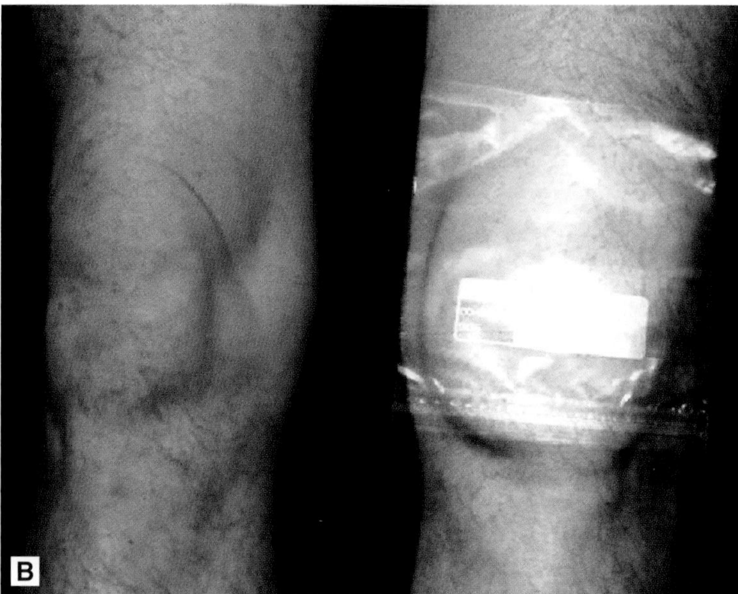

Fig. 5–11

It may be helpful to think of this reflection as analogous to a thin sandwich bag tucked under the distal quadriceps muscles, in free communication with the joint (Fig. 5–11B). This "synovial sandwich bag" can become distended with synovial fluid (or blood) due to inflammation or injury of the knee. As distention increases, the suprapatellar pouch swells in a characteristic sequence and pattern which can be readily recognized by clinicians: initial loss of the normal concavity (sulcus) at the medial side of the knee followed by visible bulging superolaterally (Fig. 5–12A) and finally gross distention of the entire suprapatellar pouch (Fig. 5–12B).

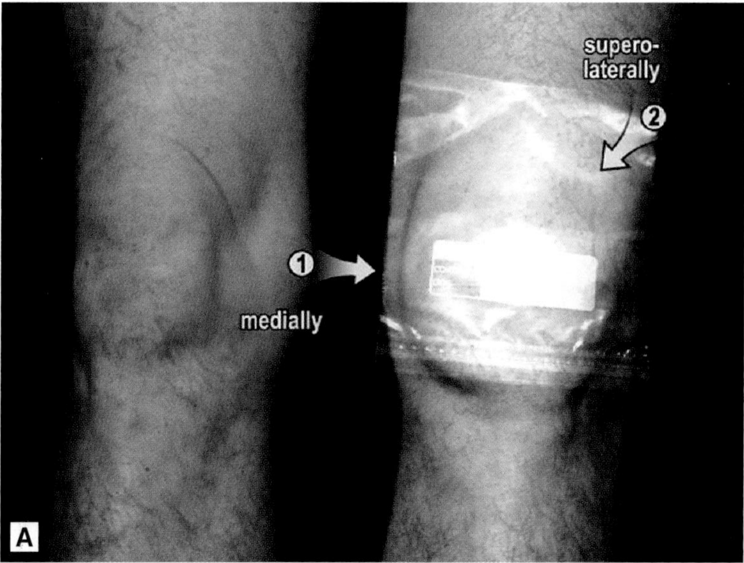

Fig. 5–12

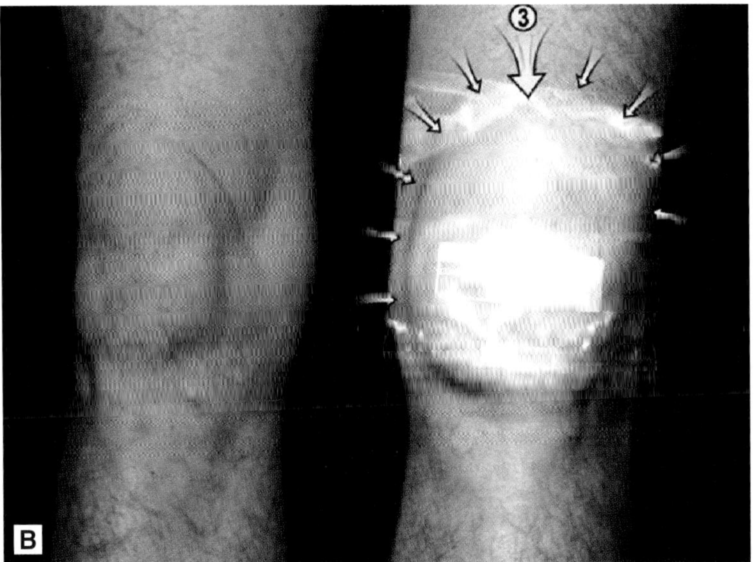

Fig. 5–12

Clinical History The patient's history is the essential first step in all musculoskeletal diagnosis and directs the focus of an appropriate physical examination. The musculoskeletal physical examination is used to confirm or refute diagnostic hypotheses generated by a thoughtful history.

Particularly useful background information includes age; occupation or recreational activities; a history of joint swelling, instability, or injury; or any prior knee problems.

Asking the patient to localize the area of maximal pain (anterior, medial, lateral, or posterior) may help with your preliminary differential diagnosis. An initial pain assessment can be well delineated with the use of the mnemonic **OPQRST**: **O** = Onset, **P** = Precipitating (and ameliorating) factors, **Q** = Quality, **R** = Radiation, **S** = Severity, **T** = Timing.

THE EXAMINATION, OVERVIEW

With the patient standing, observe the knees from the front. Inspect the skin. Note any deformity or malalignment. Next, ask the patient to squat. Note the location and severity of any pain.

Ask the patient to lie supine. Inspect the quadriceps muscles. Note any muscle atrophy. Next, inspect the knees. Note any obvious deformity or visible swelling. Inspect the prepatellar area. Identify the contour of the normal infrapatellar fat pads.

Next, check for any evidence of an effusion: inspect the knee medially, superolaterally, and superiorly. Check for the presence of a bulge sign (fluid wave) on both sides.

Next, assess the patellofemoral joint. Compress the patella in the femoral channel. Note any palpable crepitus or pain. Palpate the medial and lateral patellar facets and note any tenderness. Perform the "patellar apprehension test."

Next, assess the integrity of the ACL by performing the Lachman test. Check for the normal firm "stop" provided by an intact ACL. Note any laxity or pain. Assess the MCL by bringing the knee into partial flexion. Palpate the MCL along its length and note any tenderness. Next, stress the MCL and note any laxity or pain. Assess the LCL by having the patient cross the leg. Palpate the LCL along its length and note any tenderness. Next, stress the LCL and note any laxity or pain.

Assess the integrity of the PCL by inspecting the knee from the side and checking for a "tibial sag." Apply pressure to the anterior tibia and note any laxity or pain.

Next, palpate along the joint line and note any focal tenderness or palpable abnormality.

Assess the medial and lateral menisci by performing the McMurray maneuver. Note any palpable clicks and identify the location of any pain.

Next, palpate the insertion of the pes anserine tendon and underlying anserine bursa. Note any tenderness.

Finally, assess knee range of motion. Note any flexion contracture (deficit in full extension).

THE EXAMINATION, COMPONENT PARTS

Inspection With the patient standing, observe the knees from the front. Note any scars, rashes, or other cutaneous abnormalities. Inspect for deformity or malalignment (Fig. 5–13).

Next, ask the patient to squat down. *(If squatting is anticipated to be painful, holding the patient's hands for support during the squat may increase their confidence and cooperation.)*

Ask the patient to localize any discomfort. Identifying whether the pain is primarily anterior, medial, lateral, or posterior may provide valuable initial clues to the anatomical origin of the problem (Fig. 5–14).

Note any symptoms as the patient returns to the standing position.

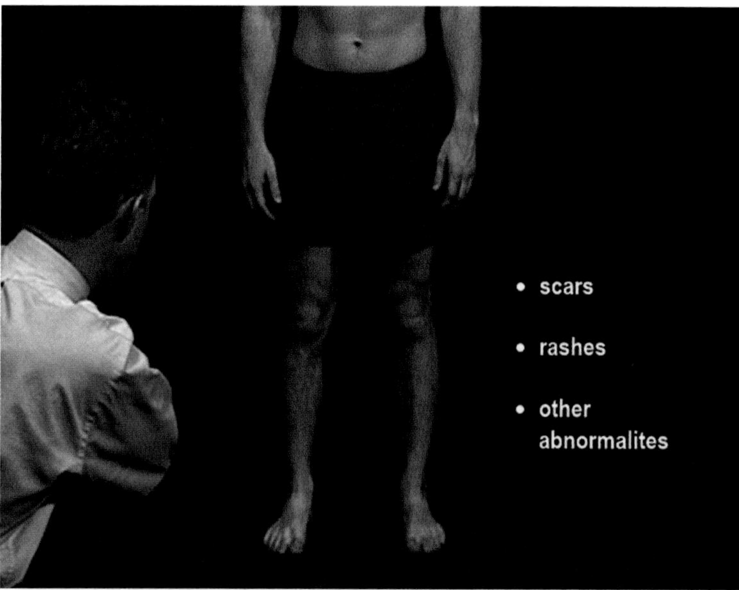

Fig. 5–13

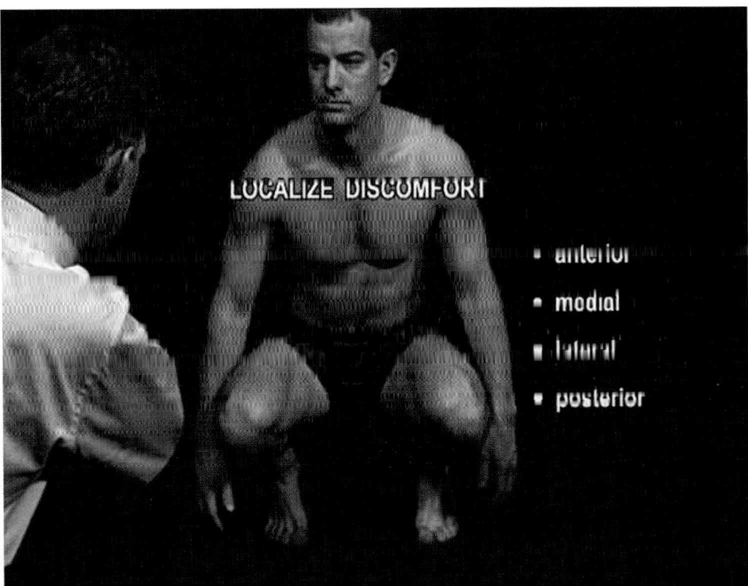

Fig. 5–14

Ask the patient to lie supine. Inspect the quadriceps muscles and check for bulk and symmetry with the quadriceps relaxed and contracted. Note any muscle atrophy (Fig. 5–15).

With the legs fully extended and the quadriceps muscles relaxed, inspect the knees and note any obvious deformity or visible swelling.

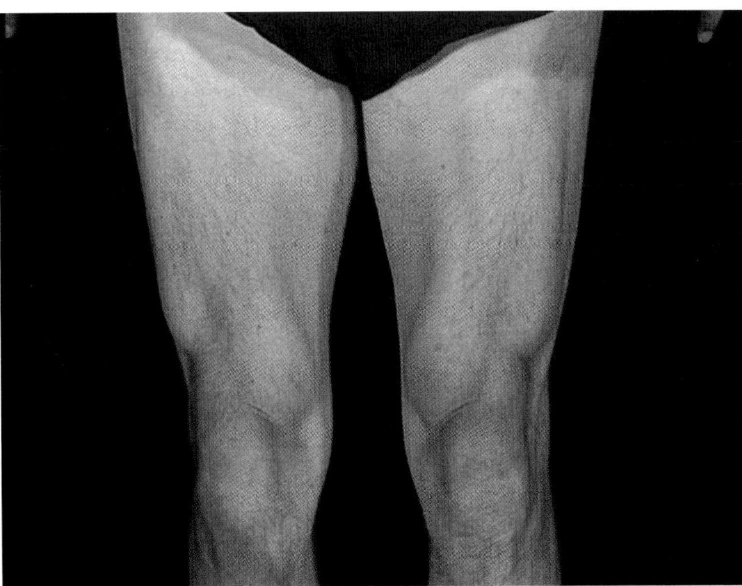

Fig. 5–15

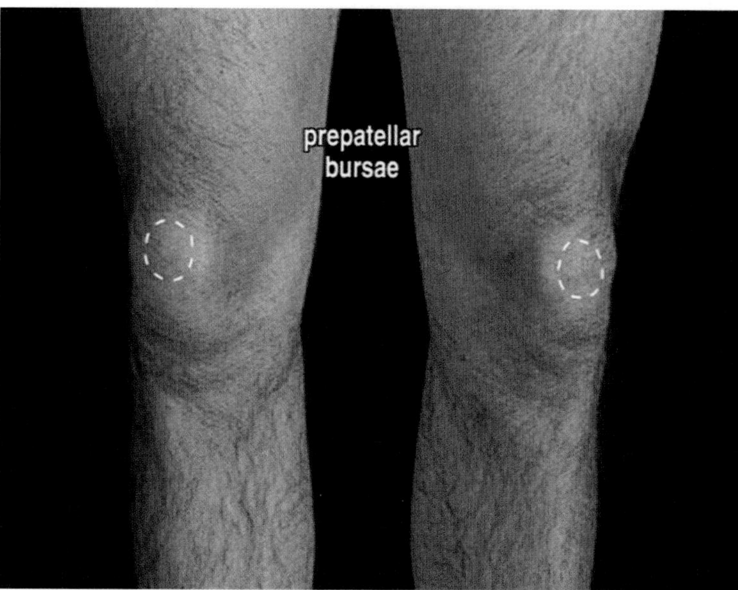

Fig. 5–16

First, examine the prepatellar region (Fig. 5–16). Swelling of the prepatellar bursa presents as visible or palpable distension directly in front of the patella. Subcutaneous nodules (rheumatoid nodules or gouty tophi) may also be found in the prepatellar bursa and may only be apparent on careful palpation.

Next, note the soft tissue prominence below the patella on either side of the patellar tendon. This is the normal infrapatellar fat pad, usually more prominent in women (and most easily seen in full knee extension) (Fig. 5–17A, B).

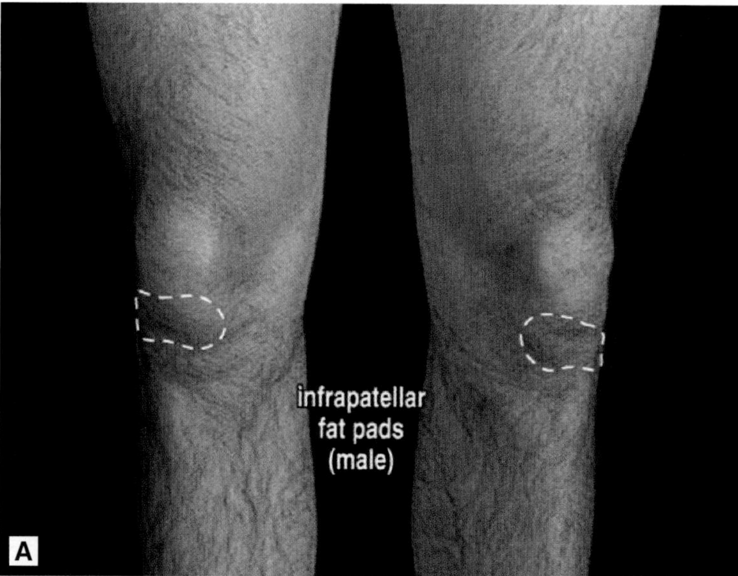

Fig. 5–17

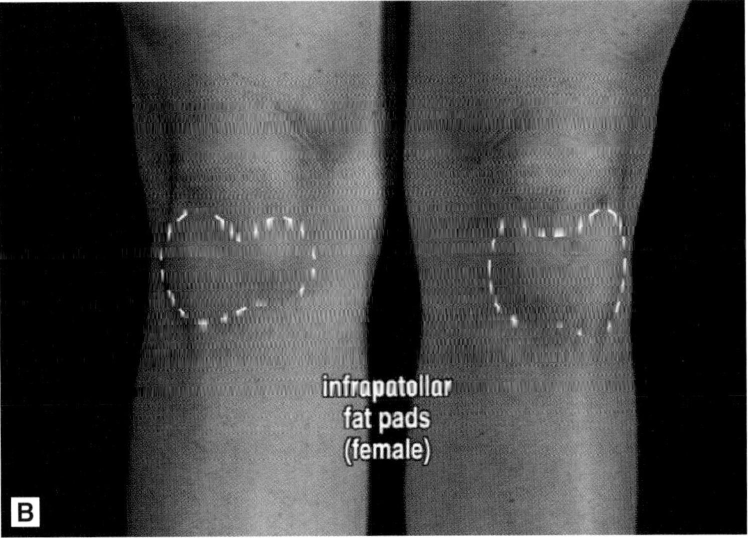

Fig. 5–17

Next, inspect the knee joint for any evidence of an effusion. A small knee effusion will cause a visible bulge medially, between the medial femoral epicondyle and the medial patella (Fig. 5–18). A moderate knee effusion will cause loss of the normal concavity at the medial joint line but will also usually result in a visible bulge superolateral to the patella. Following your initial inspection of the medial knee, check the superolateral suprapatellar region of each knee for any visible swelling.

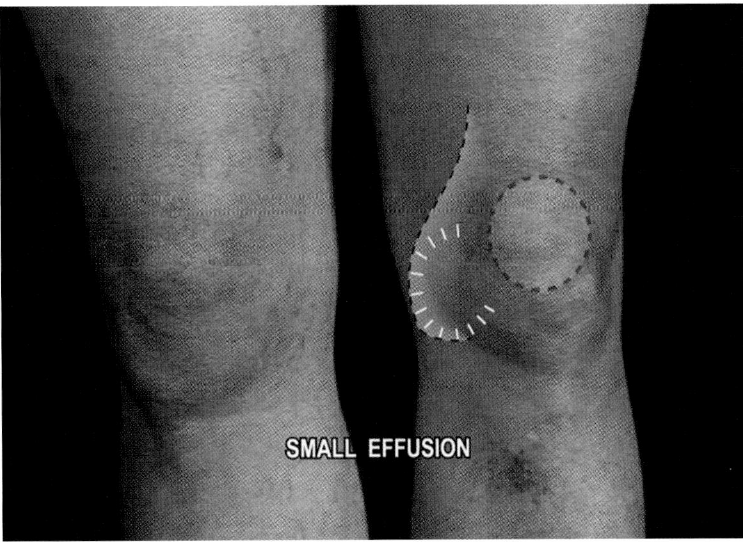

Fig. 5–18

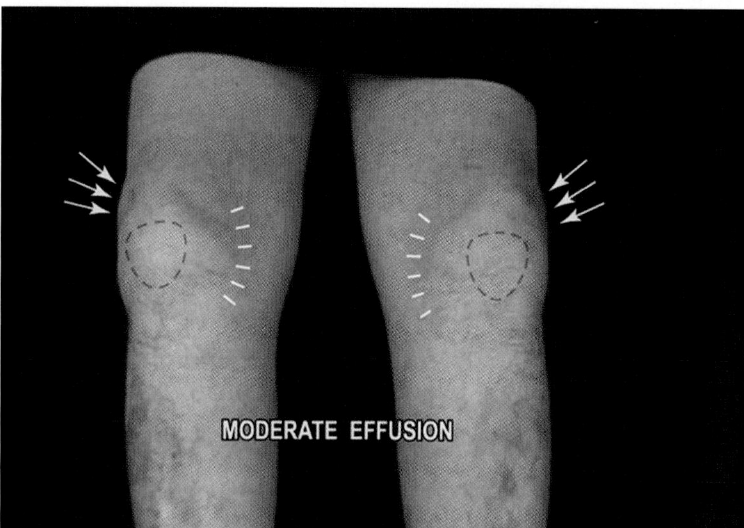

Fig. 5–19

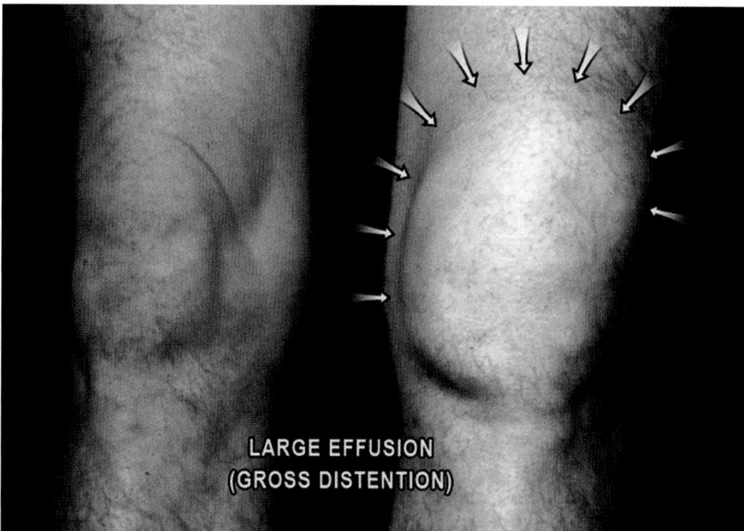

Fig. 5–20

A moderate effusion will cause a visible bulge to appear in the "bare area" distal to the vastus lateralis, as it distends with fluid accumulating in the lateral suprapatellar pouch (Fig. 5–19). A large knee effusion will not only cause loss of the normal concavity at the medial side of the knee and a visible bulge superolaterally, but will also cause visible distention of the entire suprapatellar pouch with bulging medially, superolaterally, and superiorly (Fig. 5–20).

Small Effusions A small volume of fluid will tend to pool medially, causing a slight bulge to develop where there was previously a normal concavity. A suspected small effusion can be readily confirmed by testing for a "bulge sign" (also known as a "fluid wave").

To check for a fluid wave in the patient's left knee, remain standing on the right side of the examination table and place the ring and little fingers of your right hand on the tibial tubercle. Place your right

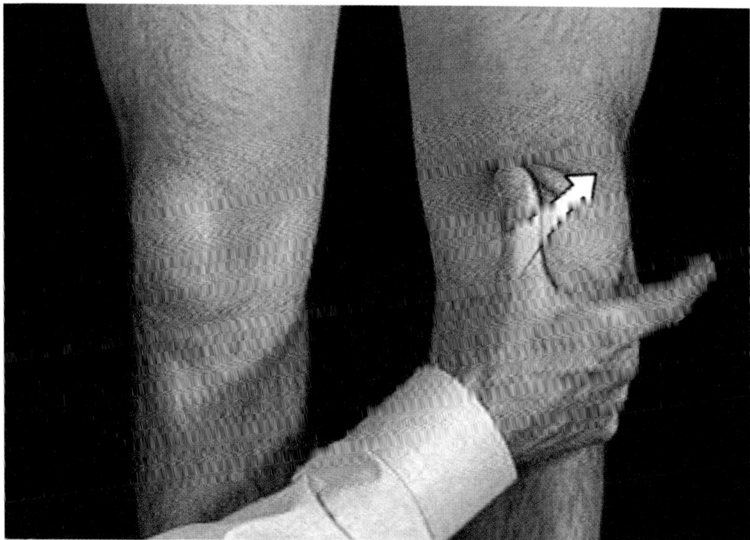

Fig. 5–21

thumb on the medial aspect of the knee just below the level of the patella and sweep your thumb in a cephalad and lateral direction, pushing any movable fluid from the medial aspect of the joint into the superolateral suprapatellar pouch (Fig. 5–21). Your right fourth and fifth fingers provide an excellent fulcrum against the tibia, as you sweep your right thumb in a superolateral direction. Keep your index finger fully extended, with your thumb and index fingers forming a backward "L," to prevent inadvertently compressing the area into which you are attempting to move the joint fluid. Any fluid which has been moved to the opposite side of the joint will accumulate in the space which lies between the superior pole of the patella and the distal vastus lateralis (Fig. 5–22). This area, the superolateral "suprapatellar pouch" of

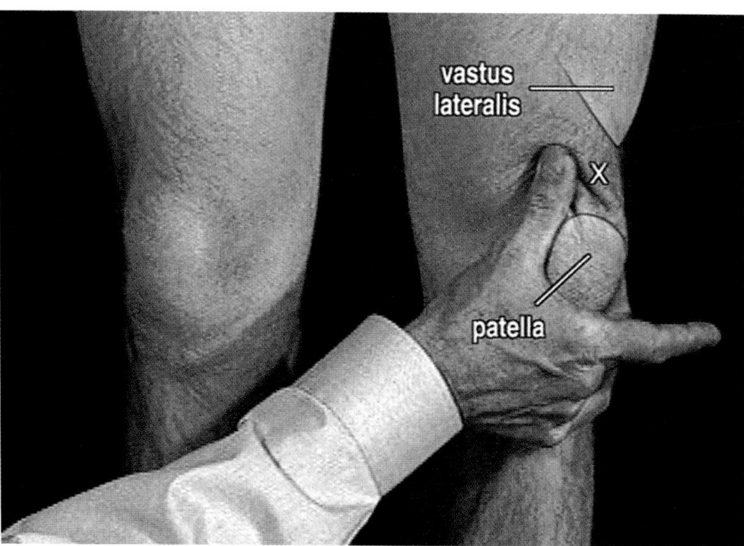

Fig. 5–22

the knee joint, can now be compressed using your right hand with your fingers fully extended (Fig. 5–23) driving any fluid back across the joint, causing a visible bulge on the medial side (Fig. 5–24).

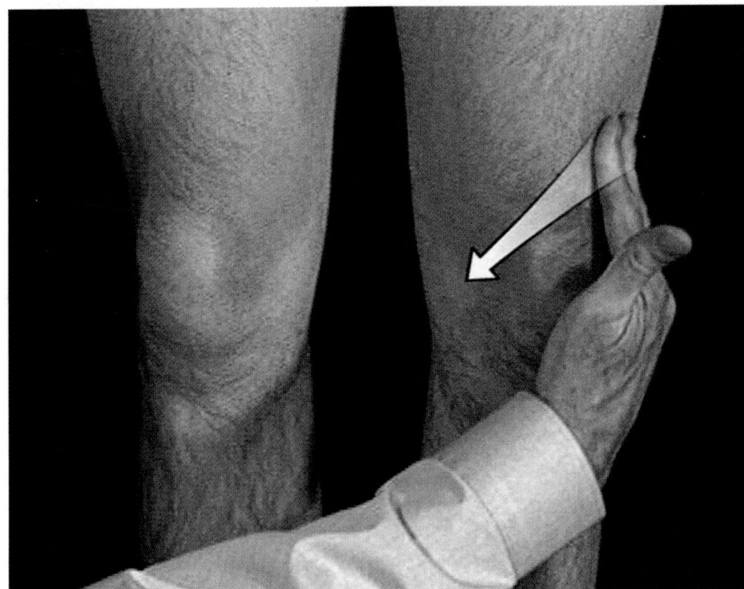

Fig. 5–23

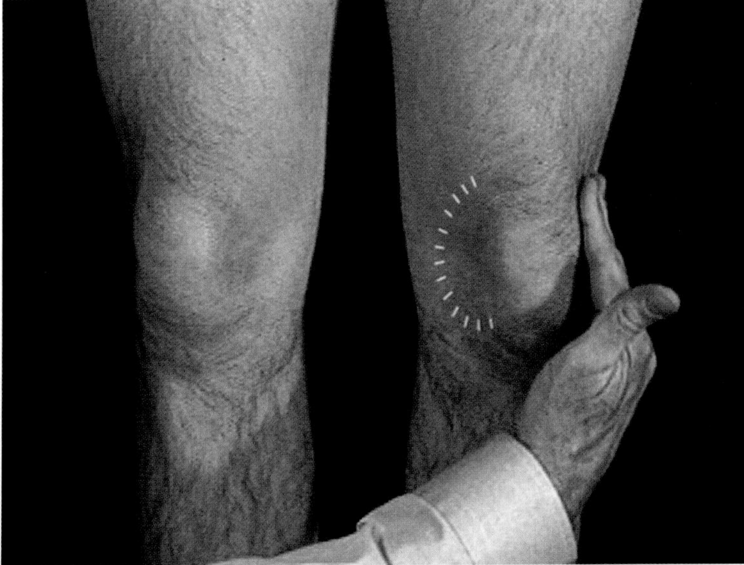

Fig. 5–24

To check for a fluid wave in the patient's right knee, remain standing on the patient's right side. Beginning just below the level of the patella, use your right or left hand with your fingers fully extended to sweep the medial surface of the right knee in a cephalad and lateral direction (Fig. 5–25).

Fluid at the medial joint line will now be compressed and driven into the superolateral suprapatellar pouch (Fig. 5–26).

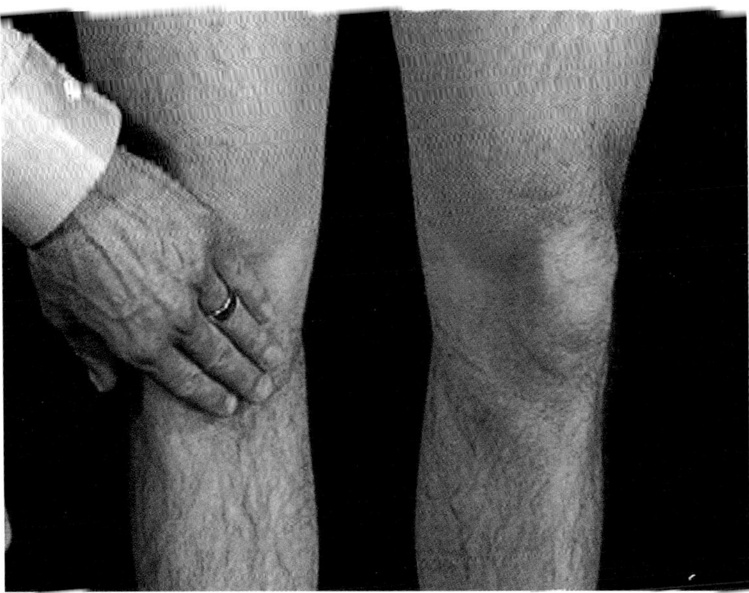

Fig. 5–25

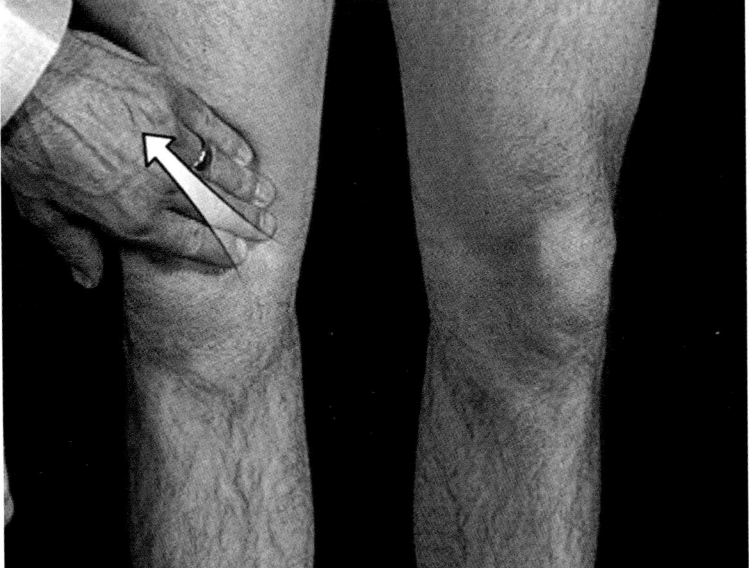

Fig. 5–26

Now use the flattened back of your right hand and compress the superolateral suprapatellar pouch. Any fluid will now be driven back across the knee and appear as a bulge on the medial side (Figs. 5–27 and 5–28). *(Although it is possible to demonstrate a fluid wave using other methods, this technique is easy to perform and yields consistent results.)*

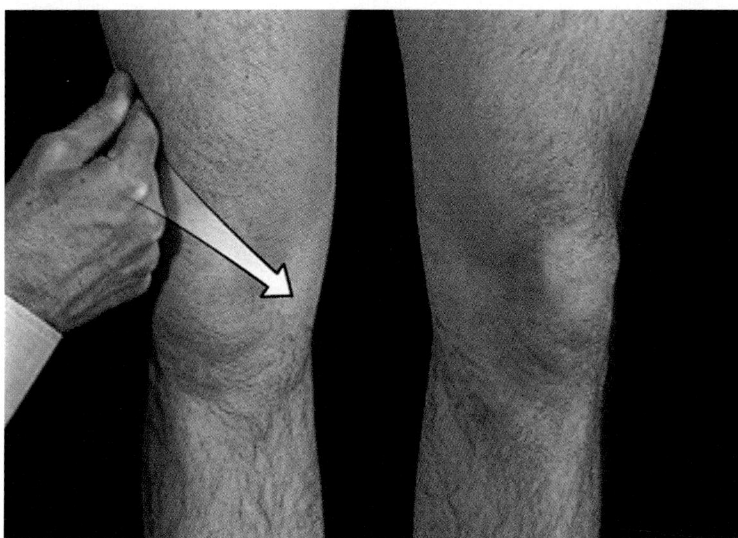

Fig. 5–27

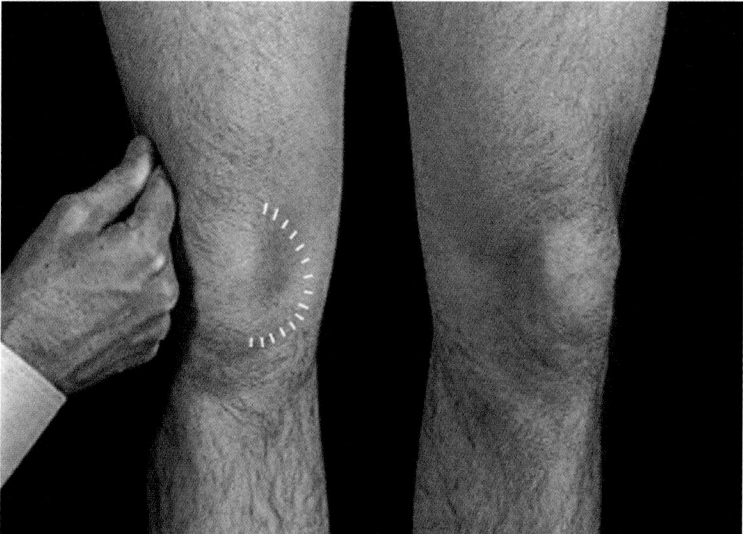

Fig. 5–28

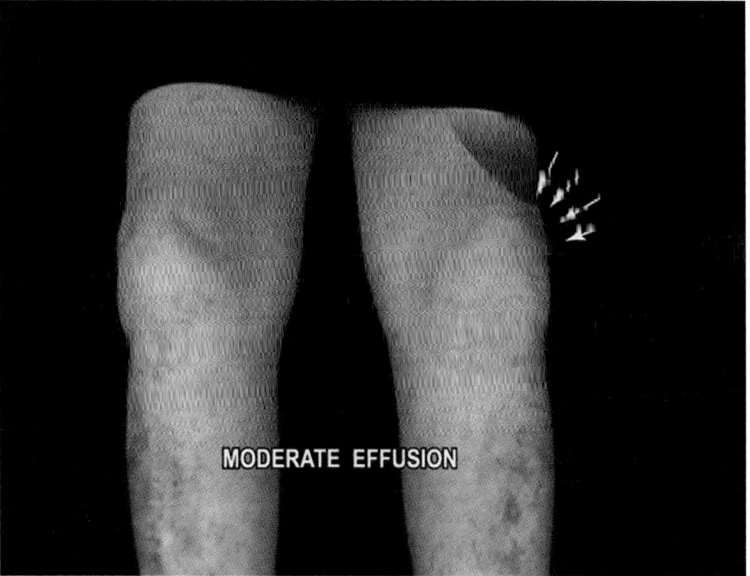

Fig. 5–29

Moderate Effusions The presence of a moderate knee effusion not only causes loss of the normal concavity at the medial joint line but also causes a visible bulge superolaterally. This bulge, in the "bare area" distal to the vastus lateralis, develops as fluid accumulates in the superolateral suprapatellar pouch (Fig. 5–29).

If a moderate effusion is suspected on visual inspection, you can confirm it by gently compressing the suprapatellar pouch with your left hand as you slide it inferiorly toward the patella. This will drive any joint fluid centrally, beneath the patella, causing the patella to "float" above the intercondylar groove (Fig. 5–30). With your left hand compressing the suprapatellar pouch medially, laterally, and superiorly,

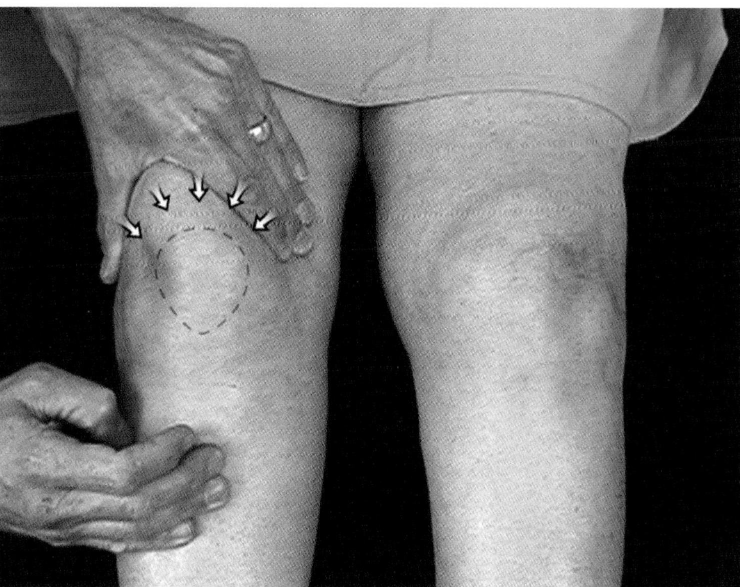

Fig. 5–30

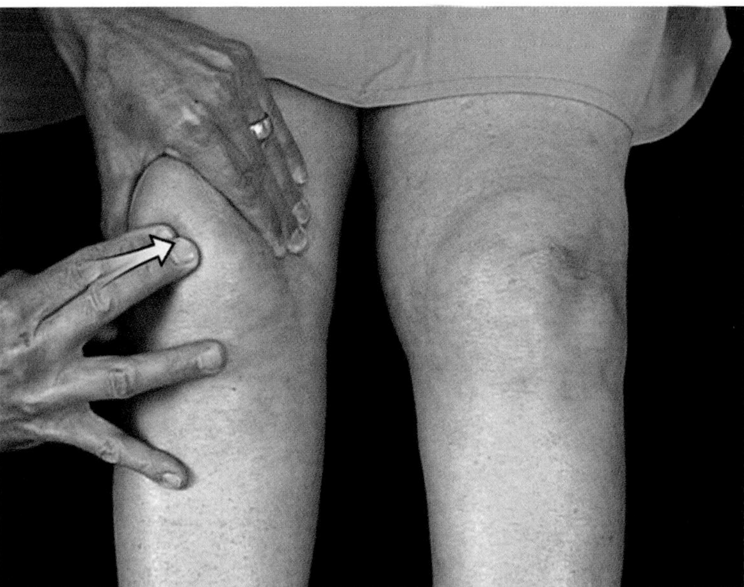

Fig. 5–31

use your right index and middle fingers to apply several rapid, downward compressions to the patella. (Fig. 5–31).

When sufficient fluid is present, you will feel a tapping or clicking sensation at the end of patellar compression, as the patella bounces off the femur (Fig. 5–32A, B). This is called a "patellar tap" or "ballotable patella." This technique is performed in the same manner on both the right and left knees.

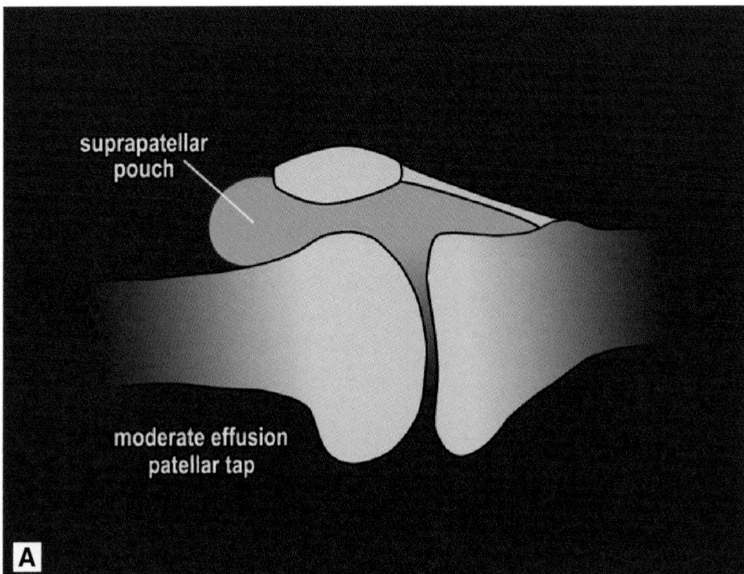

Fig. 5–32

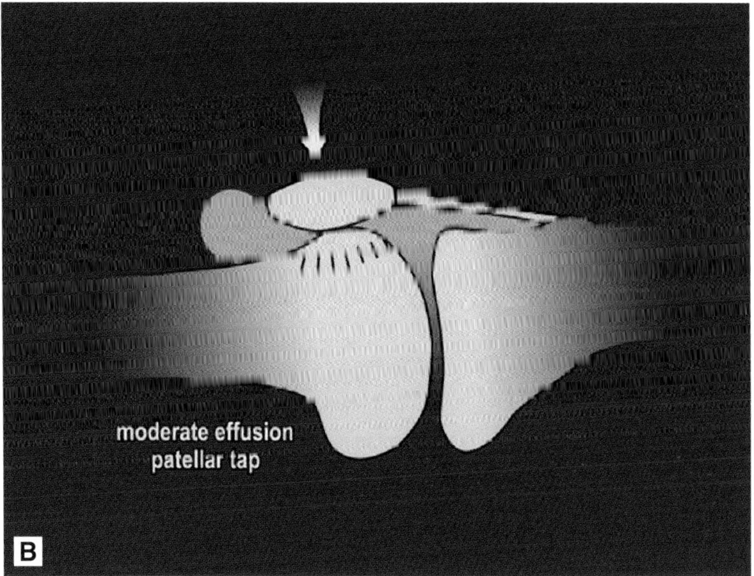

Fig. 5–32

Large Effusions If a large knee effusion is present, it is usually most obvious on visual inspection. As expected, a large volume of synovial fluid will first cause loss of the normal concavity at the medial side of the knee, followed by a visible bulge superolaterally. In addition, however, a large knee effusion will cause visible distention of the *entire* suprapatellar pouch with visible and palpable bulging medially, superolaterally, and superiorly (Fig. 5–33).

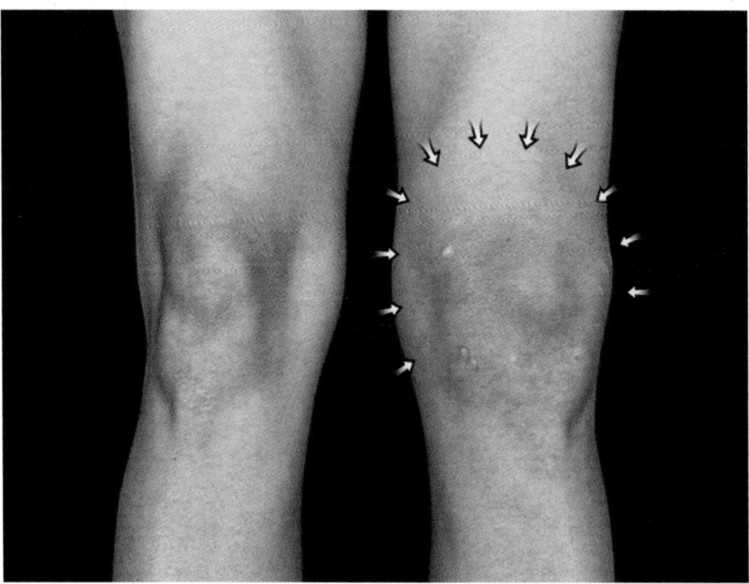

Fig. 5–33

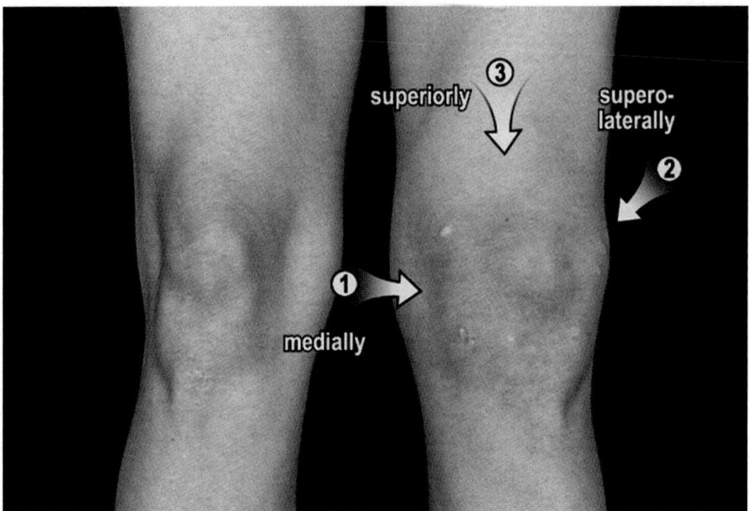

Fig. 5–34

Such gross distention usually makes it difficult to detect a fluid wave or even a ballotable patella because such a large, tense volume of fluid is present.

If you always inspect the knee in an orderly sequence, first medially, then superolaterally, and last superiorly, while comparing side to side, you will greatly improve your ability to identify knee effusions (Fig. 5–34).

Patellofemoral Joint Next, check the patellofemoral joint. With the patient's leg relaxed, apply alternating downward pressure on the superior and inferior poles of the patella, gently but firmly rocking it in the femoral groove. Note any tenderness or crepitus (Fig. 5–35A, B).

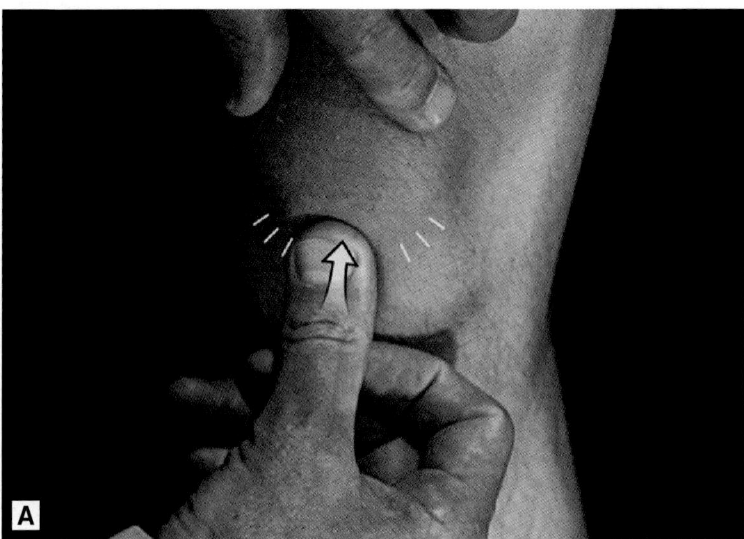

Fig. 5–35

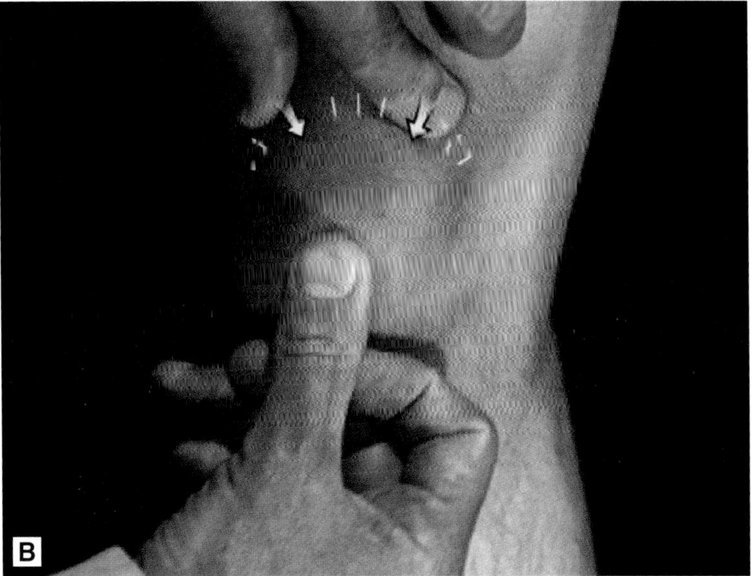

Fig. 5–35

Next, palpate the medial and lateral patellar facets to assess the undersurface of the patellae.

To examine the patient's right patella, use both thumbs to push the patella medially to expose the medial patellar facet for palpation with your index finger(s) (Fig. 5–36A, B).

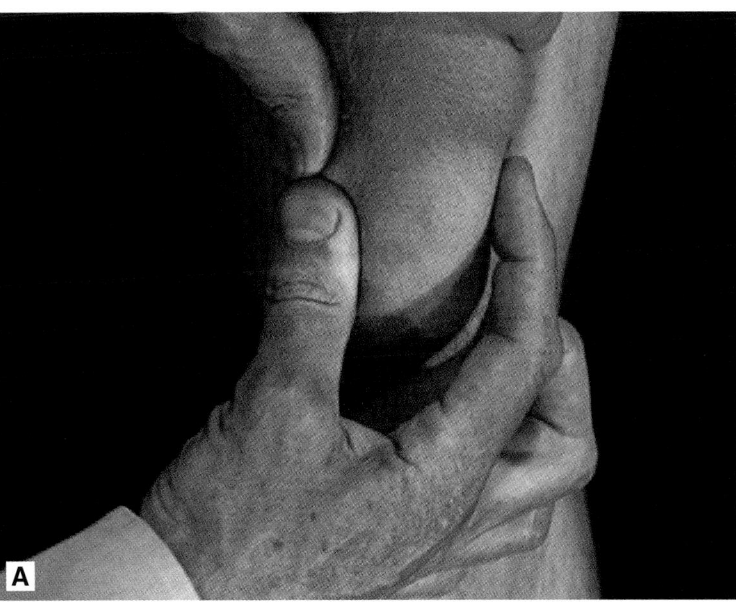

Fig. 5–36

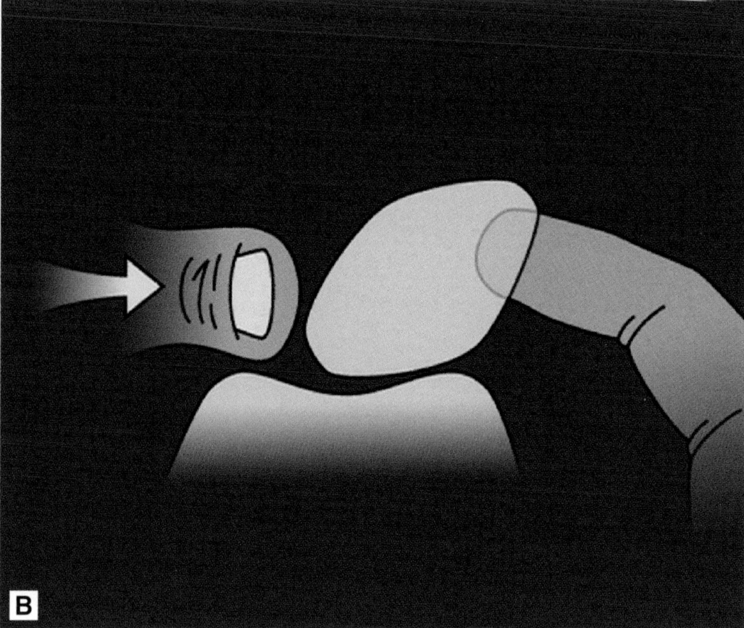

Fig. 5–36

Then, use your index fingers to pull the patella laterally to palpate the undersurface of the lateral patellar facet with your thumb(s) (Fig. 5–37A, B).

To examine the patient's left patella, use your index fingers to pull the patella medially while you use your thumb(s) to palpate the medial patellar facet. Use both thumbs to push the patella laterally to palpate the lateral patellar facet with your index finger(s).

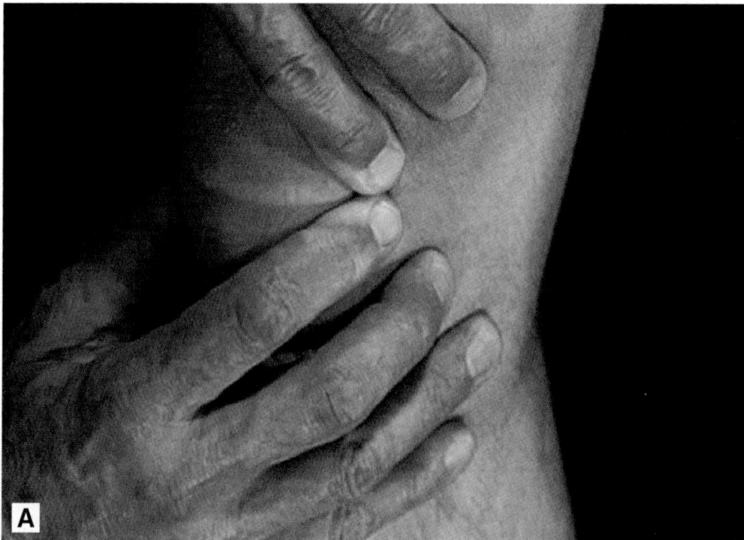

Fig. 5–37

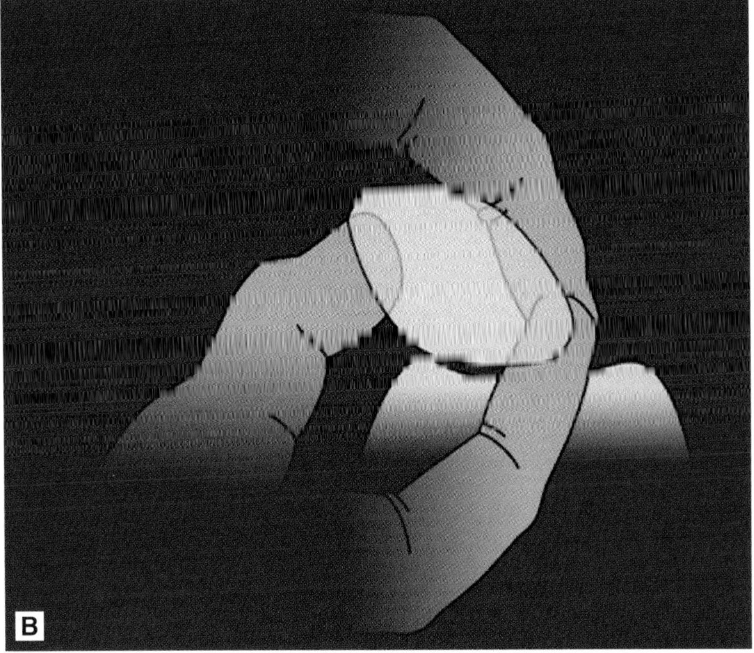

Fig. 5–37

Complete the examination by performing the "patellar apprehension test." Apply gradually increasing pressure on the medial aspect of the patella, attempting to force the patella laterally (Fig. 5–38).

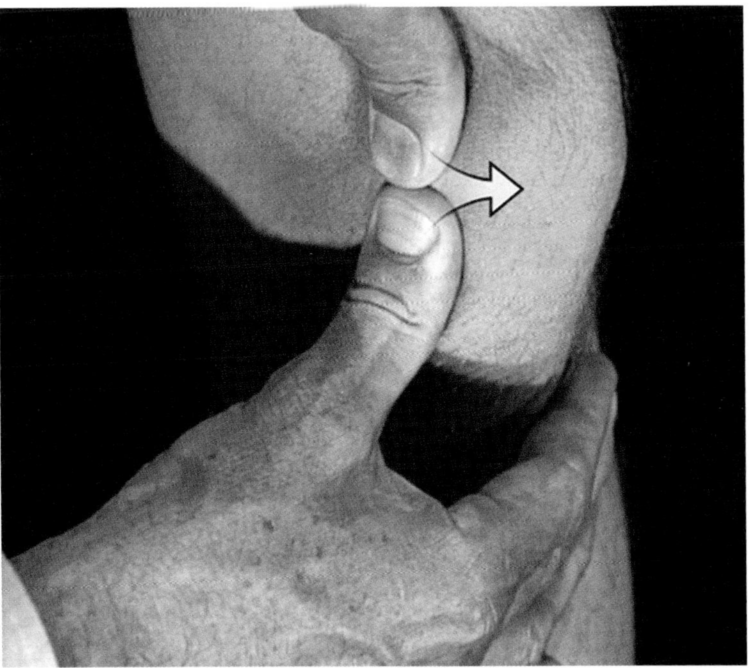

Fig. 5–38

Patients who are prone to patellar dislocation may experience apprehension during this maneuver and request that you stop (or physically grab your hand) to prevent impending patellar dislocation. Significant apprehension or patellar dislocation is considered a "positive" apprehension test.

Anterior Cruciate Ligament Now, assess the integrity of the anterior cruciate ligament (ACL).

To examine the patient's right knee, remain standing on the patient's right side. Face the patient's head while you lean your right lateral thigh against the examination table. Grasp the patient's distal femur with your left hand. Place your second through fifth fingers posteriorly several centimeters above the popliteal space, and your left thumb anteriorly several centimeters above the patella (Fig. 5–39). Next, grasp the patient's proximal tibia with your right hand. Place your second through fifth fingers several centimeters below the popliteal space and wrap your right thumb around the anterior tibia at the level of the tibial tuberosity (Fig. 5–40). Stabilize the patient's lower extremity against your right thigh. Ask the patient to relax the leg (Fig. 5–41). *(You can facilitate relaxation by having the patient lying completely flat and looking away from the examiner.)* Gently, passively "rolling" the leg while asking the patient to "relax your hip" may also help relaxation of the quadriceps muscles.

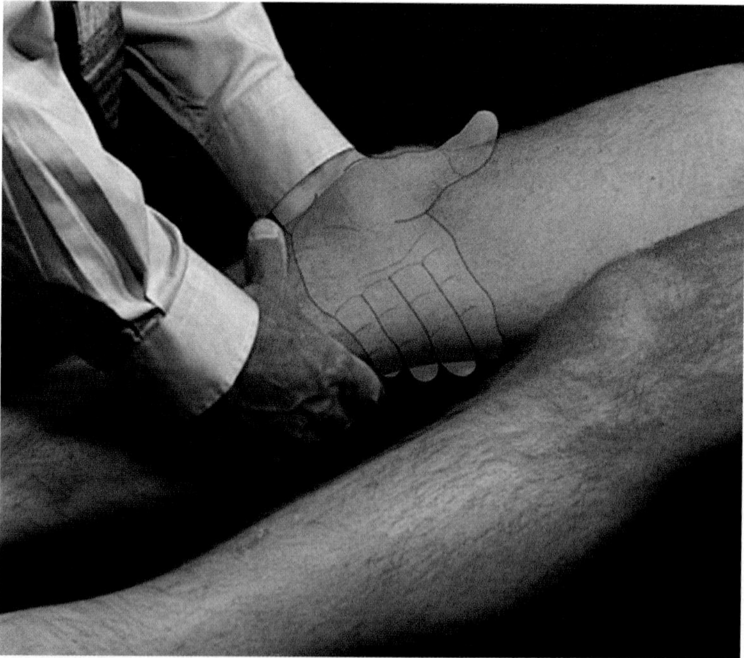

Fig. 5–39

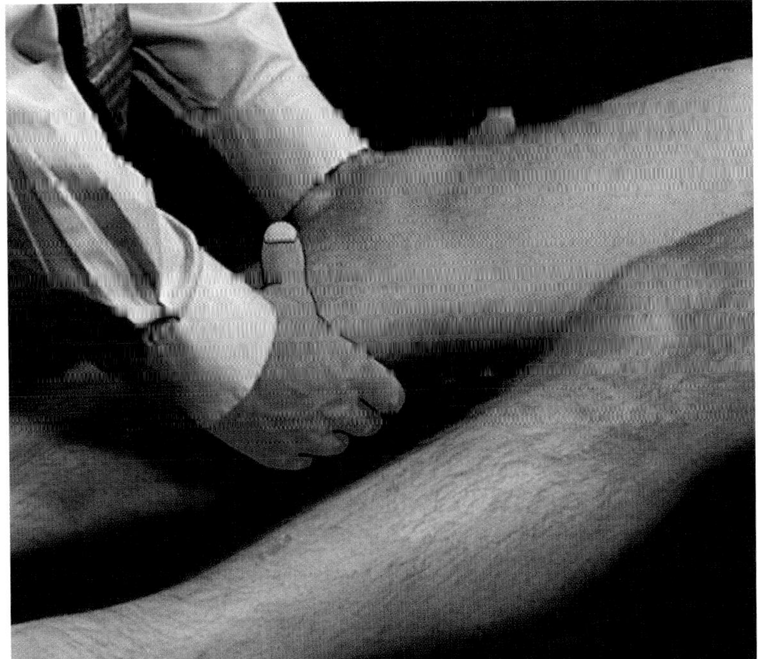

Fig. 5–40

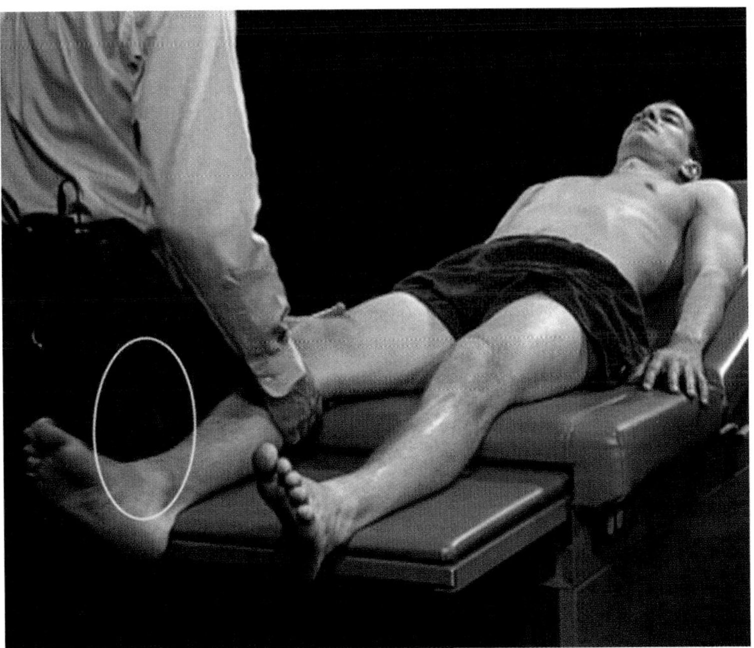

Fig. 5–41

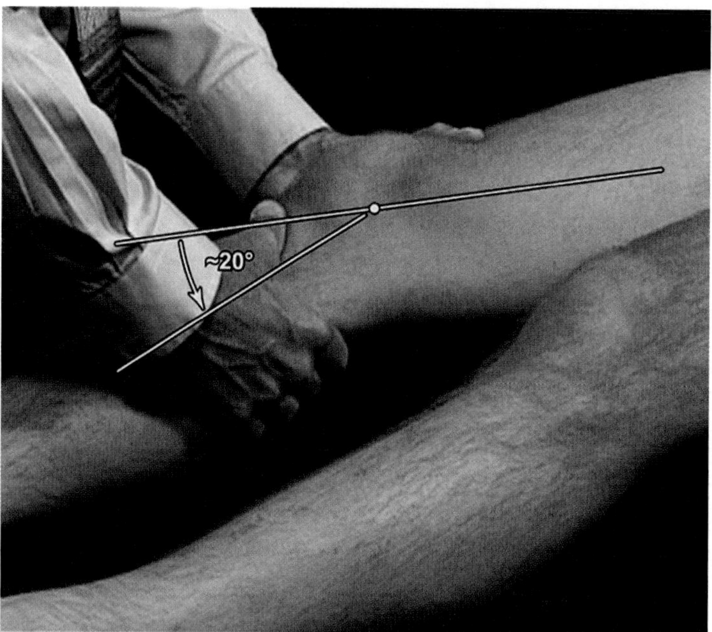

Fig. 5–42

Once your hands are in the proper position and the patient is relaxed, gradually bring the knee into ~20° to 30° of flexion while repeatedly and briskly pulling the proximal tibia forward on the distal femur (Fig. 5–42). Check for a firm "stop," the endpoint of movement provided by an intact ACL (Fig. 5–43A, B, C).

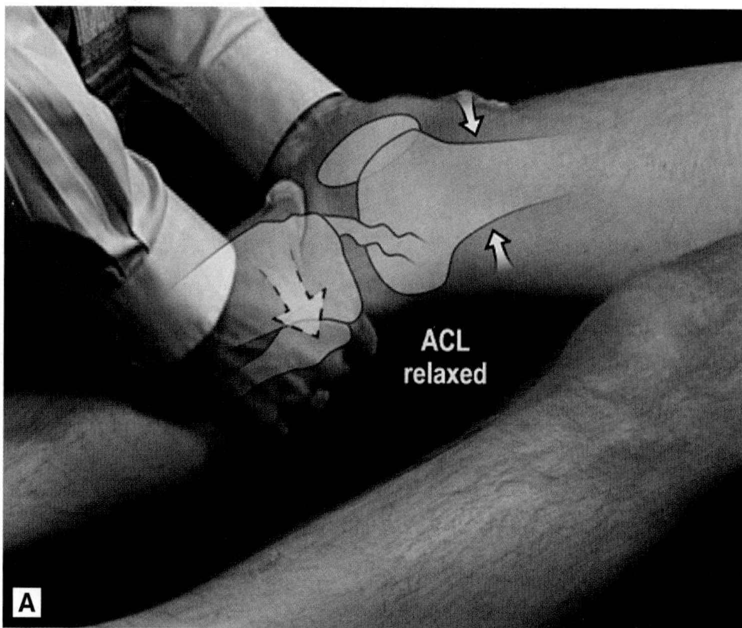

Fig. 5–43

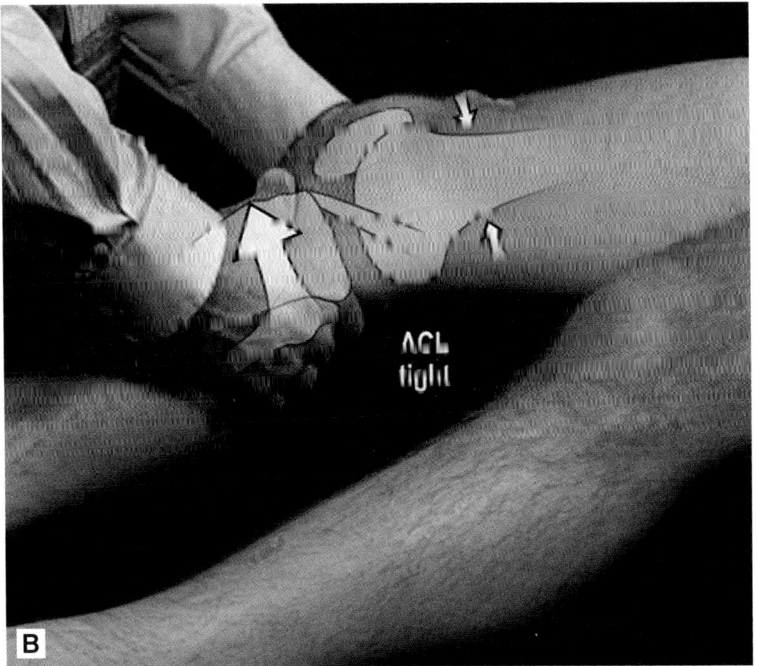

Fig. 5–43

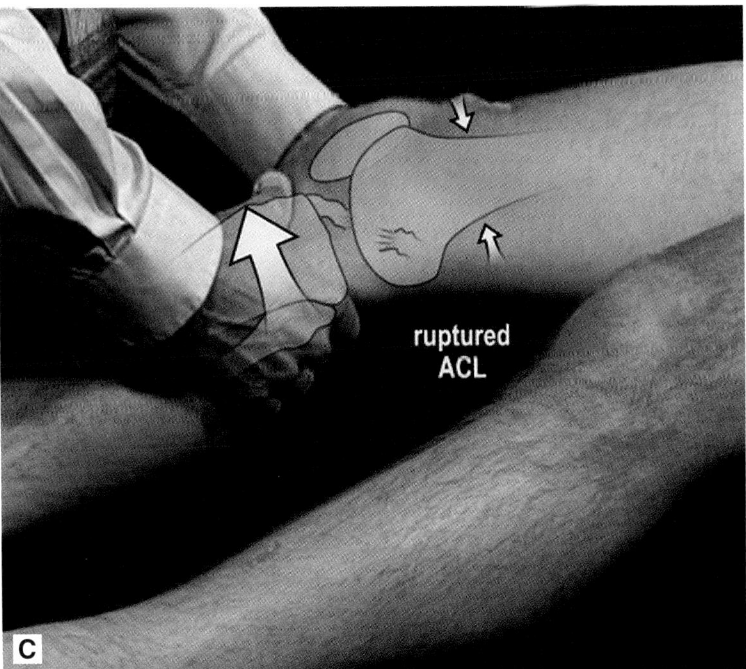

Fig. 5–43

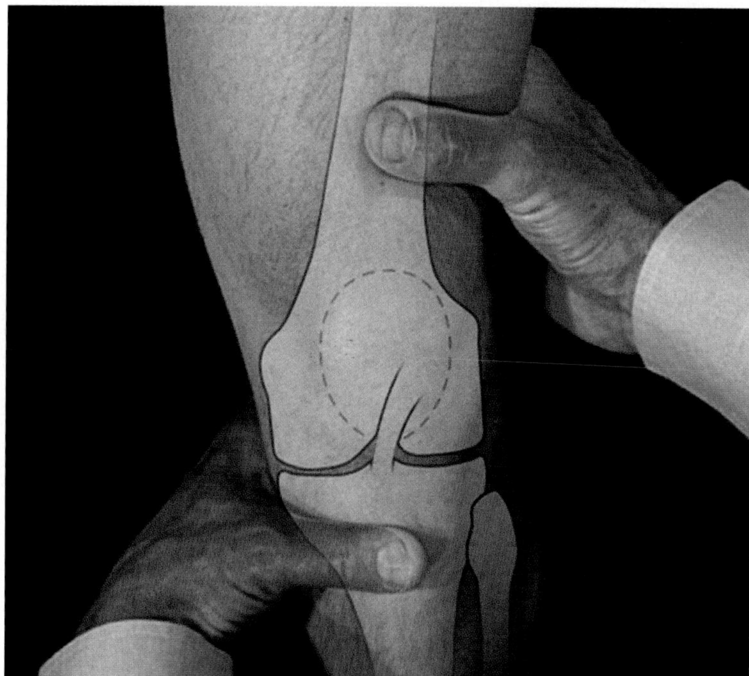

Fig. 5–44

To perform the Lachman test on the patient's left knee, stand on the left side of the examination table and use the same technique you employed with patient's right knee, but reverse your hand positions: grasp the distal femur with your right hand and the proximal tibia with your left hand (Fig. 5–44).

The appropriate technique for the Lachman test involves firm stabilization of the distal femur with one hand (with downward pressure from your thumb) while simultaneously, firmly, and rapidly pulling forward on the tibia with the other hand. After pulling forward on the tibia, it is important to release your traction briefly, allowing the tibia and femur to return to their neutral positions with the ACL fully relaxed. Perform these movements in several rapid cycles, while checking for the normal firm "stop" provided by an intact ACL. The normal endpoint of movement should first become apparent at ~20° of flexion. As you continue this maneuver and slowly bring the knee into greater flexion, this firm endpoint will disappear, as elements of the knee capsule tighten, restraining movement and obscuring the distinct contribution of the ACL.

The Lachman test has replaced the insensitive "anterior drawer test" as a means of assessing the integrity of the ACL. (The anterior drawer test, performed at 90° of knee flexion, primarily stresses the knee joint capsule rather than the ACL; Fig. 5–45.)

An alternative method for performing the Lachman test may be helpful in patients who are particularly large-framed or where there is a significant mismatch between the size of the examiner's hands and the patient's lower extremity.

To perform a "modified" Lachman on the patient's right knee, stand at the side of the examination table and place your left knee under the patient's right knee (Fig. 5–46). Stabilize the distal femur by using your left hand to press down on the distal thigh, several centimeters above the patella. With your right hand, grasp the proximal tibia and pull firmly and rapidly forward. Check for a firm endpoint of movement, indicating an intact ACL.

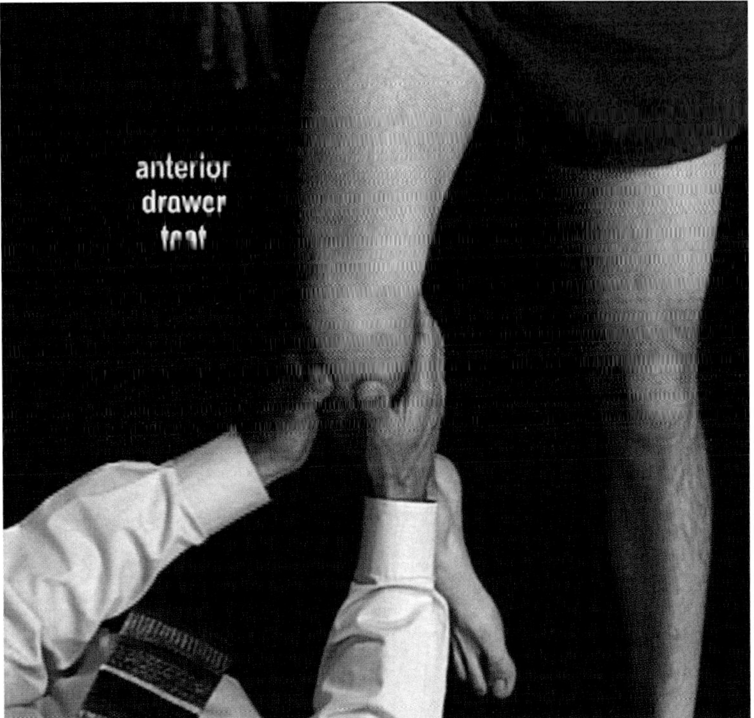

Fig. 5–45

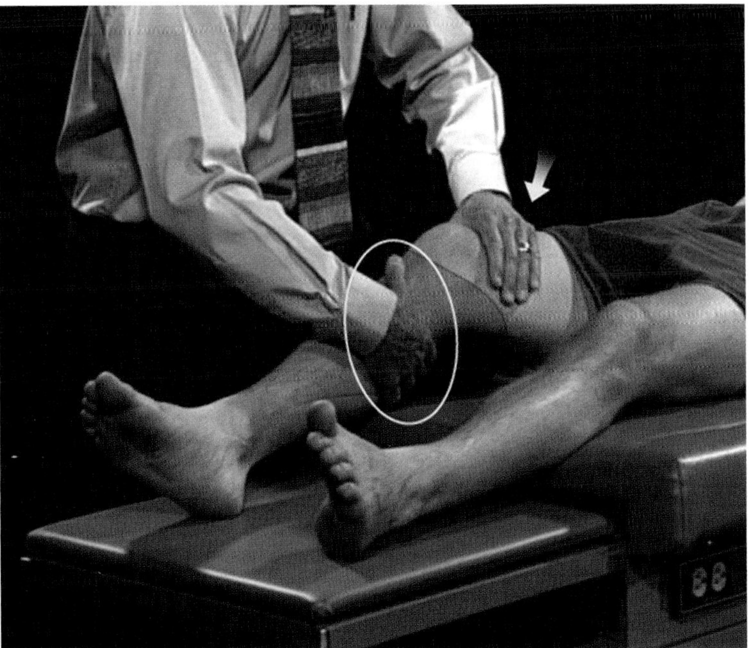

Fig. 5–46

To perform a modified Lachman on the patient's left knee, stand on the left side of the examination table and use the same technique employed with the patient's right knee, but reverse your knee and hand positions. (Place your right knee under the patient's left knee, your right hand on the patient's distal left femur, and your left hand on the proximal tibia; Fig. 5–47.)

Mastering the technique of successfully and reproducibly performing the Lachman test will require practice (Fig. 5–48). Children or small-framed adults can be ideal for practicing this technique and increasing your confidence.

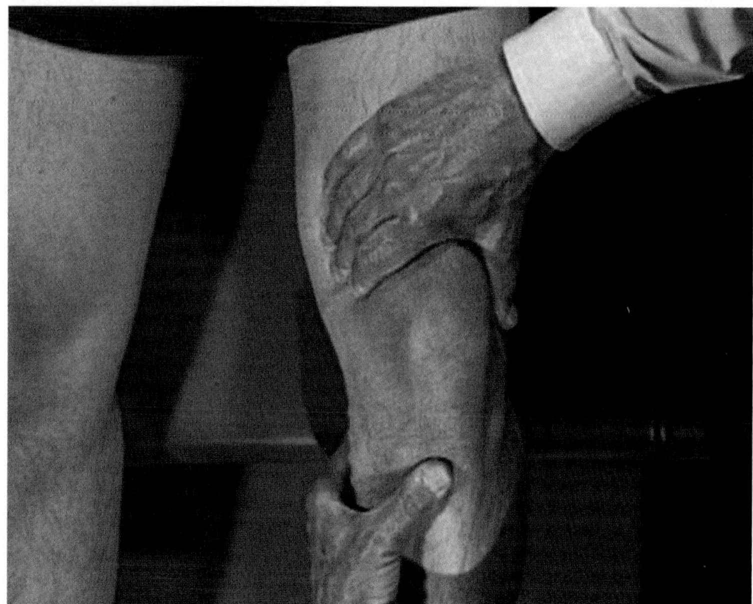

Fig. 5–47

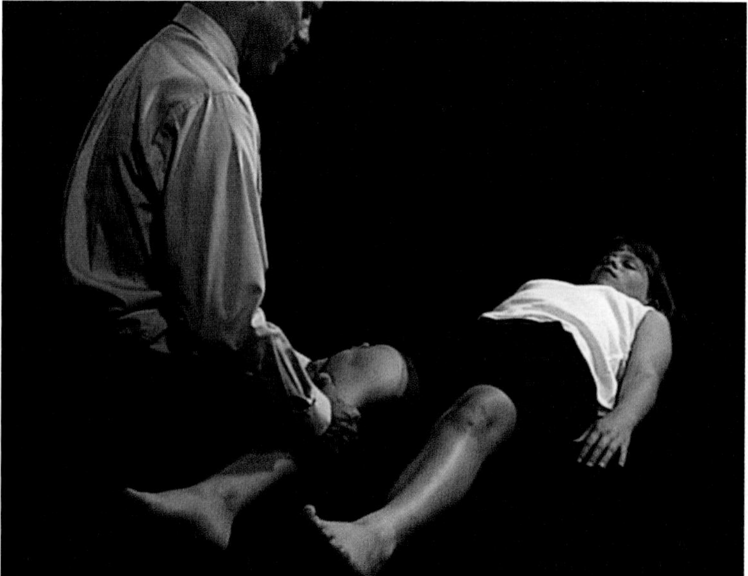

Fig. 5–48

Medial Collateral Ligament With the knee flexed, identify the anteromedial joint line, then move your fingers posteriorly and palpate the medial aspect of the knee between the medial femoral epicondyle and the tibial plateau. Your fingers are now over the medial collateral ligament (MCL), a broad, thin ligament connecting the distal femur and proximal tibia. Palpate the MCL along its length. Note any tenderness (Fig. 5–49A, B).

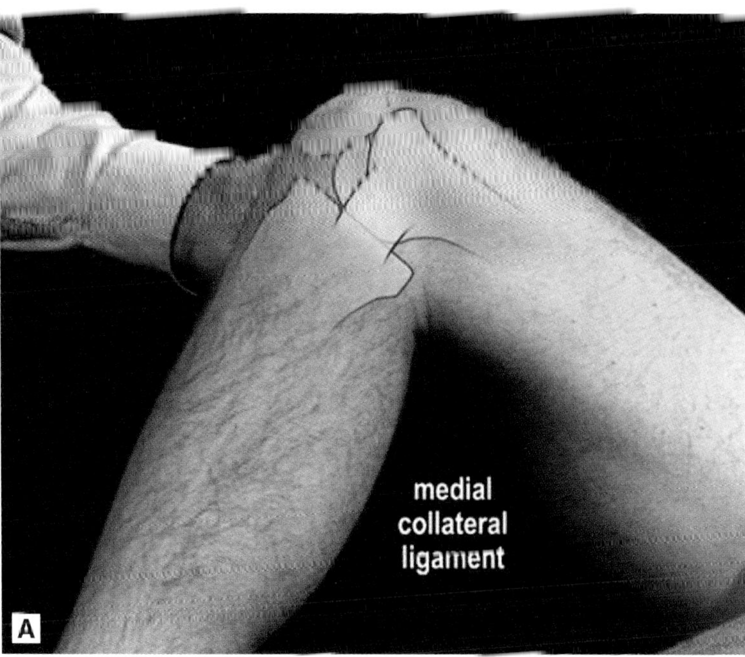

Fig. 5–49

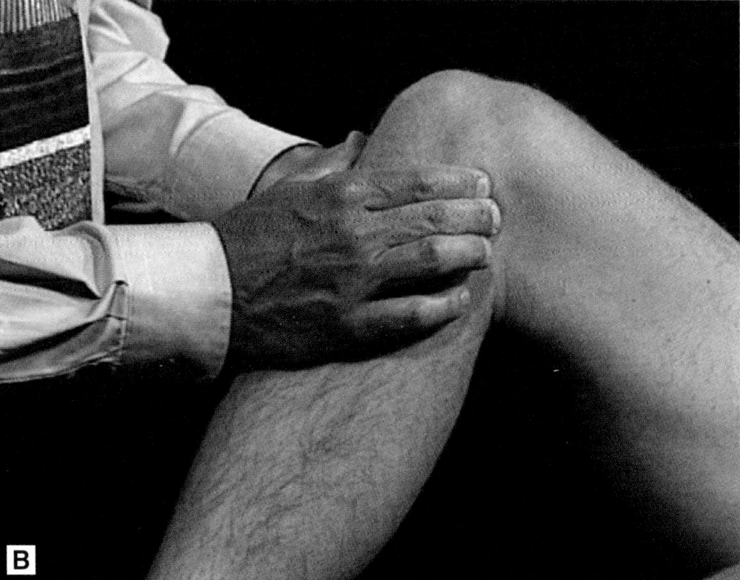

Fig. 5–49

Next, stress the MCL: place your left hand under the patient's knee at the level of the distal femur and grasp the femoral epicondyles.

To assess the right MCL, take the patient's foot in your right hand while you flex the knee to ~30° (Fig. 5–50).

Apply a valgus stress to the tibia by pulling the foot and ankle toward you (Fig. 5–51).

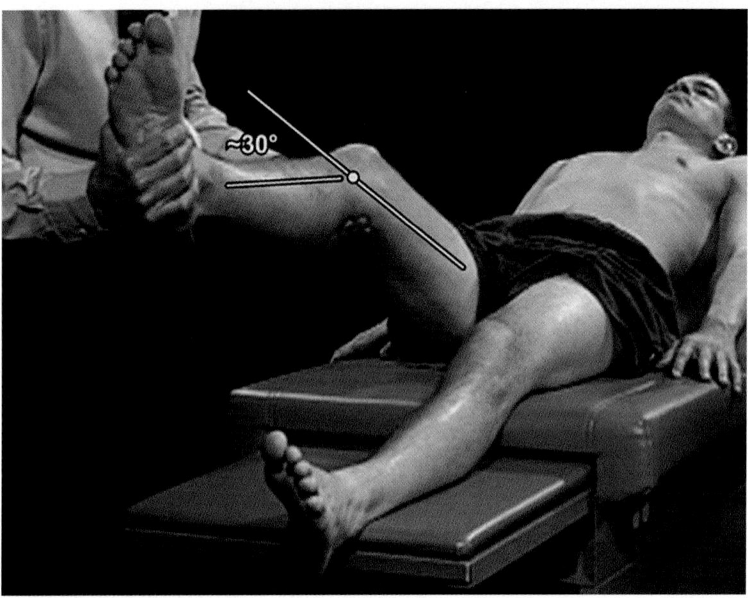

Fig. 5–50

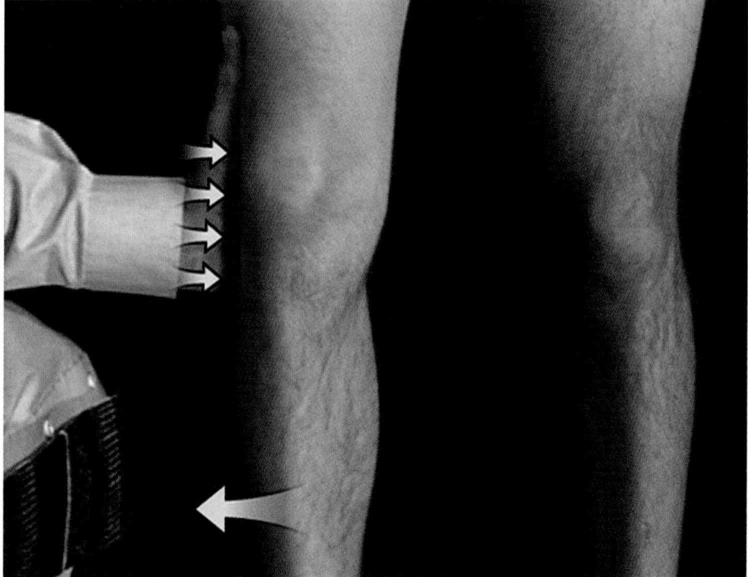

Fig. 5–51

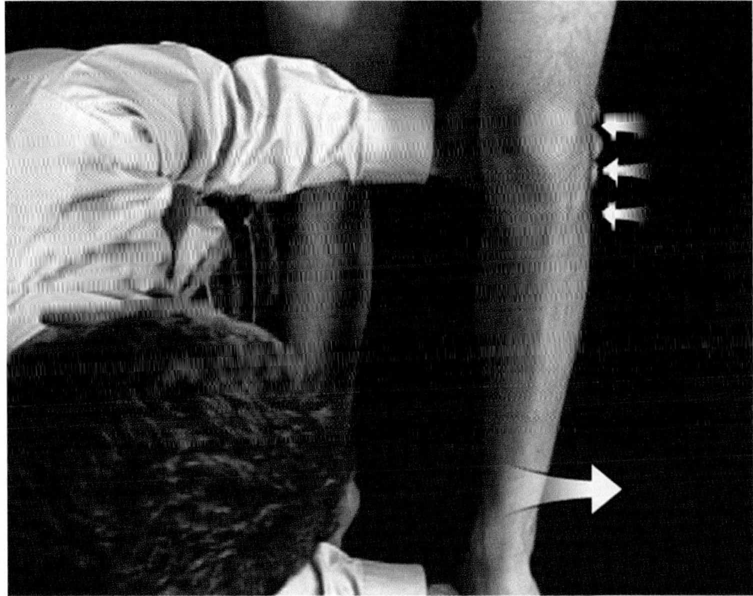

Fig. 5–52

To assess the left MCL, use the same technique but apply a valgus stress to the tibia by pushing the foot and ankle away from you (Fig. 5–52).

These maneuvers isolate and stress the MCLs. Note any pain or laxity.

Lateral Collateral Ligament To assess the integrity of the lateral collateral ligament (LCL), have the patient cross the leg (placing the ankle on the opposite leg, with the hip in abduction and external rotation) (Fig. 5–53). This position facilitates palpation of the LCL, which can now be felt as a tight

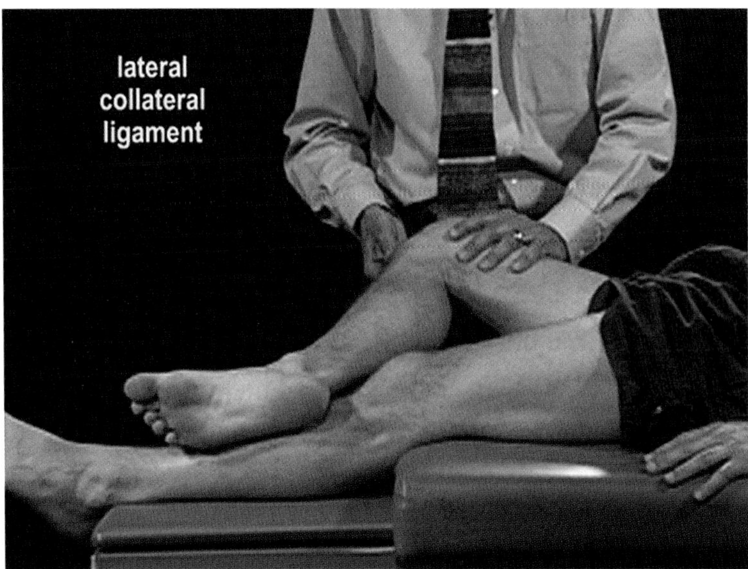

Fig. 5–53

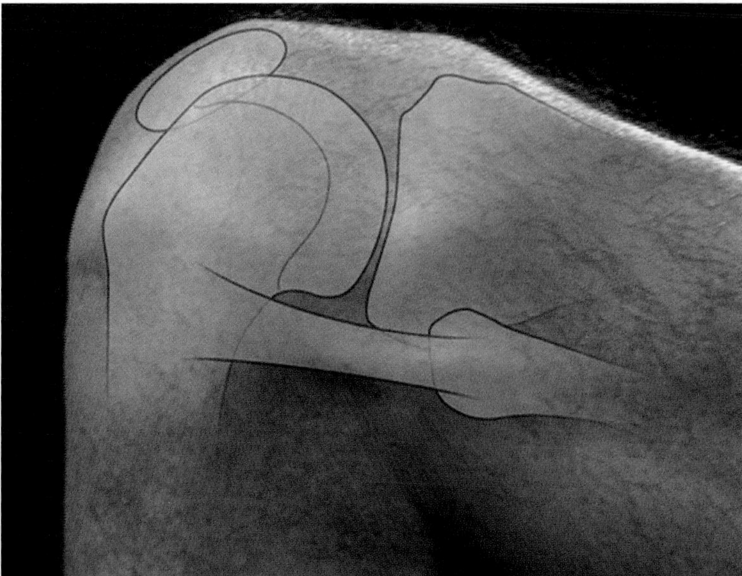

Fig. 5–54

"pencil-like" cord, connecting the lateral femoral epicondyle and proximal fibula and tibia (Fig. 5–54). Begin palpation at the head of the fibula and palpate proximally to the ligament's insertion on the lateral femoral epicondyle. Note any tenderness (Fig. 5–55). Next, stress the LCL: place your left hand under the patient's knee at the level of the distal femur and grasp the femoral epicondyles.

To assess the right LCL, take the patient's foot in your right hand while you flex the knee to ~30° (Fig. 5–56). Apply a varus stress to the tibia by pushing the foot and ankle away from you.

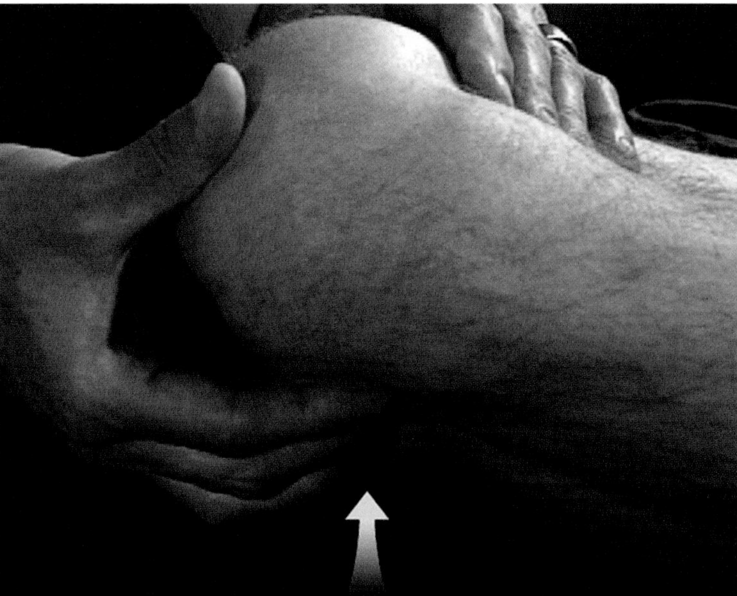

Fig. 5–55

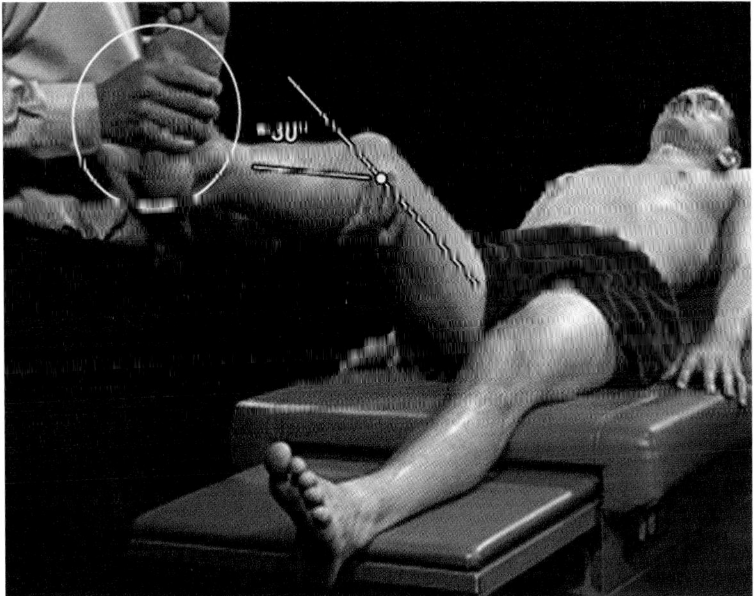

Fig. 5–56

To assess the left LCL, use the same technique but apply a varus stress to the tibia by pulling the foot and ankle toward you (Fig. 5–57). These maneuvers isolate and stress the LCLs.

Note any pain or laxity.

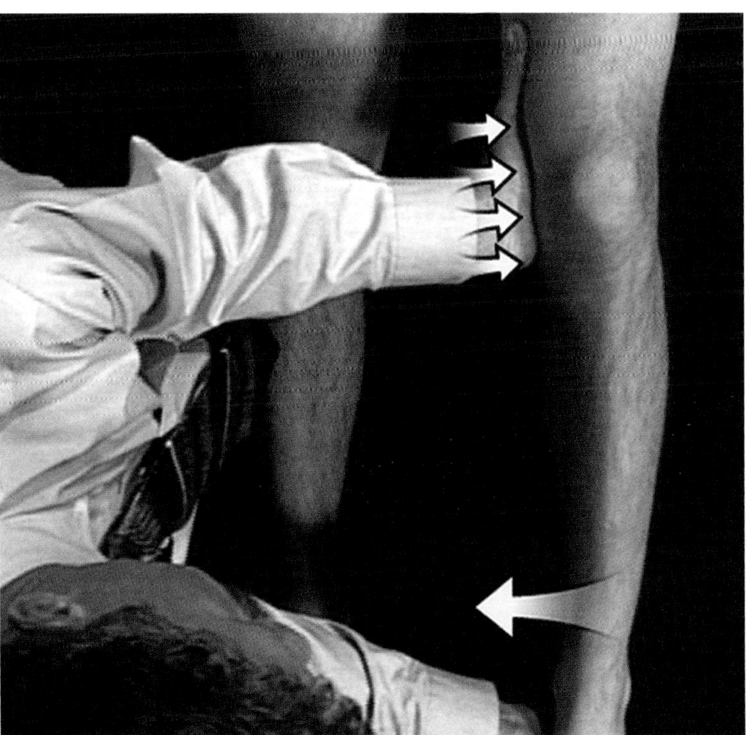

Fig. 5–57

Posterior Cruciate Ligament Now, with the patient still lying supine, move the knee into 90° of flexion, with the patient's feet flat on the examination table (Fig. 5–58). Inspect the knee from the side and note any posterior displacement of the tibia on the femur in the resting position, a so-called "tibial sag" (Fig. 5–59).

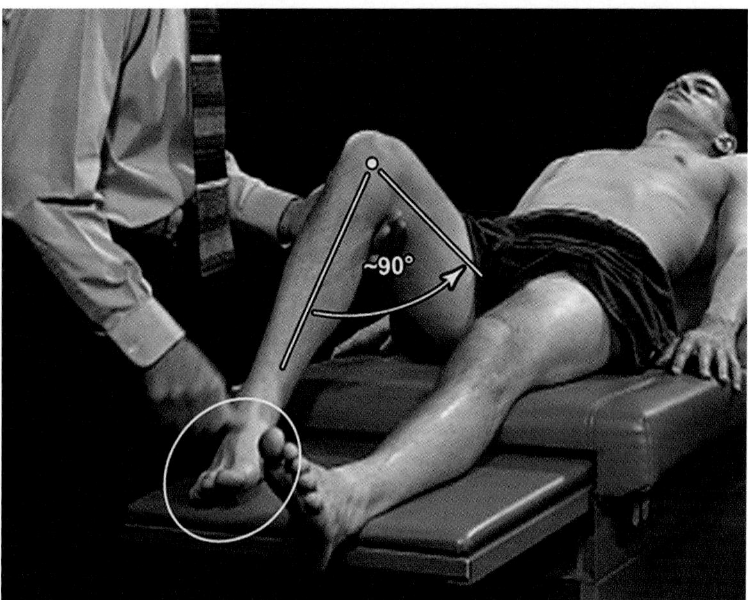

Fig. 5–58

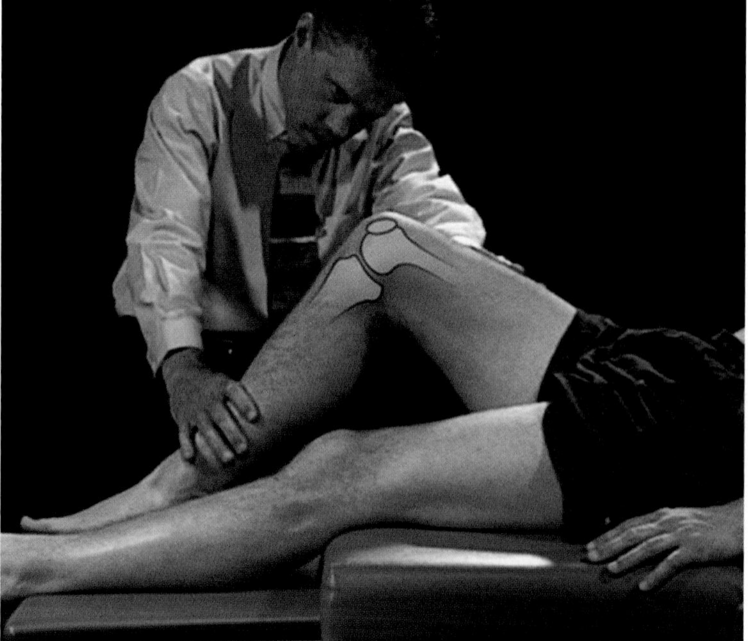

Fig. 5–59

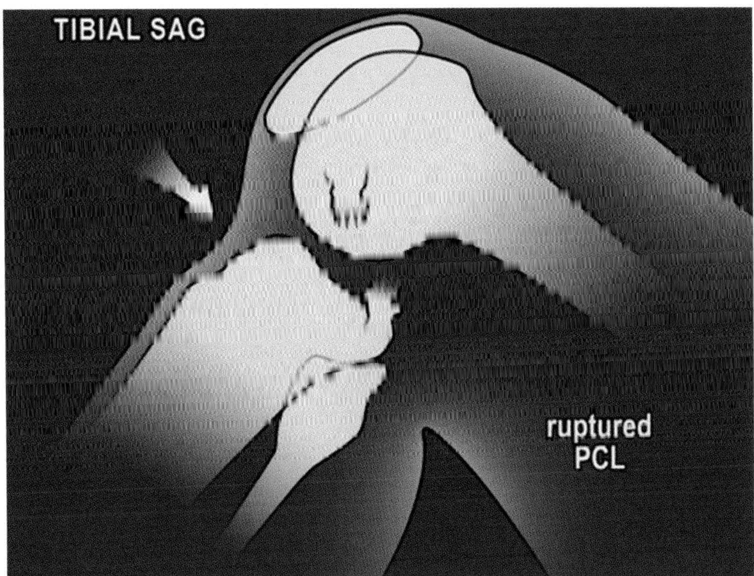

Fig. 5–60

A ruptured PCL will cause the tibia to fall posteriorly, creating an indentation below the patella when compared to the other side (Fig. 5–60).

Complete assessment of the PCL by applying pressure to the anterior tibia. Note any pain or laxity.

Knee Joint Line With the knee still in ~70° to 90° of flexion, palpate carefully along the joint line and note any focal tenderness or palpable abnormality (Fig. 5–61).

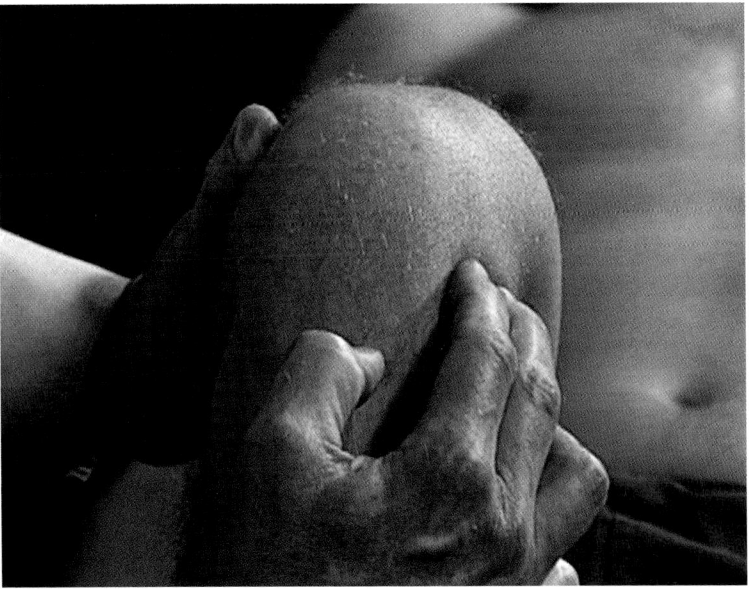

Fig. 5–61

Meniscal Cartilages (McMurray Maneuver) To assess the medial and lateral menisci, grasp the patient's heel with your right hand and position the center of the heel in your palm. Wrap your fingers around the calcaneus, firmly cupping the heel in your hand. Position the plantar surface of the patient's foot to rest against your forearm. This position will facilitate your control of the lower extremity and will minimize patient discomfort, especially in individuals with ankle edema or venous stasis (Fig. 5–62).

Next, spread your left thumb and index finger (with your palm facing the patient's head) and place them along the joint line for palpation during the McMurray maneuver (Fig. 5–63).

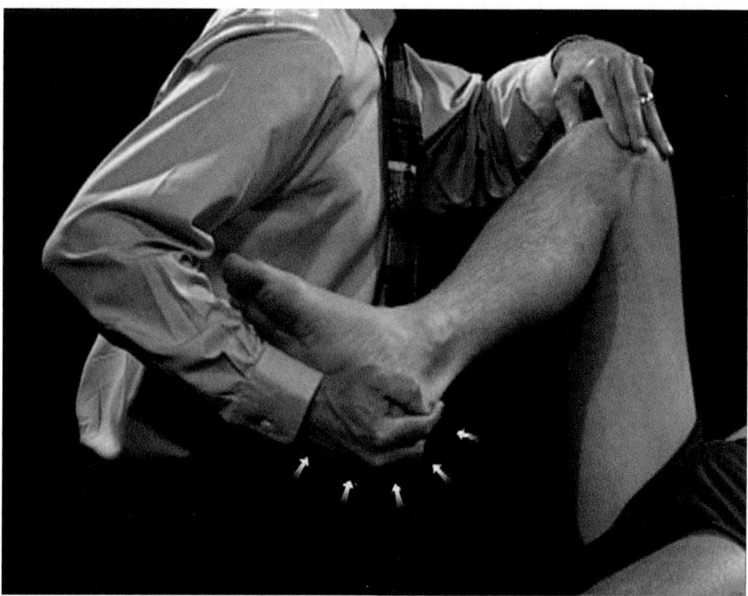

Fig. 5–62

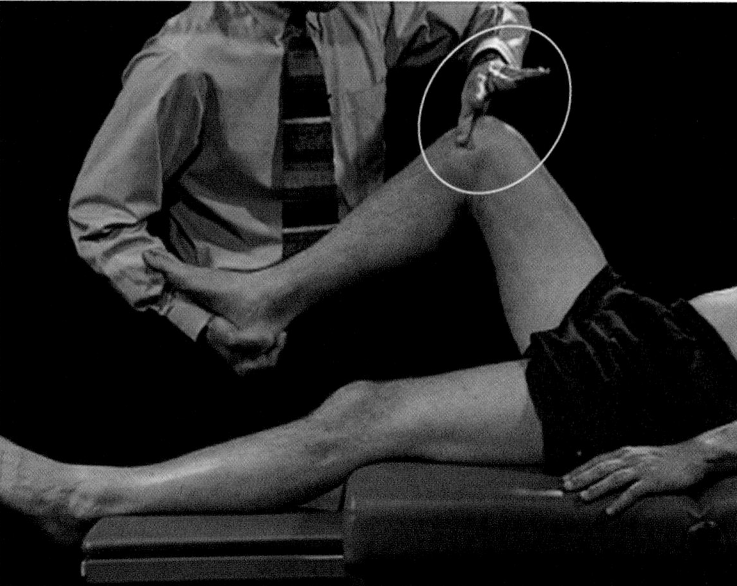

Fig. 5–63

To stress the medial and lateral menisci, take the knee through several cycles of deep flexion and partial extension. Deep flexion should bring the patient's heel nearly to the buttock, and extension should bring the knee out to nearly 90° of flexion (Fig. 5–64A, B)

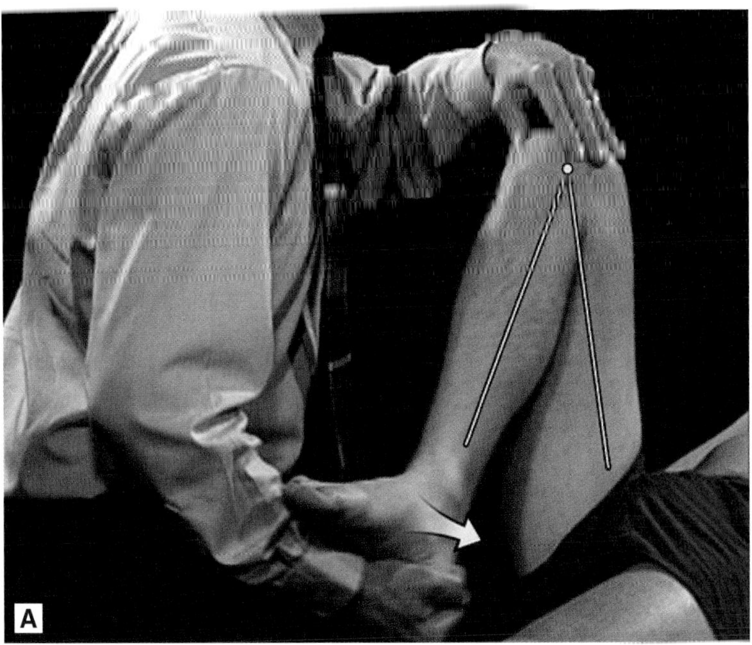

Fig. 5–64

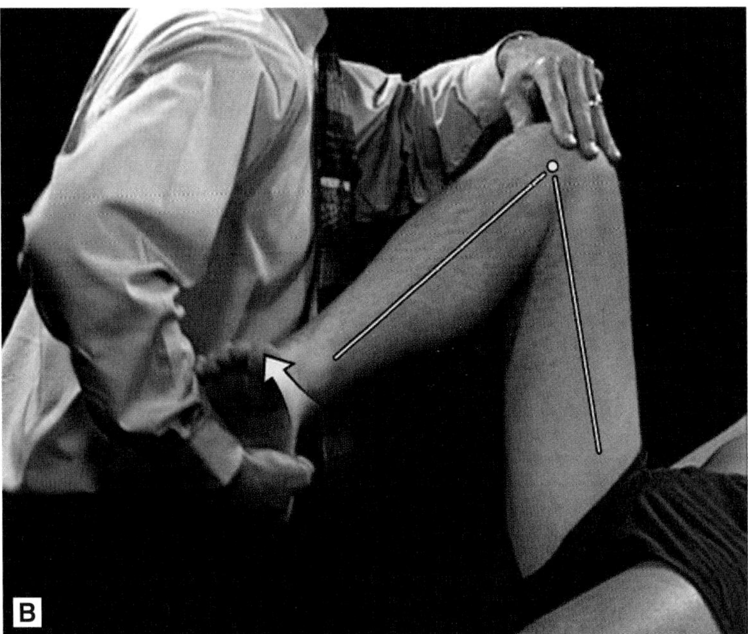

Fig. 5–64

Swing the heel in "horseshoe-shaped" arcs of flexion and extension (Fig. 5–65 A, B). while supplying alternating inversion and eversion torque to the tibia (Fig. 5–66A, B). Note any palpable clicks or pain.

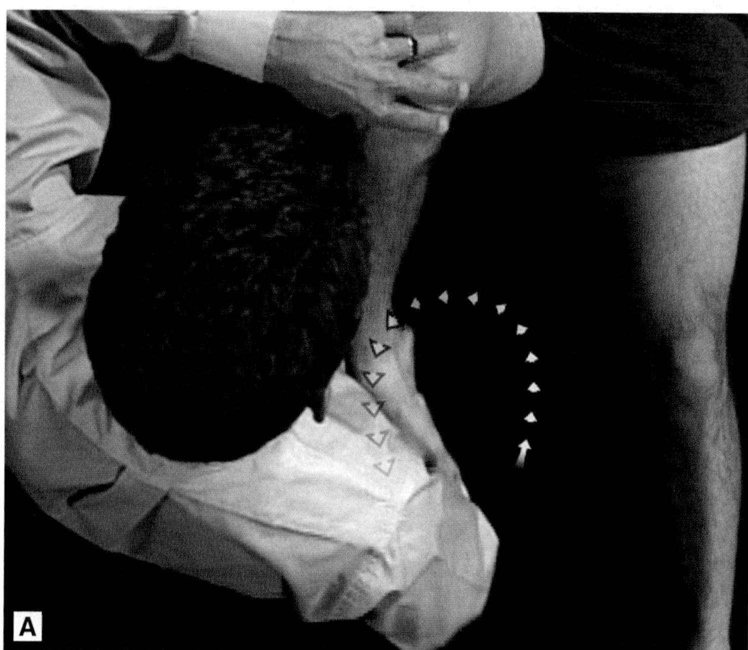

Fig. 5–65

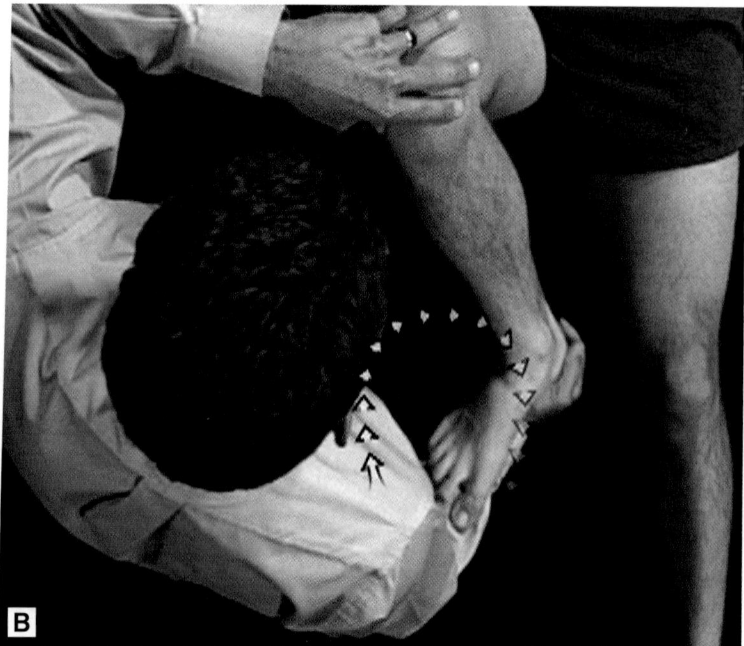

Fig. 5–65

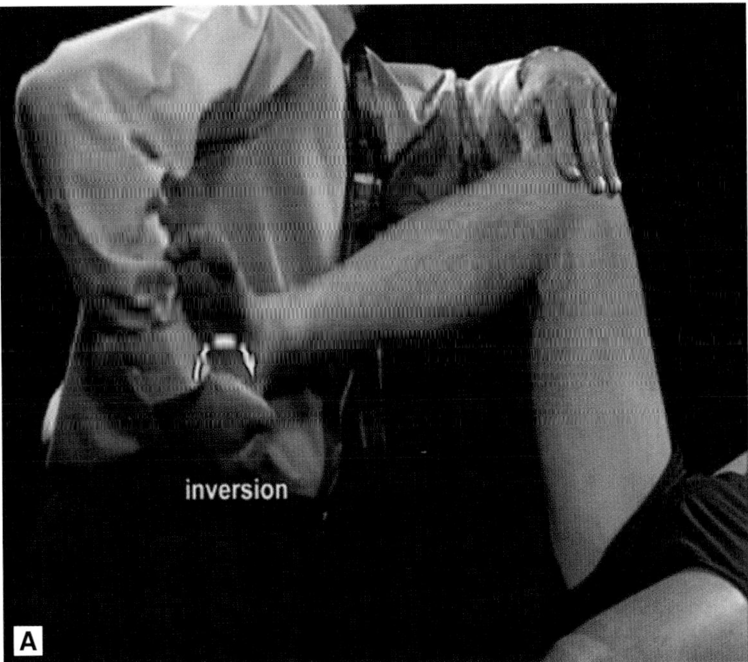

Fig. 5–66

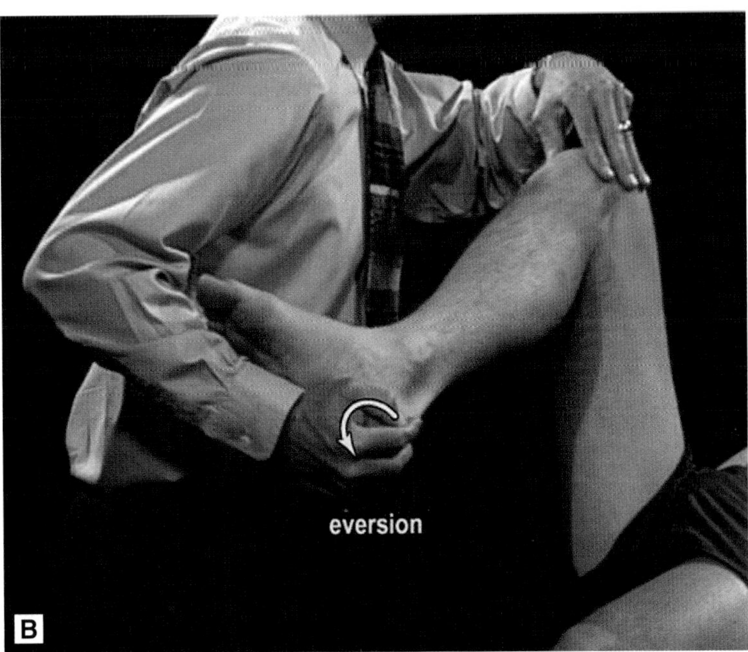

Fig. 5–66

After several cycles of flexion and extension, bring the knee into full extension while maintaining a firm inversion torque on the tibia (as though you were "screwing in" the tibia) (Fig. 5–67A). Note any medial or lateral joint pain or clicks.

Repeat the same sequence while maintaining a firm eversion torque on the tibia (as though "unscrewing" the tibia) (Fig. 5–67B). Again, note any pain or clicks.

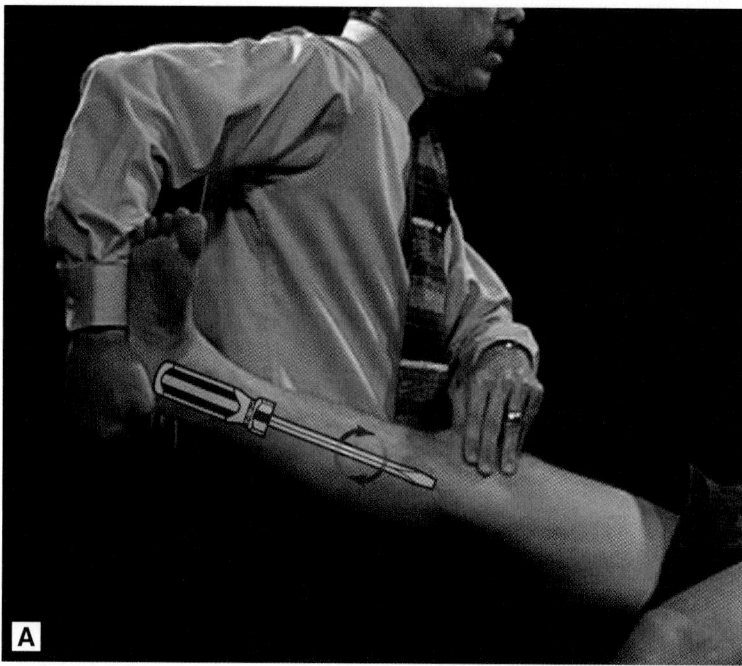

Fig. 5–67

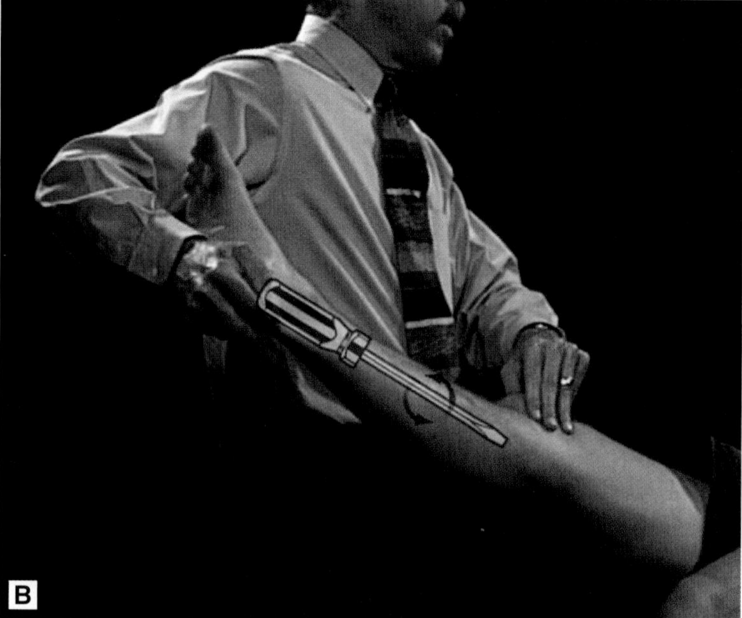

Fig. 5–67

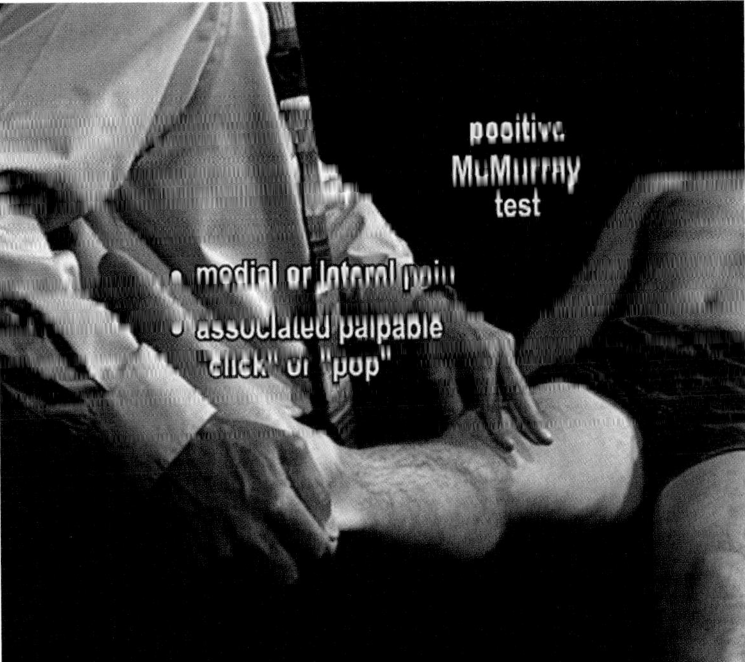

Fig. 5–68

The McMurray test requires relaxation and cooperation on the part of the patient and careful attention to proper technique on the part of the examiner. It is important that you keep your left thumb and index finger on the joint line to detect any palpable clicking or popping during this maneuver. It is equally important for the patient to report whether there is medial or lateral joint line pain during the manipulation. Reproduction of medial or lateral pain, sometimes associated with a click or pop, is considered a "positive" McMurray test (Fig. 5–68).

Anserine Bursa Next, palpate the flare in the proximal tibia medial to the tibial tuberosity. This is the region of the insertion of the pes anserine tendon and the underlying anserine bursa (Fig. 5–69A, B). Note any tenderness, indicating anserine bursitis or tendinitis. (*Anserine bursitis/tendinitis is frequently associated with exquisite tenderness but no visible or papable swelling.*)

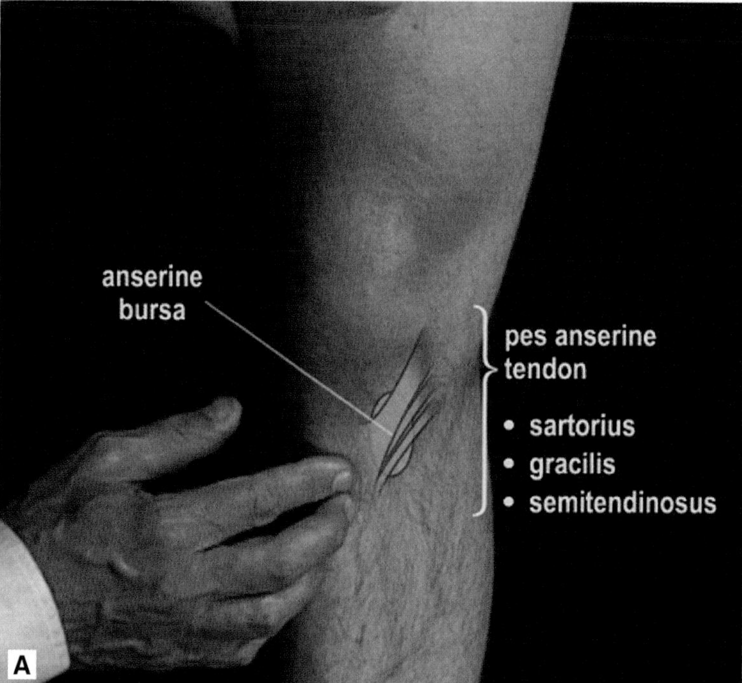

Fig. 5–69

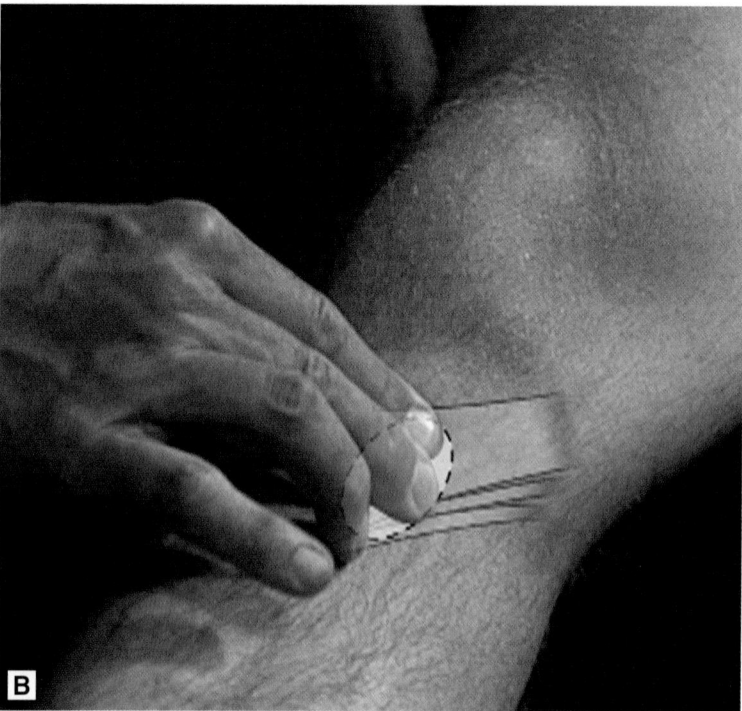

Fig. 5–69

Knee Flexion and Extension Finally, assess knee range of motion. Full flexion should bring the calf muscle against the posterior thigh (Fig. 5–70A). Full extension returns the joint to the outstretched anatomical position (0°). While holding the leg off the table, look carefully for any flexion contracture (deficit in full extension) (Fig. 5–70B).

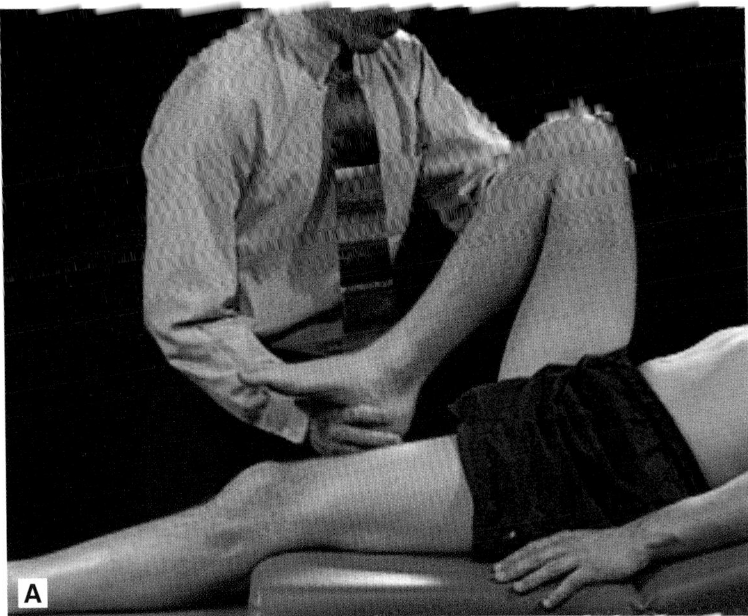

Fig. 5–70

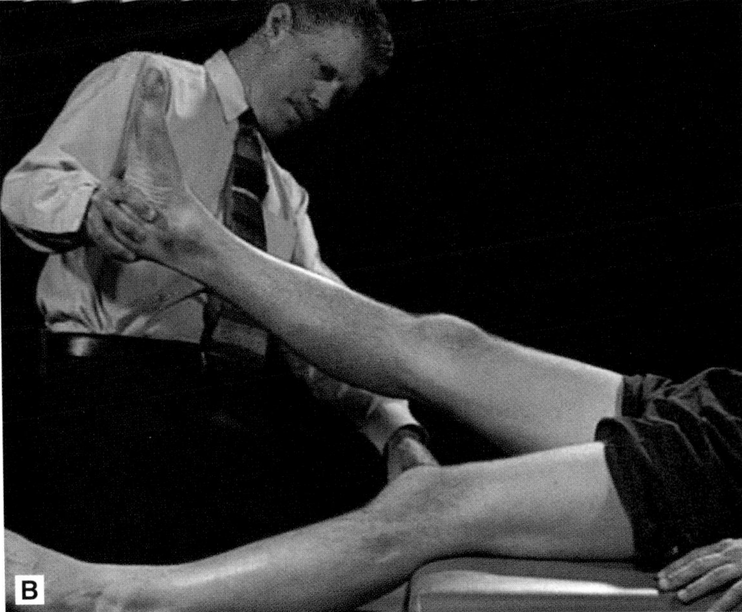

Fig. 5–70

RMSE OF THE KNEE
Practice Checklist

Patient standing

____Observe from front: check alignment

Patient squat

____Ask the patient to squat down and observe

Patient lying supine

____Inspect quadriceps (resting and contracted)
____Inspect prepatellar bursa
____Inspect medial, superolateral, and suprapatellar regions
____Check for fluid wave (bulge sign) or ballotable patella
____Compress patella in femoral groove
____Palpate medial and lateral patellar facets
____Perform patellar apprehension test (push/pull patella laterally)
____Check ACL (Lachman test)
____Check MCL
____Check LCL
____Check PCL (inspection and posterior drawer)
____Palpate joint line
____Check menisci (McMurray maneuver)
____Palpate anserine bursa (pes anserinus tendon insertion)
____Flex and extend knee

COMMON KNEE PROBLEMS

- Arthritis of the knee
- Patellofemoral pain
- Prepatellar bursitis
- Collateral ligament tear (sprain)
- Cruciate ligament tear (sprain)
- Meniscal tears
- Anserine bursitis

Arthritis of the Knee The patient's age, sex, and clinical history provide some of the most important clues to diagnosis. Pain, stiffness, crepitus, and swelling may all be indicators of knee arthritis. Physical examination findings provide additional helpful information: patellofemoral crepitus and cool effusions (osteoarthritis), cool to warm effusions (rheumatoid arthritis, crystalline arthritis, and psoriatic arthritis), and warm to very warm effusions with or without cutaneous erythema (crystalline arthritis and septic arthritis).

Patellofemoral Pain Syndrome Patellofemoral pain is characterized by diffuse, aching, anterior knee pain which increases with activities that load the patellofemoral joint: ascending or descending stairs, kneeling and squatting, or after prolonged sitting (car rides or movies). More common in women than men, it is usually not associated with swelling or a history of prior injury. Physical examination is marked by anterior knee pain on squatting and significant tenderness to palpation of the patellar facets. The origin of patellofemoral pain is multifactorial, but relative weakness/deconditioning of the quadriceps muscles (especially the vastus medialis) may play an important role in many patients.

Prepatellar Bursitis Swelling of the prepatellar bursa can result from chronic, frictional irritation of the bursa (low-grade inflammatory bursitis) from excessive kneeling; entry of bacteria into the bursal space (septic bursitis) via broken skin directly over or distal to the bursa; crystalline inflammation (gouty bursitis); or direct trauma to the anterior patella (hemorrhagic bursitis). Low-grade bursal inflammation will present as a well-defined swelling, directly anterior to the patella. High-grade inflammation in the bursa may spread into the adjacent subcutaneous tissues, severely distorting normal surface anatomy. Patients with prepatellar bursitis of any severity are able to lie with the knee in full extension (an important clue that the knee joint itself is not the primary site of pathology).

Collateral Ligament Tear (Sprain) The collateral ligaments are the primary stabilizers of the knee against valgus (MCL) and varus (LCL) stresses. MCL injury may occur if sudden force is applied to the lower extremity, driving the tibia laterally into abduction (valgus). LCL injury (less common than MCL injury) may occur if sudden force is applied to the lower extremity, driving the tibia medially into adduction (varus). Injury to the MCL or LCL (external stabilizers) may occur alone or in association with injury to the anterior or posterior cruciate ligaments and/or meniscal cartilages (internal stabilizers).

Cruciate Ligament Tear (Sprain) The cruciate ligaments are the primary stabilizers of the knee against anterior (ACL) and posterior (PCL) stresses, preventing translation of the tibia on the femur. ACL injury may result from a sudden rotational (twisting) or hyperextension (acute "back knee") injury, causing the ligament to tear. This is usually accompanied by sudden severe knee pain and giving way, and the early development of a hemorrhagic knee effusion. ACL tears are frequently associated with meniscal tears and MCL injury (so called "terrible triad").

Injury to the PCL (much less common than ACL injury) may result in a stretching injury (sprain) or rupture (tear). PCL injury may result from a sudden force applied to the anterior tibia driving it posteriorly with the knee in flexion. PCL tears are uncommonly seen in isolation, usually occurring in combination with significant injury to the ACL and/or collateral ligaments. Assessment for possible ligament tears should be performed in anyone presenting with knee pain after an acute injury.

Meniscal Tears The medial and lateral menisci are shock-absorbing, internal-stabilizing fibrocartilages which may be torn as the result of acute traumatic injury or chronic degeneration.

Acute meniscal tears usually result from a significant rotational (twisting) injury, most often associated with acute pain and the later development of stiffness and swelling with subsequent mechanical symptoms of popping, clicking, clunking, or locking of the knee.

Chronic degenerative tears may occur with no recalled injury or minimal trauma and are frequently associated with underlying knee osteoarthritis in older individuals.

Meniscal injury may occur alone or in combination with ligamentous injuries.

Anserine Bursitis Mild to severe medial knee pain and limping may result from inflammation of the pes anserine bursa. This small bursa lies underneath the insertion site of the sartorius, gracilis, and semitendinosus muscles on the anteromedial flare of the proximal tibia. Anserine bursitis is more frequently seen in women than men, characterized by exquisite local tenderness to palpation of the bursa (despite the absence of visible swelling), and is commonly associated with underlying early osteoarthritis of the medial compartment of the knee.

6

The Regional Musculoskeletal Examination of the Neck

INTRODUCTION

The *regional musculoskeletal examination* (RMSE) of the **neck** is designed to build on the sequences and techniques taught in the SMSE and GMSE. It is intended to provide a comprehensive assessment of structure and function combined with special testing to permit you to evaluate common, important musculoskeletal problems of the neck seen in an ambulatory setting. The skills involved require practice and careful attention to technique. However, they can be learned and mastered on normal individuals.

CLINICAL UTILITY

The RMSE of the neck is clinically useful as the initial examination in individuals whose history clearly suggests an acute or chronic neck problem: neck-predominant spinal pain or upper extremity–predominant pain (possible cervical nerve root irritation). With practice, a systematic, efficient RMSE of the neck can be performed in ~3 to 4 minutes.

Furthermore, the RMSE of the neck provides the foundation for learning additional, more refined diagnostic techniques through your later exposure to orthopedic surgeons, rheumatologists, physiatrists, physical therapists, and others specifically involved in the diagnosis and treatment of neck problems.

OBJECTIVES

This instructional program will enable you to identify important anatomical features, functional relationships, and common pathologic conditions involving the neck. Essential content includes

- Structural and functional anatomy
- Cervical spine range of motion
- (Myofascial) trigger points and (fibromyalgia) tender points
- Suspected nerve root irritation
- Suspected cervical myelopathy

Most importantly, this program will prepare you to perform an organized, integrated, and clinically useful RMSE of the neck.

ESSENTIAL CONCEPTS

Structural and Functional Anatomy The cervical spine consists of seven vertebrae, increasing progressively in size from C1 to C7.

C1 and C2 deserve special comment because they have unique features (Fig. 6–1). C1 (**atlas**) lacks a vertebral body but consists of anterior and posterior arches and two cup-shaped lateral masses (Fig. 6–2A). Just as in Greek mythology, Atlas was forced to bear the weight of the world on his shoulders, so the cervical atlas (C1) bears the skull on its "shoulders" (lateral masses; Fig. 6–2B), each

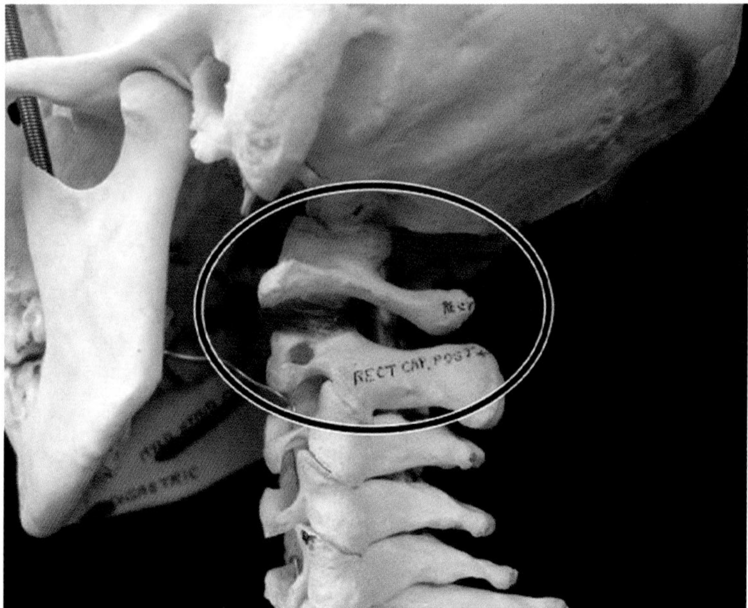

Fig. 6–1

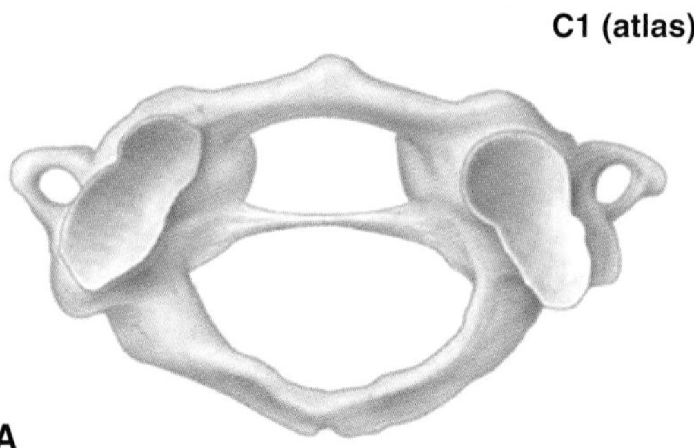

Fig. 6–2. (Modified with permission from Lawry GV, Kreder HJ, Hawker G, Jerome D. Fam's Musculoskeletal Examination and Joint Injection Techniques, 2nd ed. Mosby/Elsevier, 2010, p. 105.)

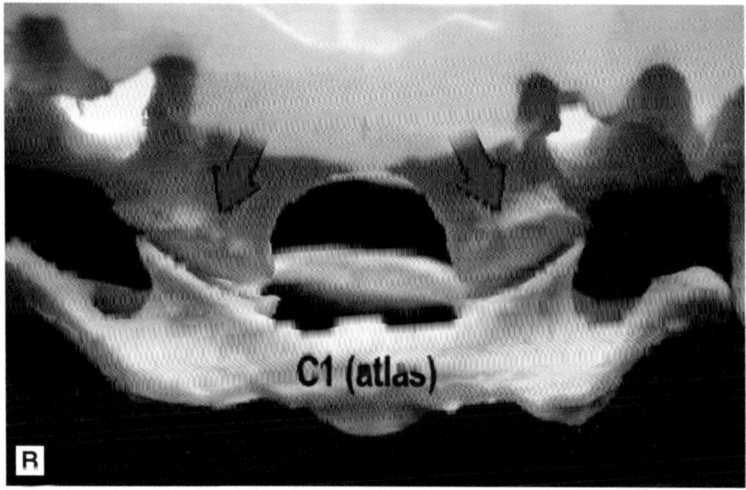

Fig. 6–2

articulating with the occipital condyles on either side of the foramen magnum at the **atlantooccipital joints** (Fig. 6–3A, B). These joints make small contributions to flexion and extension (nodding) and lateral flexion.

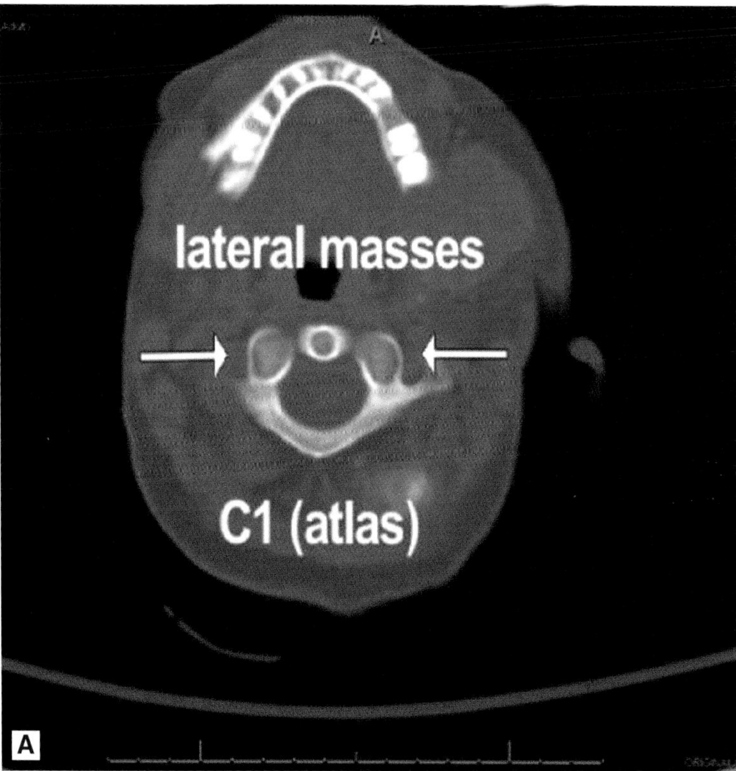

Fig. 6–3

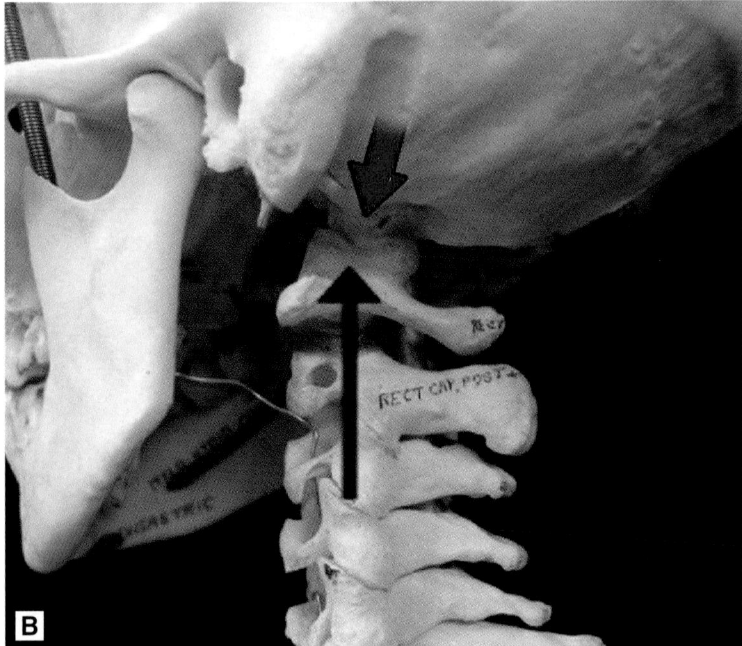

Fig. 6–3

C2 (**axis**) has a vertebral body anteriorly and from it a fingerlike peg projects superiorly (Fig. 6–4A, B). This bony process called the *odontoid* or *dens* (dont and dens from Latin for tooth) sits snuggly against the anterior arch of the atlas. The two are held together by the fibrous transverse ligament, which runs

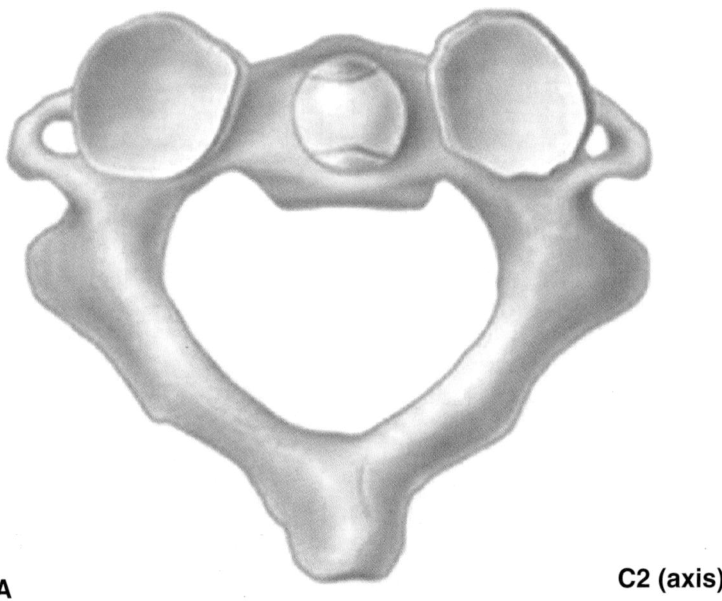

Fig. 6–4. (Modified with permission from Lawry GV, Kreder HJ, Hawker G, Jerome D. Fam's Musculoskeletal Examination and Joint Injection Techniques, 2nd ed. Mosby/Elsevier, 2010, p. 105.)

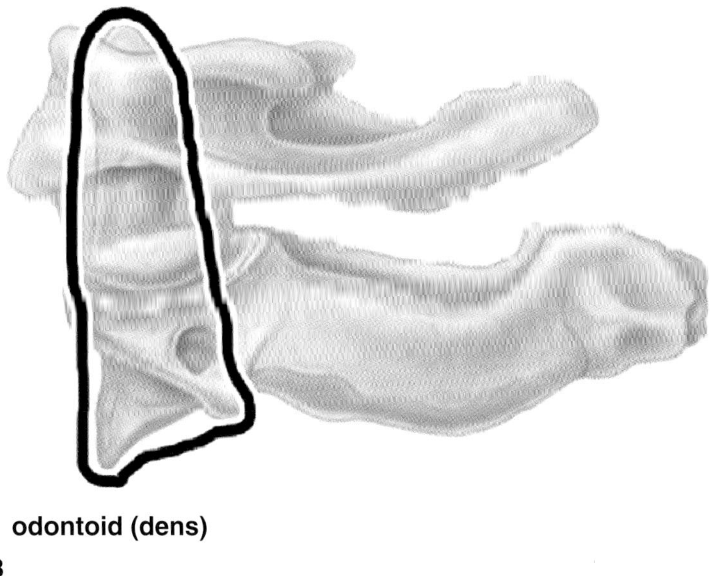

Fig. 6–4. (Modified with permission from Lawry GV, Kreder HJ, Hawker G, Jerome D. Fam's Musculoskeletal Examination and Joint Injection Techniques, 2nd ed. Mosby/Elsevier, 2010, p. 105.)

behind the odontoid process (Fig. 6–5). About 50° of rotation of the cervical spine occurs at the **atlantoaxial joint** (C1-C2).

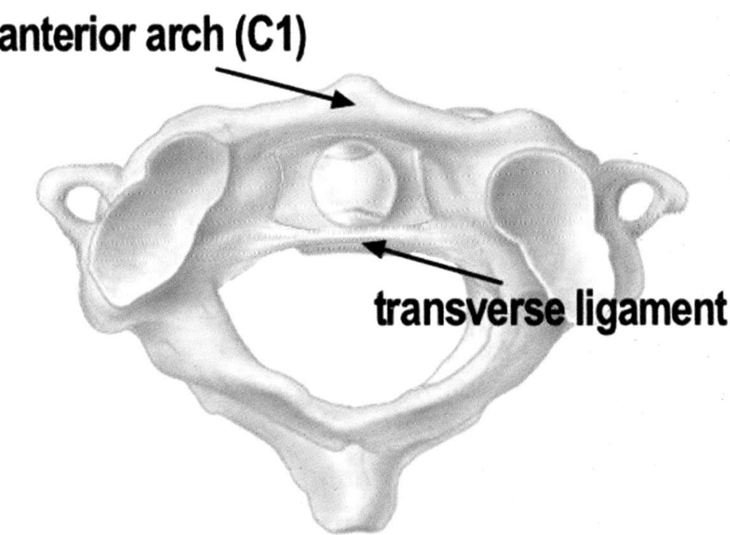

Fig. 6–5. (Modified with permission from Lawry GV, Kreder HJ, Hawker G, Jerome D. Fam's Musculoskeletal Examination and Joint Injection Techniques, 2nd ed. Mosby/Elsevier, 2010, p. 105.)

C3 through C7 are more typical vertebrae and possess an anterior weight-bearing element, the **vertebral body**, and posterior elements, including the neural arch and facet joints (Fig.6–6A through C).

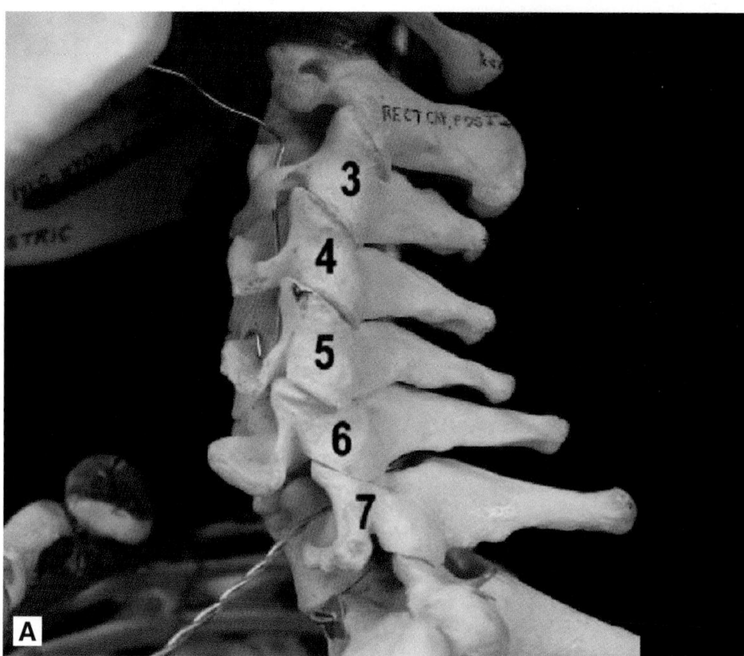

Fig. 6–6

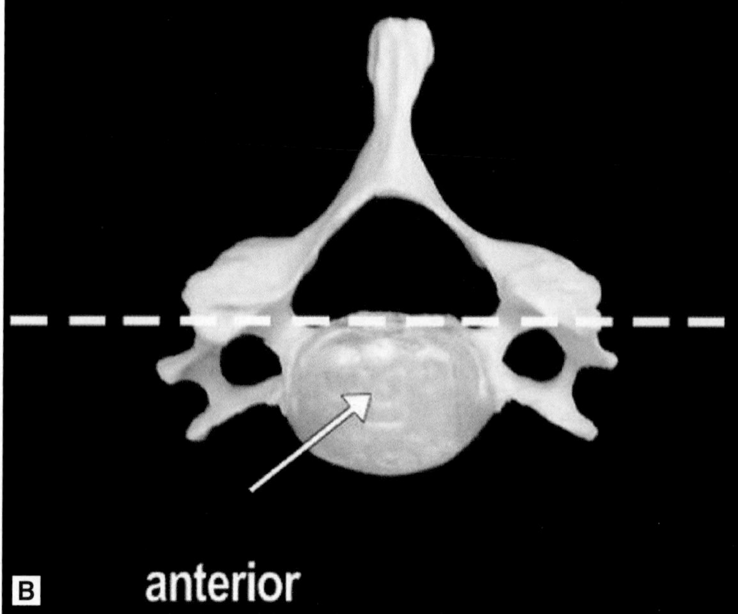

Fig. 6–6

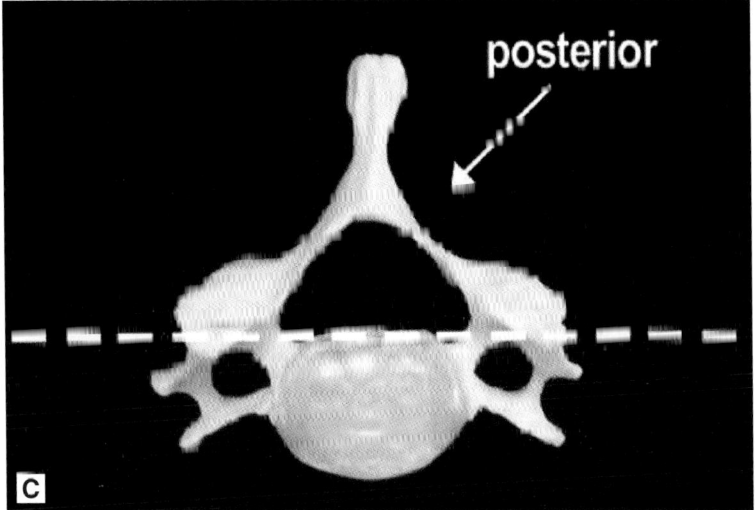

Fig. 6–6

The neural arch is made up of two **pedicles** attached to the vertebral body and two **laminae** which fuse in the midline to form the **spinous process** (Fig. 6–7A through C).

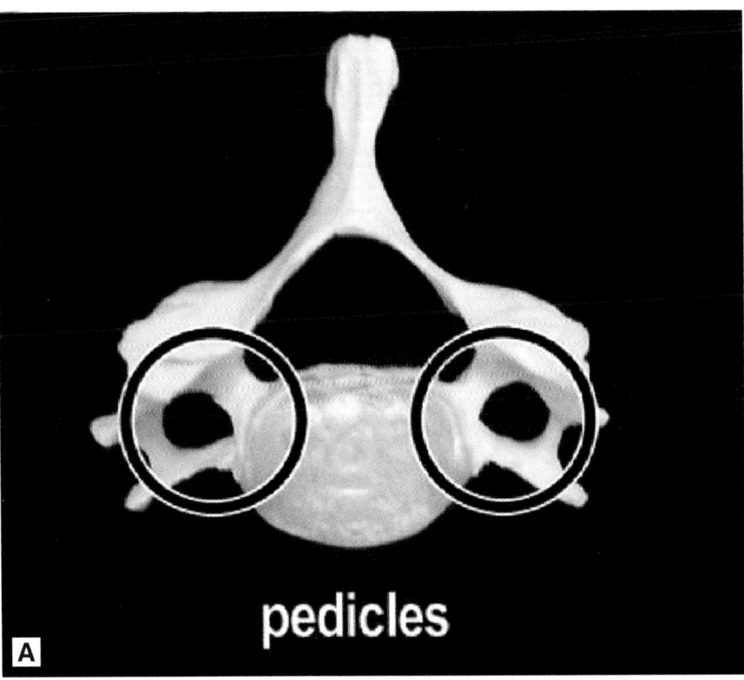

Fig. 6–7

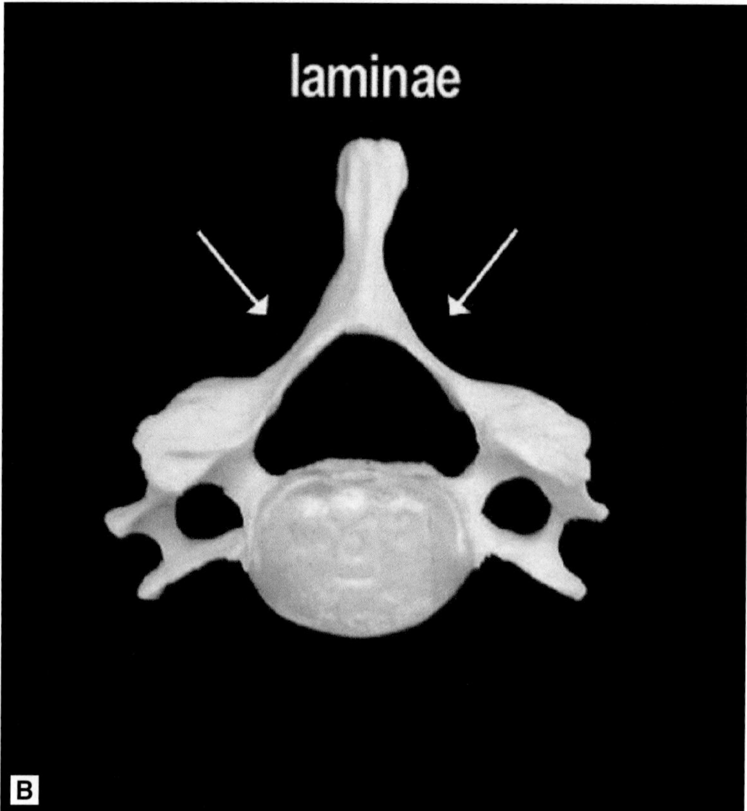

Fig. 6–7

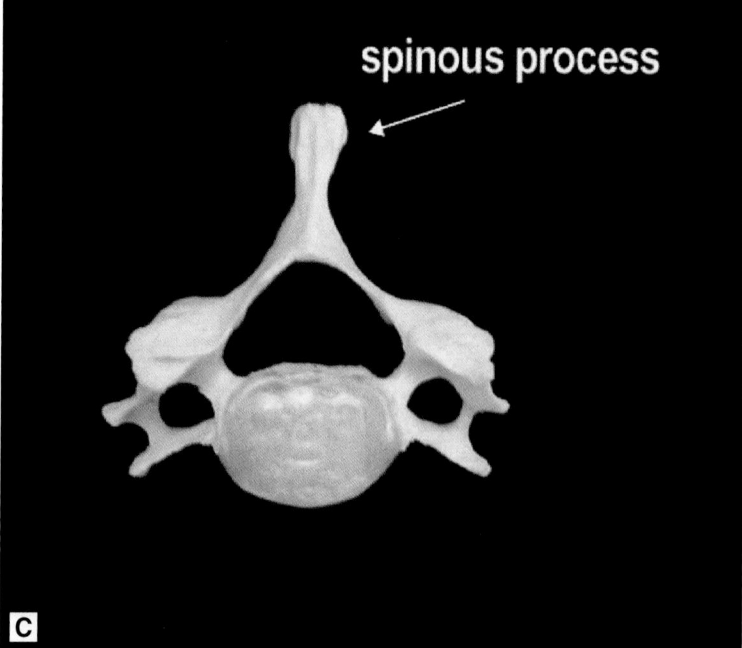

Fig. 6–7

Three pairs of bony processes project from each arch close to the junction of the pedicles and laminae: two transverse processes, two superior articular processes, and two inferior articular processes (Fig. 6–8A through C).

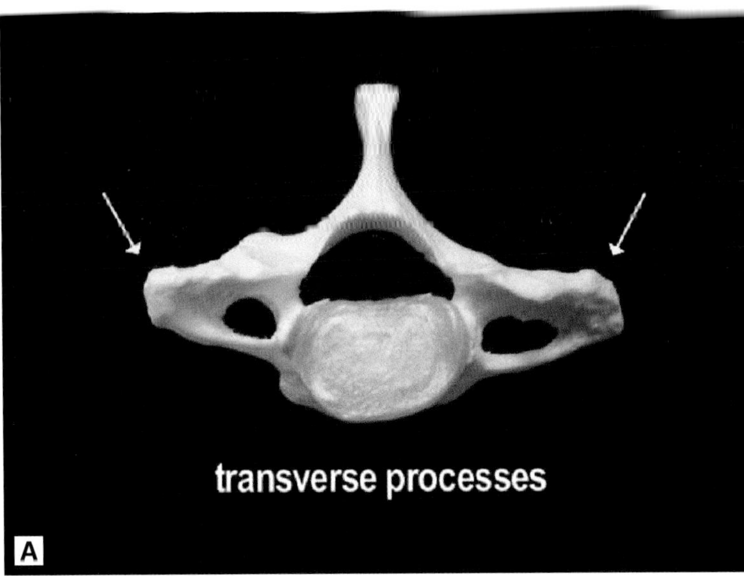

Fig. 6–8

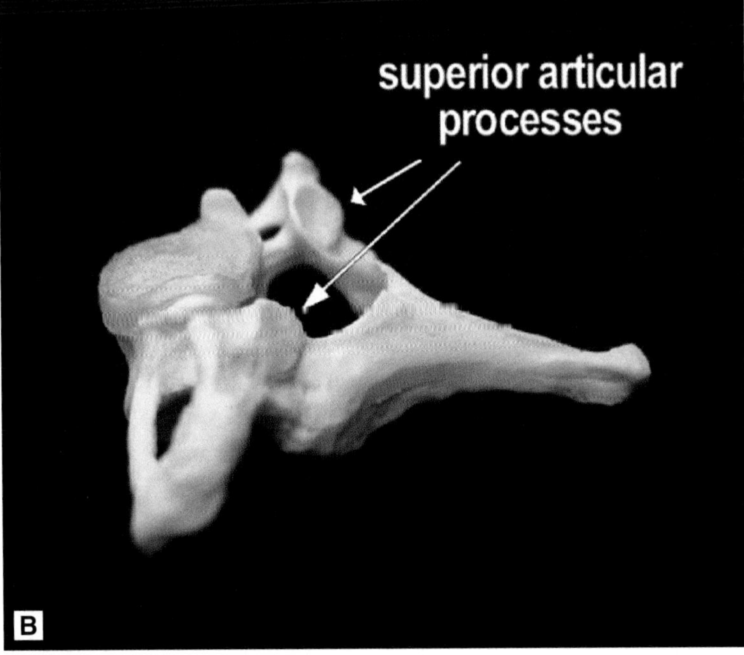

Fig. 6–8

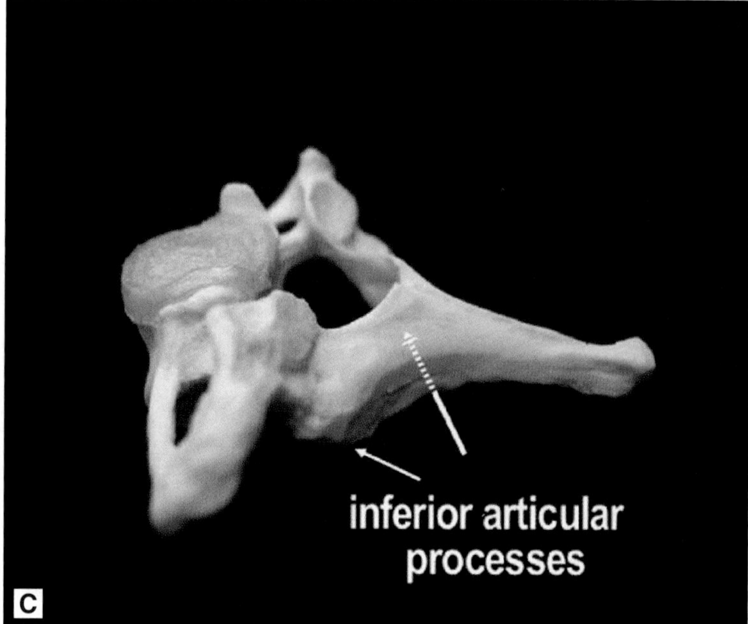

Fig. 6–8

Together, the superior and inferior articular processes form the **facet (apophyseal) joints**. These "stacking joints" allow movements at the spine and prevent forward sliding of one vertebra on another (Fig. 6–9A, B).

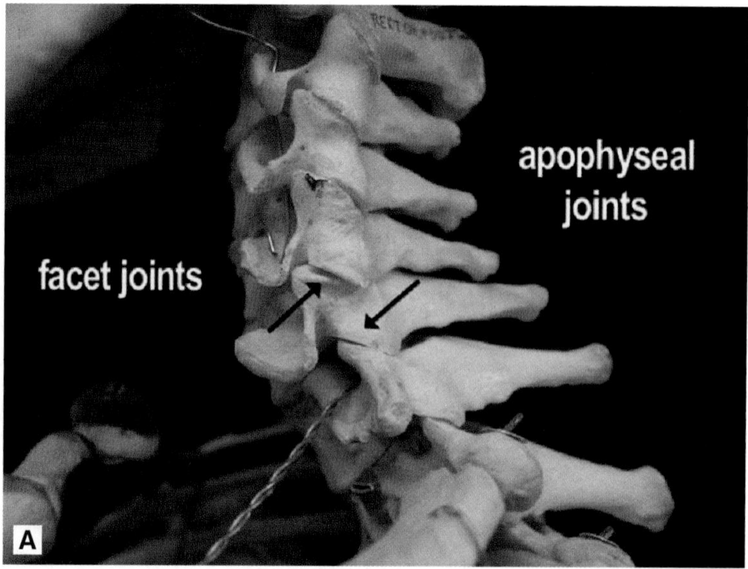

Fig. 6–9

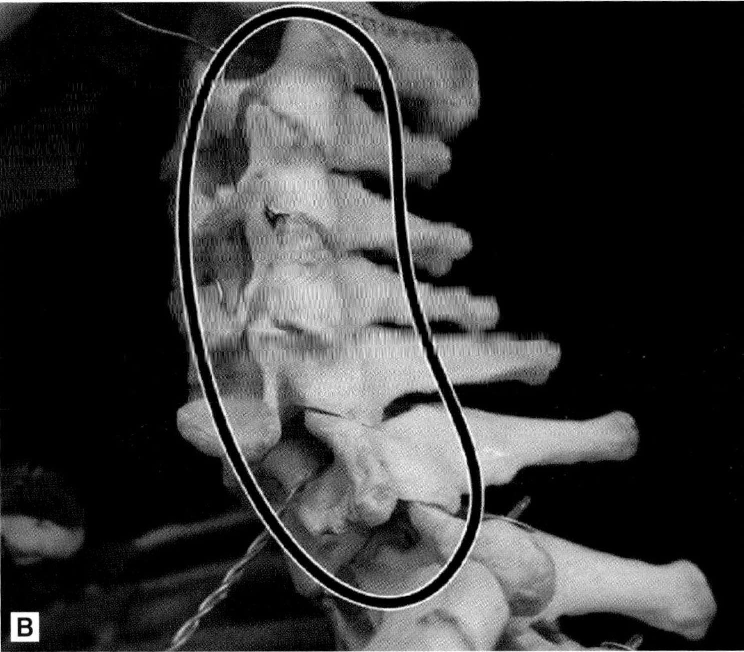

Fig. 6–9

In addition, C3 through C7 frequently have unique bony projections posteriorly and laterally from the superior end plate of each vertebra which articulate with the beveled inferolateral surface of the vertebra above to form the **uncovertebral joints of Luschka** (Fig. 6–10A, B).

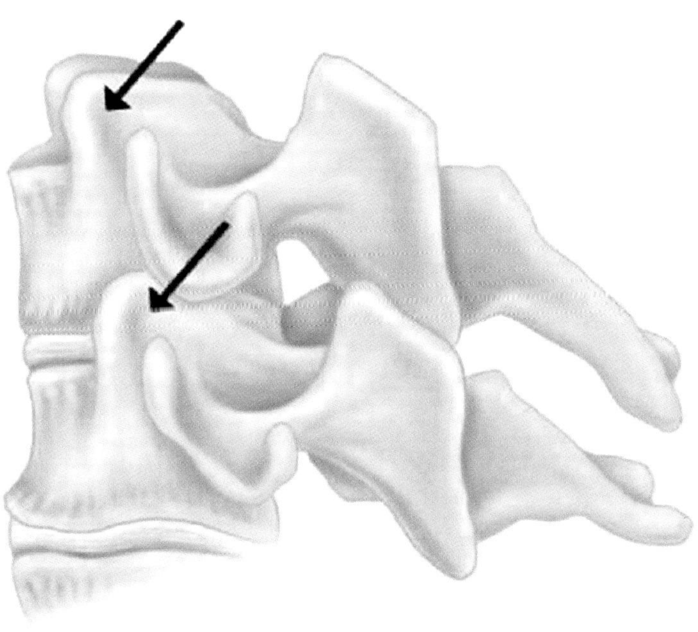

Fig. 6–10. (Modified with permission from Lawry GV, Kreder HJ, Hawker G, Jerome D. Fam's Musculoskeletal Examination and Joint Injection Techniques, 2nd ed. Mosby/Elsevier, 2010, p.105.)

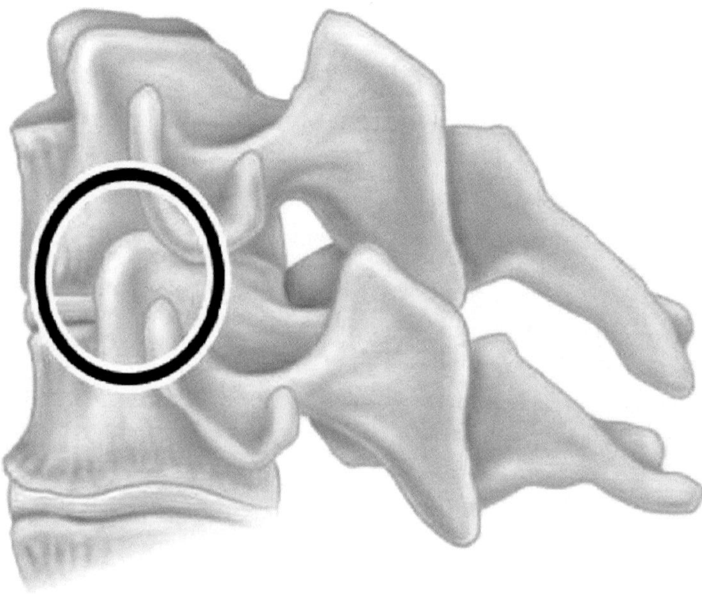

Fig. 6–10. (Modified with permission from Lawry GV, Kreder HJ, Hawker G, Jerome D. Fam's Musculoskeletal Examination and Joint Injection Techniques, 2nd ed. Mosby/Elsevier, 2010, p.105.)

These joints permit greater movements at the cervical spine compared with the thoracic and lumbar spine, and also provide lateral stability to the diskovertebral complex, forming a barrier to extrusion of disk material posterolaterally.

The C3 through C7 vertebrae allow cervical spinal flexion, extension, lateral bending, and rotation. In the resting neutral position, the posterior process of C7 (**vertebra prominens**) is palpable in the midline at the base of the neck.

Clinical History and Examination The patient's history is the essential first step in all musculoskeletal diagnosis and directs the focus of an appropriate physical examination. Particularly useful background information includes age; occupation and recreational activities; a history of injury or arthritis; and any prior neck problems.

An initial pain assessment can be well delineated with the use of the mnemonic **OPQRSTU**: where **O** = Onset; **P** = Precipitating and ameliorating factors; **Q** = Quality; **R** = Radiation; **S** = Severity; **T** = Timing; and **U** = Urinary or upper motor neuron symptoms.

Once pain characteristics are established, additional historical features may help focus the diagnostic evaluation.

Is there evidence of major trauma or injury?

Is there evidence of neurologic compromise requiring surgical consultation?

Is there an underlying serious systemic disease?

Is there social or psychological distress that may amplify, prolong, or complicate the pain?

Most neck pain is attributed to muscle and/or ligamentous strain, facet joint arthritis, intervertebral disk herniation, or other miscellaneous causes. However, despite advances in imaging and neurodiagnosis, the etiology of most acute and chronic neck pain is complex and frequently poorly understood.

The thrust of a brief, focused history should inquire about risk factors pointing to fracture, malignancy, infection, underlying visceral or systemic disease, or the need for urgent surgical consultation. The musculoskeletal physical examination of the neck should be focused and used to confirm or refute diagnostic hypotheses generated by a focused, but thoughtful history.

Acute uncomplicated idiopathic neck and low back pain accounts for the vast majority of spinal pain seen in clinical practice. A focused clinical history and physical examination is important, and in the absence of serious underlying conditions, a diagnosis of acute nonspecific neck or low back pain can be made.

A definitive anatomic diagnosis cannot be made in as many as 85% of patients presenting with acute neck or low back pain, but up to two-thirds of such patients have resolution of their symptoms in 4 to 8 weeks.

Fortified by this information, the clinician is able to direct subsequent management efforts at reassurance and resumption of normal functional activity rather than extensive and expensive (and frequently misleading) imaging studies.

THE EXAMINATION, OVERVIEW

Observe the patient's posture, movement, and behaviors throughout the history and the physical examination.

With the patient seated, observe the resting posture and alignment of the cervical spine. Note any resting asymmetry or deformity and inspect for the normal resting cervical lordosis. Next, inspect the skin. Note any scars or rashes.

Palpate the inion (greater occipital protuberance), then palpate inferiorly along the spinous processes from C2 to the mid-thoracic spine and note any tenderness. Assess for tender points or trigger points by palpating the suboccipital muscle insertions, the mid to upper trapezius, the supraspinatus, and medial scapular borders on each side.

Assess neck flexion by asking the patient to touch the chin to the chest. Assess neck extension by asking the patient to look up at the ceiling. Observe right and left rotation by asking the patient to place the chin on each shoulder. Assess lateral flexion (or lateral bending) by asking the patient to incline the ear toward each shoulder.

If indicated from the history or physical, also perform an RMSE of the shoulders.

If indicated from the history or physical, perform special testing for possible nerve root irritation or signs of cervical myelopathy.

Assess biceps, brachioradialis, and triceps reflexes. Test muscle strength of deltoids (resisted shoulder abduction), biceps (resisted elbow flexion), triceps (resisted elbow extension), and interossei (spreading fingers against resistance). Now, assess sensation to light touch and/or pin prick over the lateral deltoid, thumb and index finger, middle finger, and ring and little fingers.

Rotate and extend the cervical spine while providing gentle/firm pressure to the patient's occiput (Spurling maneuver). If radicular pain or symptoms are present, note whether patient obtains relief by placing the ipsilateral distal forearm on the occiput (abduction relief sign).

Assess for possible upper motor neuron signs. Flick the tip of the patient's middle finger and note any involuntary flexion of thumb and index finger (Hoffman sign). Next, check knee and ankle reflexes. Note any hyperreflexia. Check for ankle clonus. Assess for extensor plantar reflexes (Babinski sign). Observe the patient's gait for a broad base or unsteadiness.

If clinically indicated from the patient's history, consider cervical spine pain referral from pulmonary, cardiac, or other visceral sources.

THE EXAMINATION, COMPONENT PARTS

Observation and Inspection Carefully observe the patient's posture, movement, and behaviors during the history and physical examination. This provides an important opportunity to observe function and range of motion at a time when the patient is unaware that such observations are being made.

Clearly establishing yourself as the patient's advocate throughout the history and physical examination facilitates communication and enhances your ability to obtain essential information.

With the patient seated, note the resting posture and alignment. Note any asymmetry or deformity and inspect for the normal resting cervical lordosis (Fig. 6–11).

Next, inspect the skin both anteriorly and posteriorly and note any scars from prior surgery or significant injury. Note any rashes, particularly vesicles characteristic of herpes zoster.

Palpation Palpate the greater occipital protuberance (inion) while gently supporting the head. Note any tenderness. Next, palpate the spinous processes. Begin below the occiput at C2 and palpate inferiorly to the upper thoracic spine. Note any focal tenderness (Fig. 6–12).

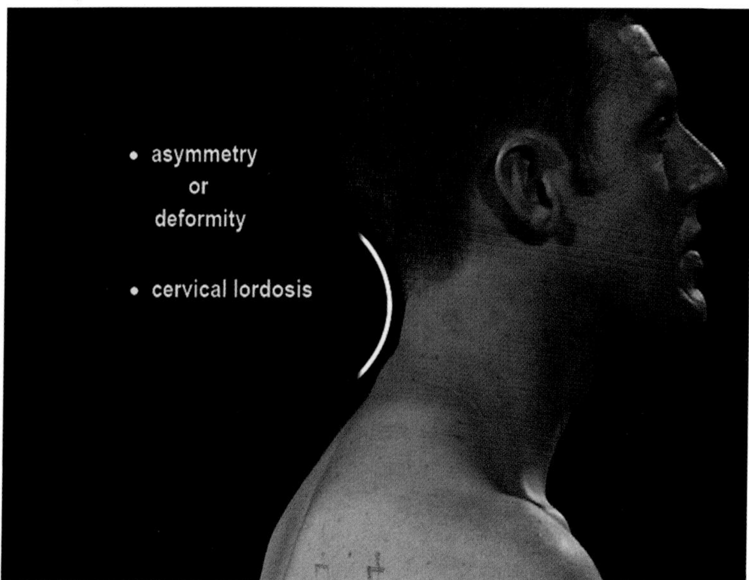

Fig. 6–11

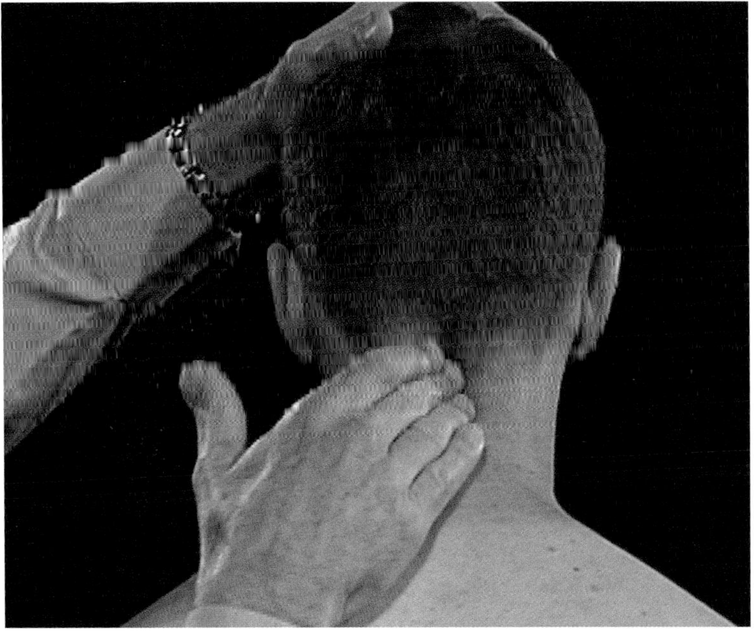

Fig. 6–12

Next, ask the patient to identify any focal tender areas they may have already recognized. Palpate this/these area(s) to assess for discrete myofascial trigger points (Fig. 6–13A).

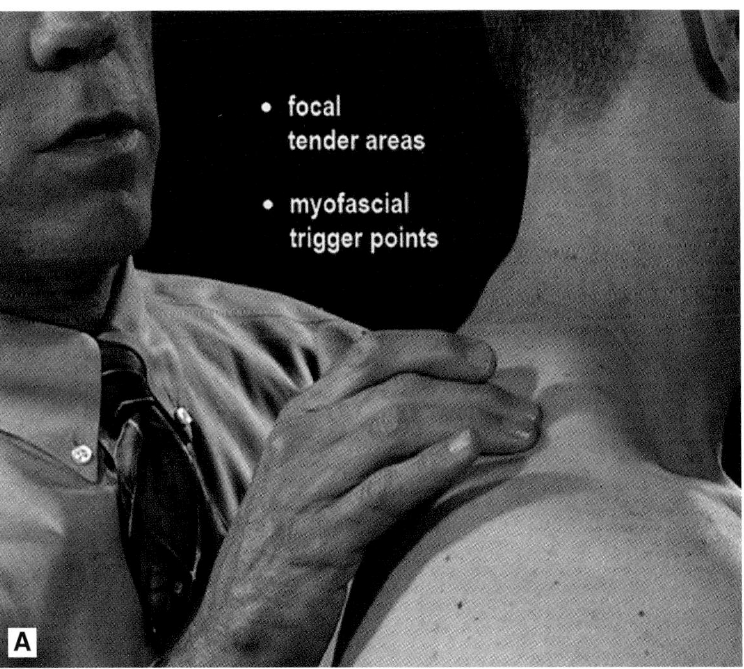

Fig. 6–13

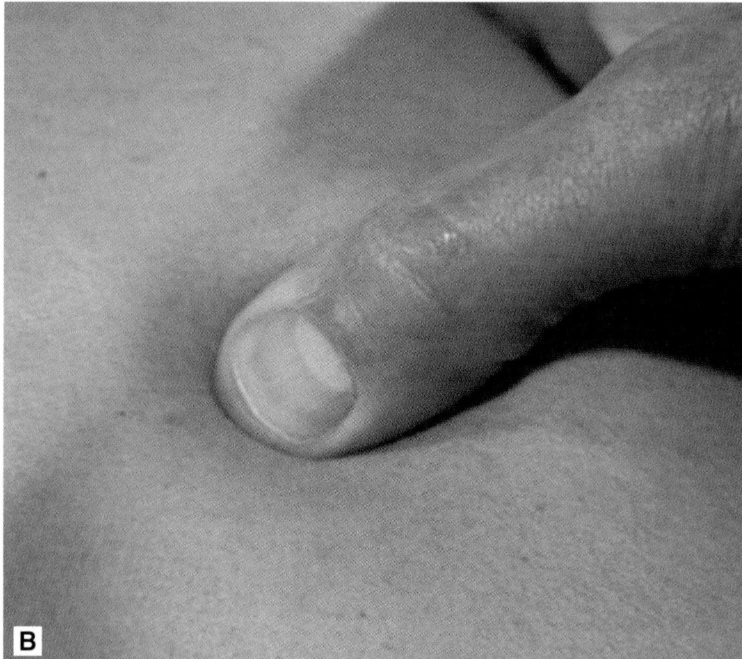

Fig. 6–13

Apply sufficient pressure to blanch your fingernails (~5 lb of pressure) (Fig. 6–13B). Note whether this reproduces the patient's complaints.

Palpate the suboccipital muscle insertion sites on either side of the greater occipital protuberance, the mid to upper trapezius at the base of the neck, the mid-supraspinatus and along the medial scapular border (Fig. 6–14A through D).

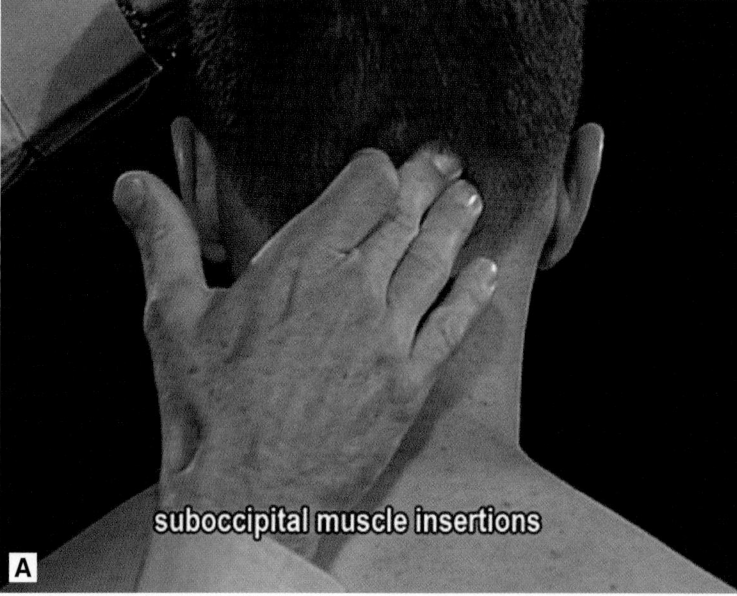

Fig. 6–14

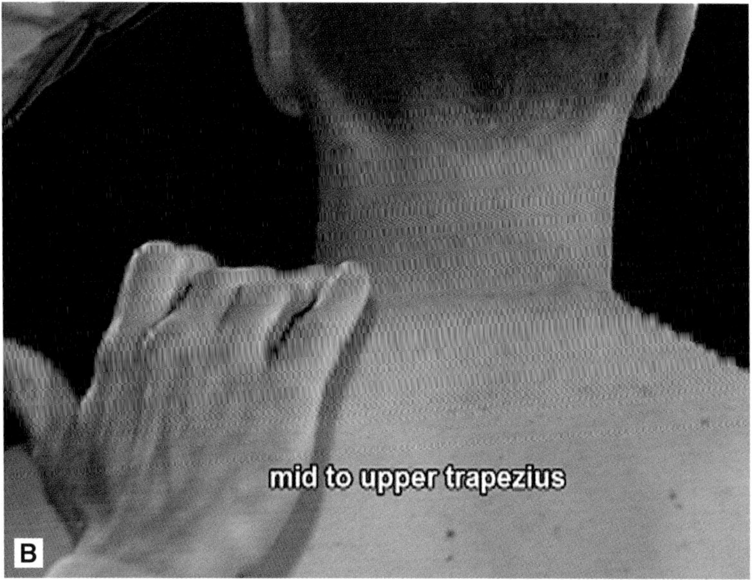

Fig. 6–14

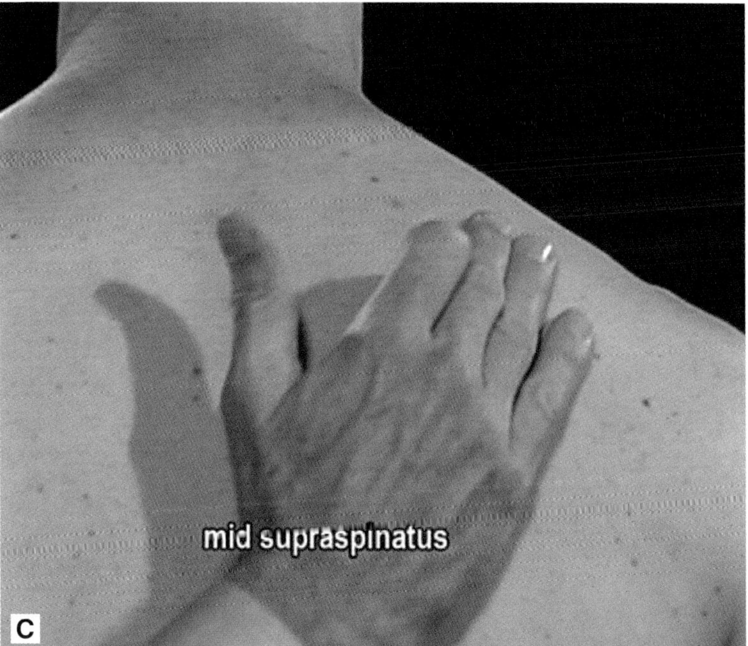

Fig. 6–14

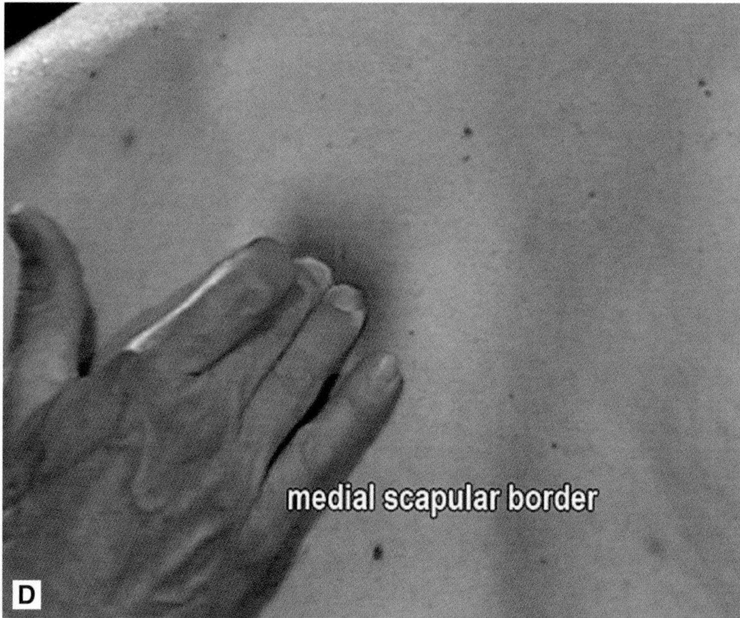

Fig. 6–14

If multiple tender points are identified in the cervical region, complete your assessment for possible fibromyalgia with a complete tender point examination (Fig. 6–15A, B).

Widespread sensitivity to light touch of superficial soft tissues over the neck (excluding prior scars) may indicate significant psychological distress.

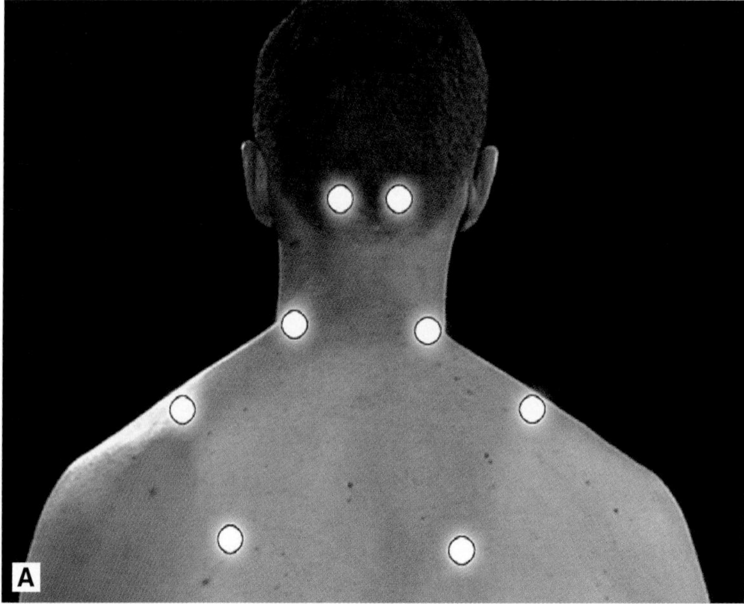

Fig. 6–15

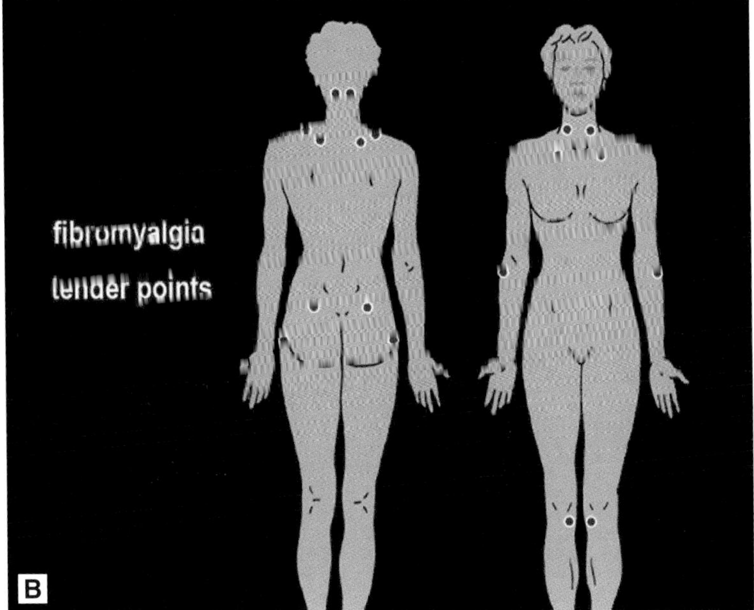

Fig. 6–15

Range of Motion Next, observe cervical range of motion. Assess neck flexion by instructing the patient to place his chin on the chest. Normal flexion should permit the chin to touch the upper sternum (Fig. 6–16A).

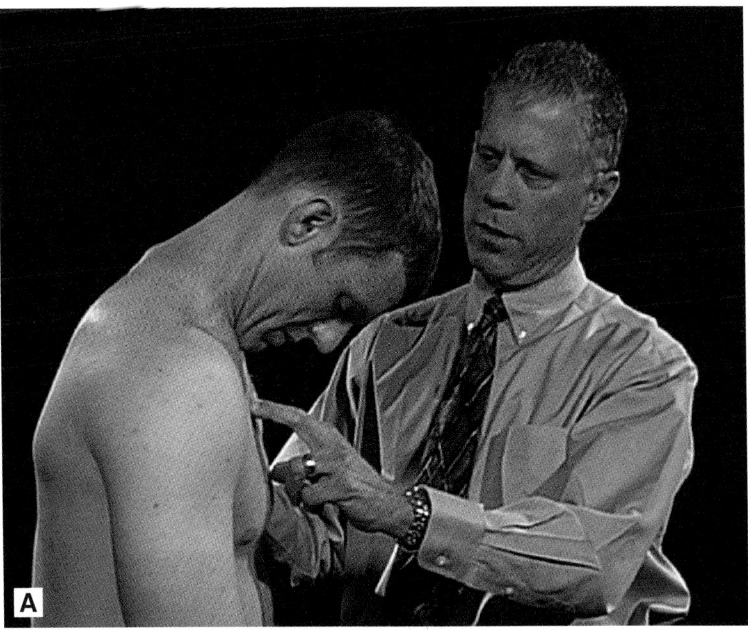

Fig. 6–16

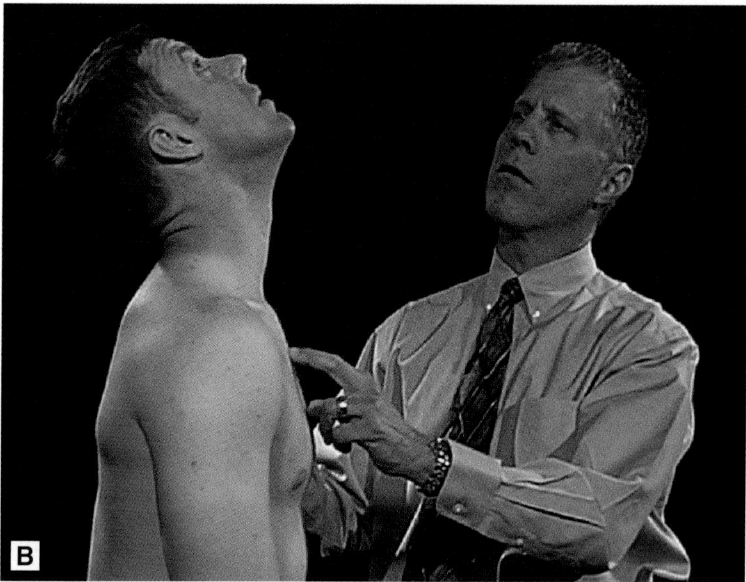

Fig. 6–16

Next, assess neck extension by asking the patient to look up at the ceiling (Fig. 6–16B). Normal extension should bring face nearly parallel to the ceiling.

Observe right and left rotation by asking the patient to place his chin on each shoulder. Normal cervical rotation should permit the chin to touch the top of each shoulder (Fig. 6–16C, D).

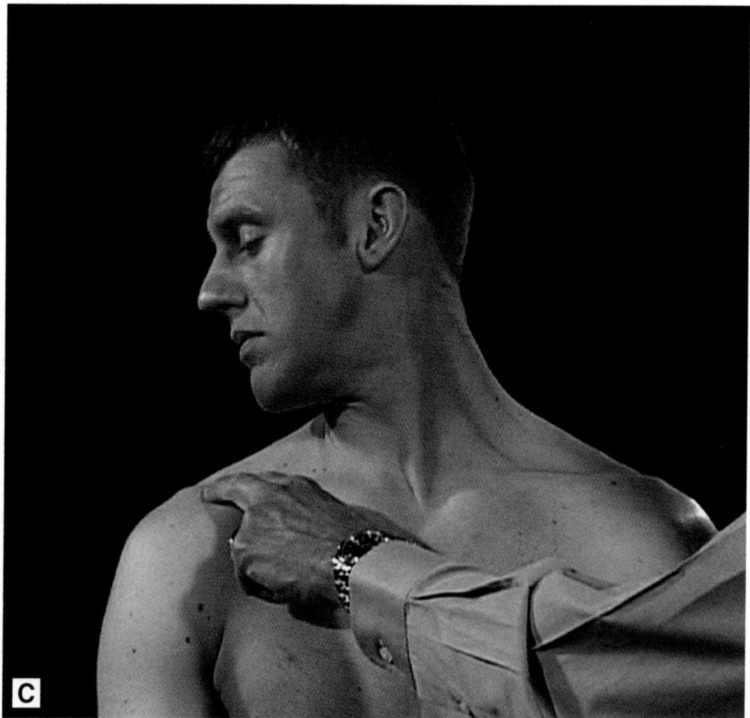

Fig. 6–16

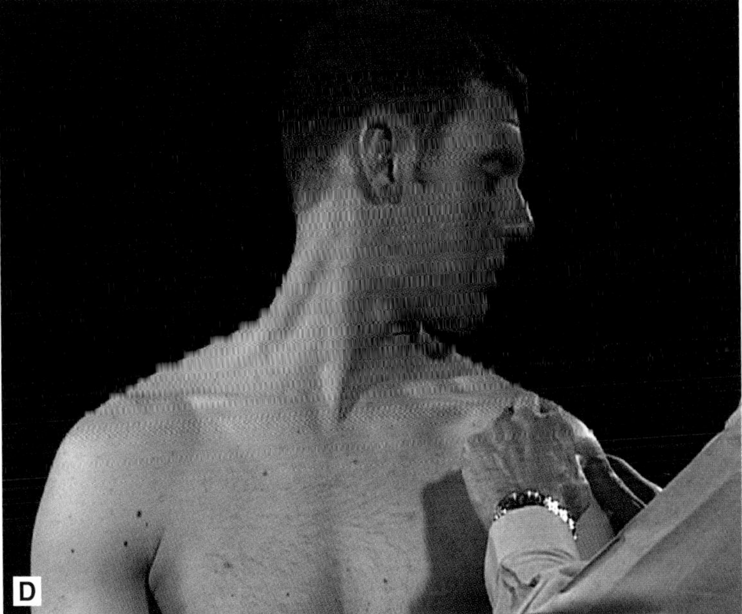

Fig. 6–16

Assess lateral flexion (lateral bending) by asking the patient to incline his ear toward each shoulder. Normal lateral flexion permits lateral deviation of the head to ~30° to 45° (Fig 6–16E, F). Note the location of any pain produced during active range of motion.

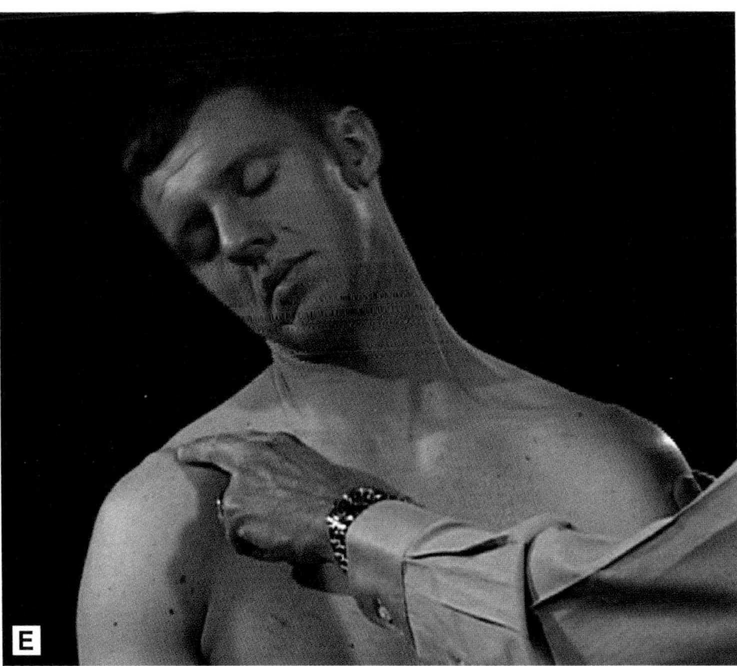

Fig. 6–16

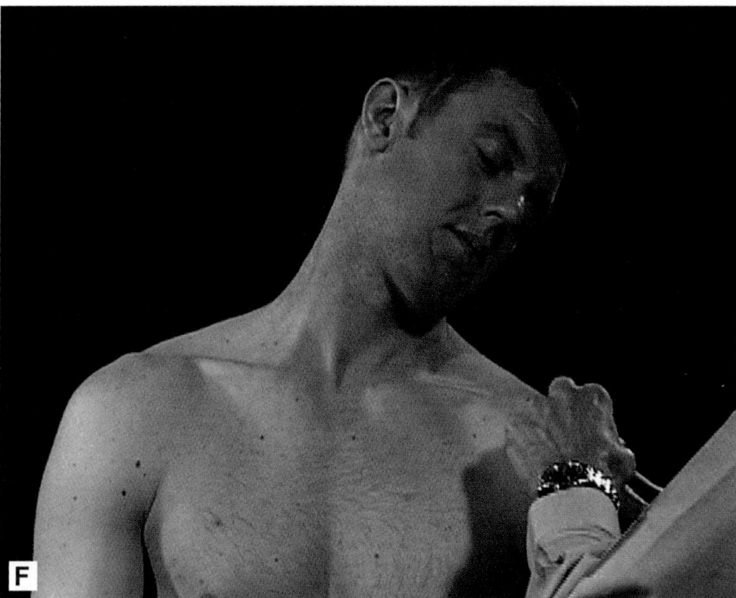

Fig. 6–16

If active ROM is limited but does not reproduce the patient's pain, adding gentle, passive (examiner-initiated) force to assist in attempted completion of flexion, extension, or rotation may reproduce the patient's symptoms (suggesting the neck as the site of origin of the pain) (Fig. 6–17A, B).

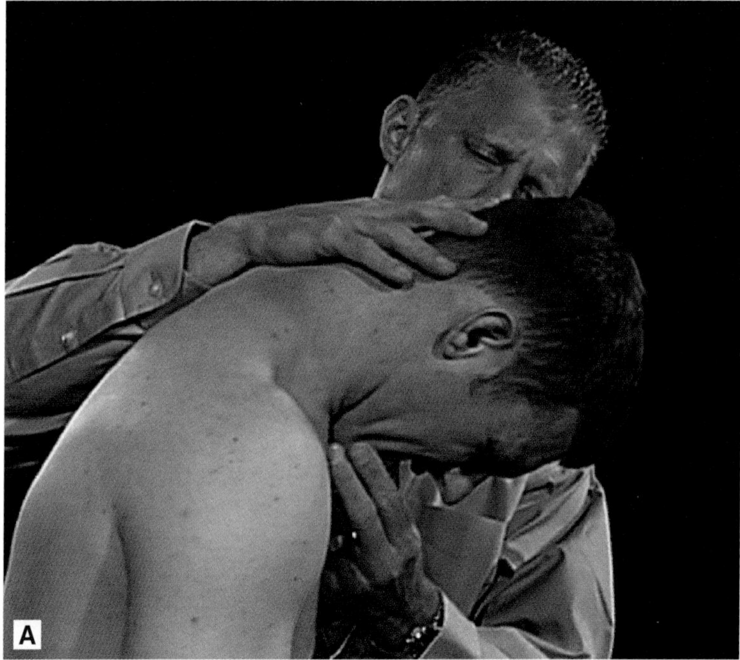

Fig. 6–17

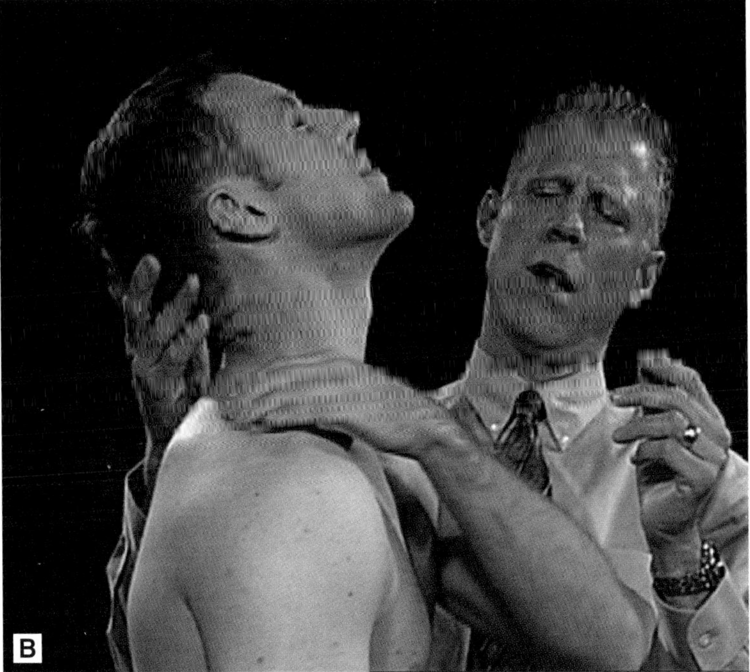

Fig. 6–17

In patients presenting with nonradiating neck pain and no historical features suggesting neurologic, visceral, or systemic disease, no further physical examination may be necessary (Fig. 6–18).

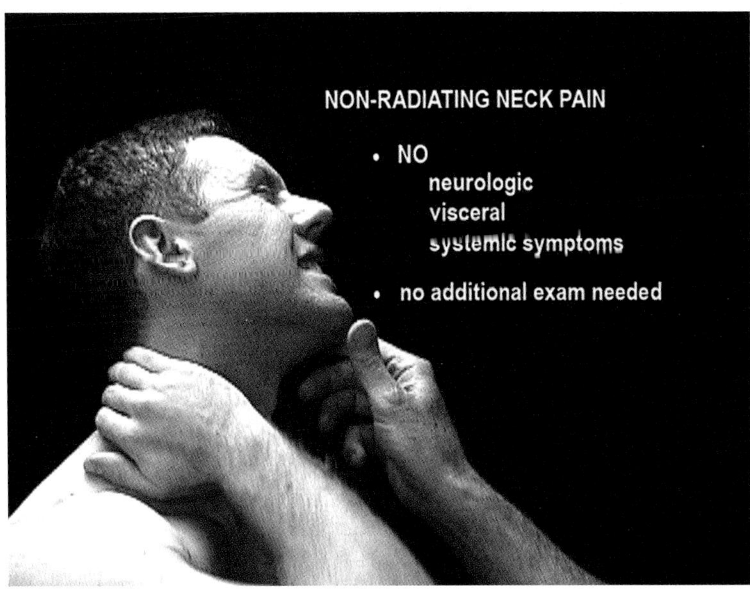

Fig. 6–18

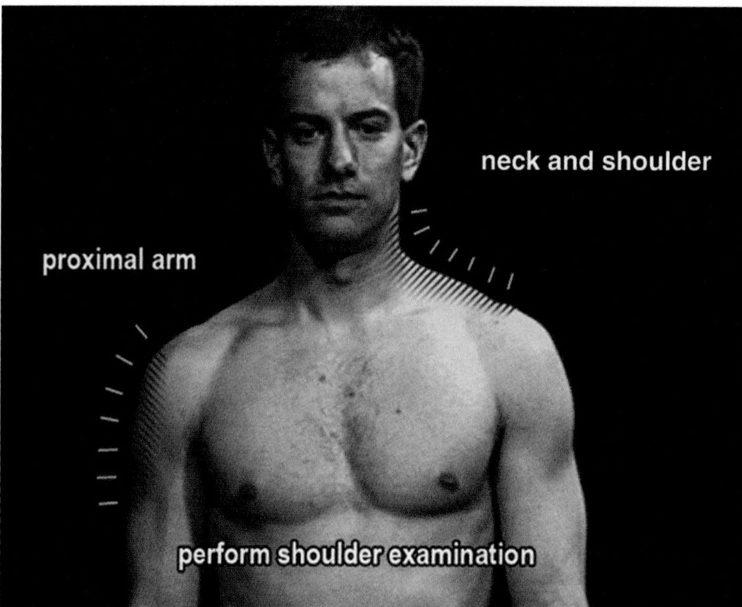

Fig. 6–19

Special Testing

Shoulders In patients presenting with neck and shoulder or proximal arm pain, a regional examination of the shoulder is also indicated (Fig. 6–19).

Special Testing

Suspected Nerve Root Irritation If cervical nerve root irritation is suspected (neck plus upper limb pain), assess upper extremity reflexes, strength, and sensation. With the patient seated and relaxed, check biceps (C5), brachioradialis (C6), and triceps reflexes (C7) bilaterally (Fig. 6–20A through C).

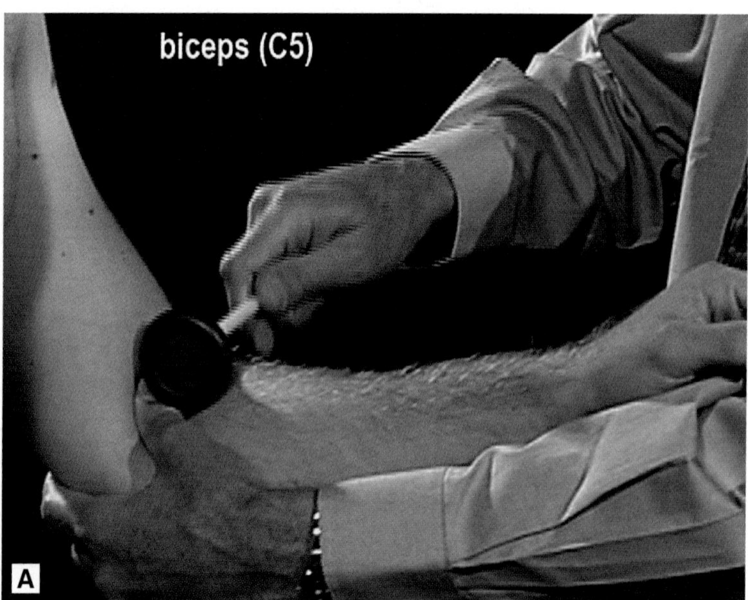

Fig. 6–20

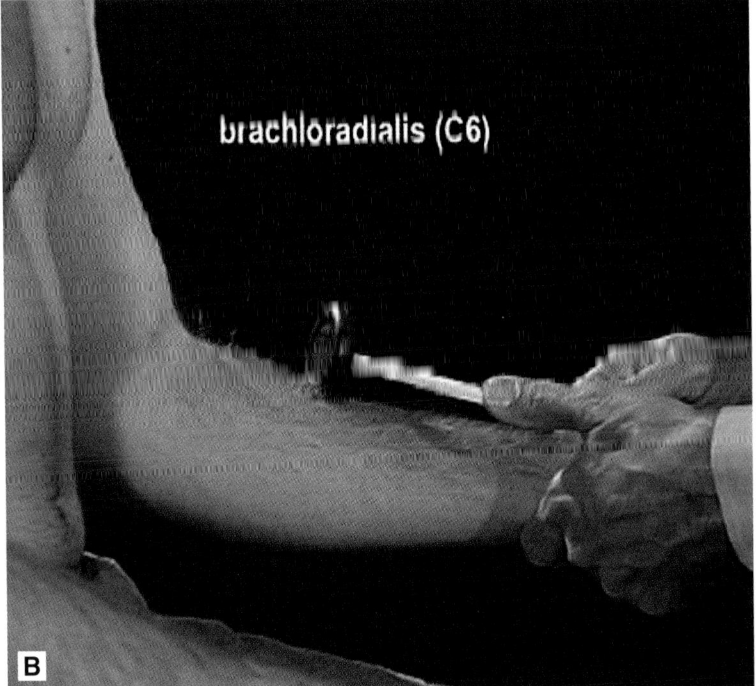

Fig. 6–20

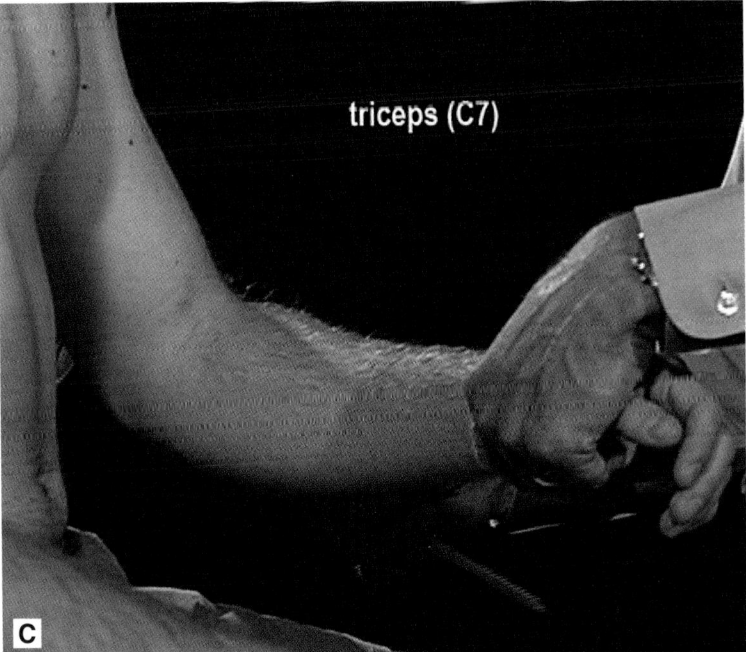

Fig. 6–20

Assess deltoid muscle strength (C5) by simultaneous resisted shoulder abduction. Place the patient's shoulders at ~ 45° of abduction and ask him to resist when you apply pressure over the elbows, driving the arms in toward the body (Fig. 6–21A, B). Next, assess biceps muscle strength (C6). Move the

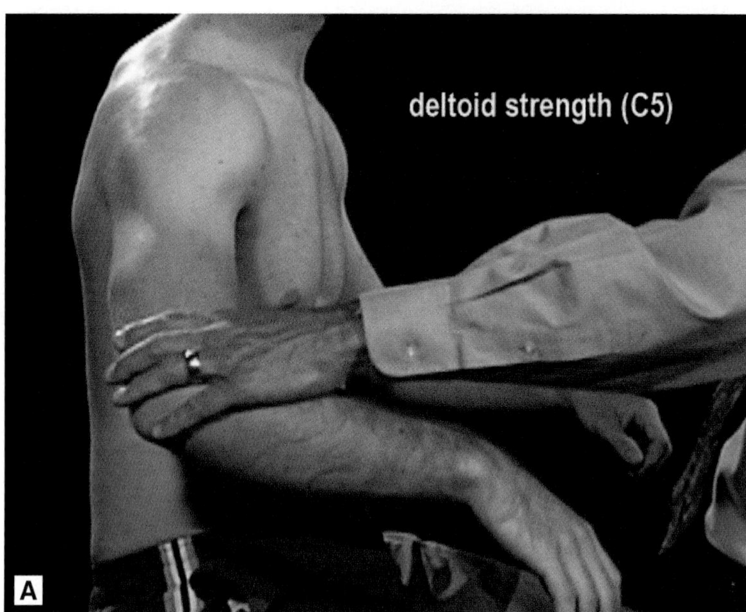

Fig. 6–21

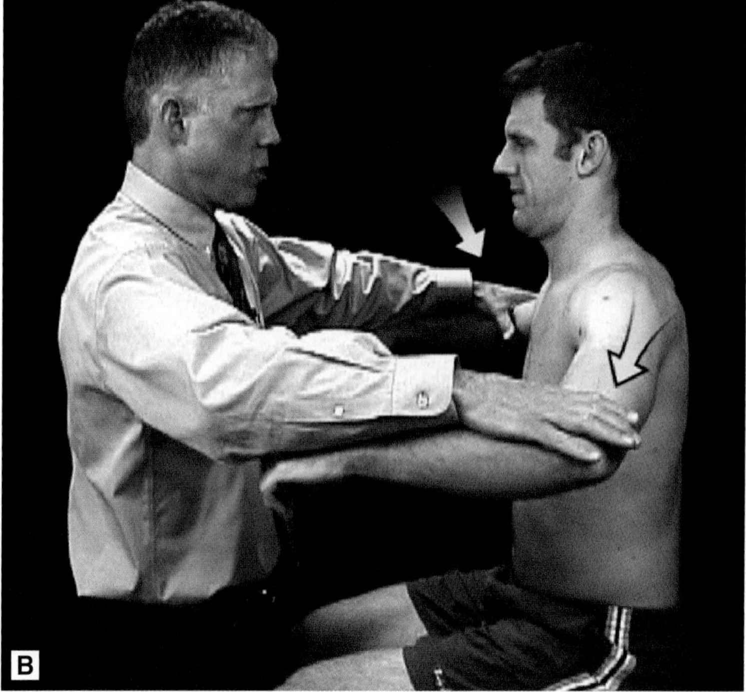

Fig. 6–21

patient's elbow into 90° of flexion. Place one hand under the olecranon (for support) and ask the patient to resist when you attempt to pull his forearm into extension (Fig. 6–22A, B).

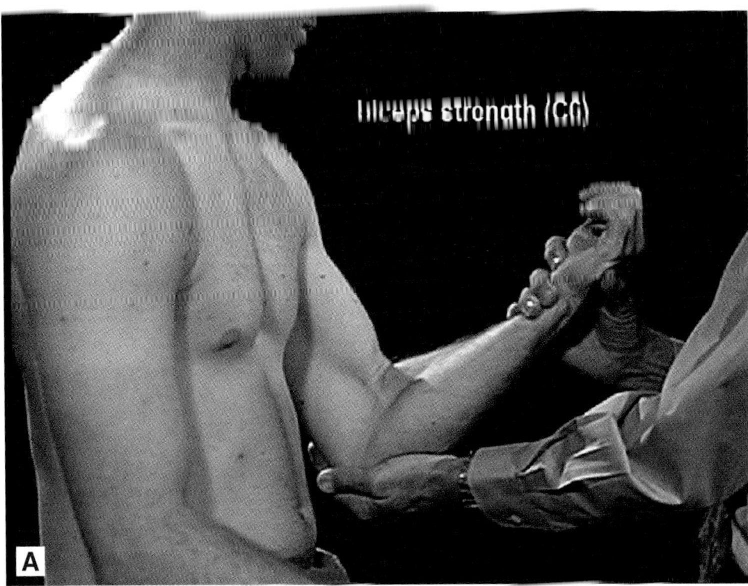

Fig. 6–22

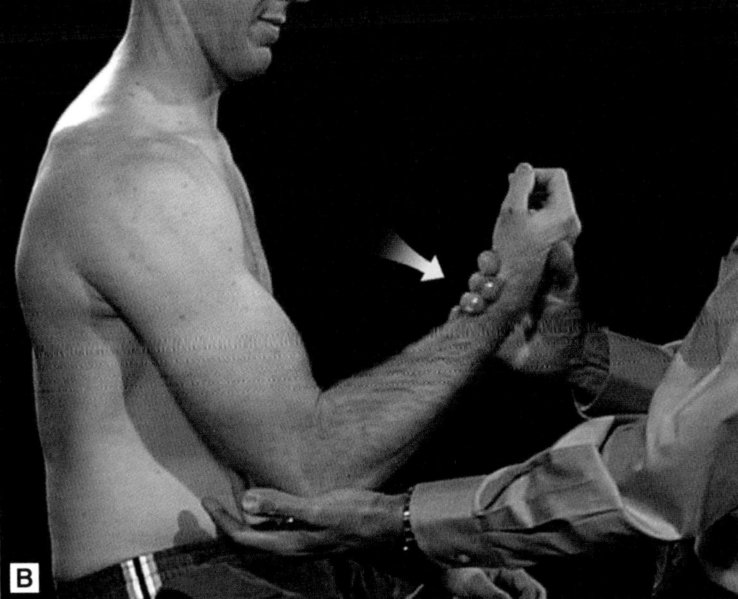

Fig. 6–22

Now, assess triceps (C7) muscle strength with the patient's elbow still at 90° of flexion. Ask the patient to resist when you apply force at the wrist, attempting to push the forearm in toward the biceps (Fig. 6–23A, B).

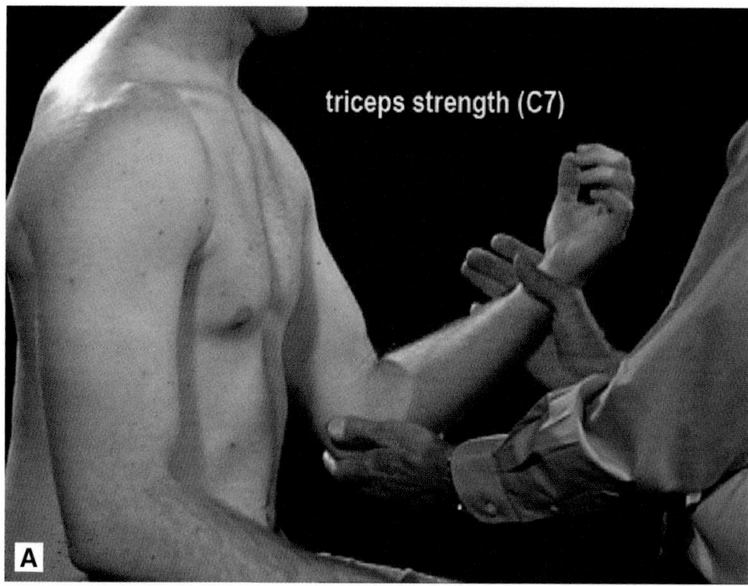

Fig. 6–23

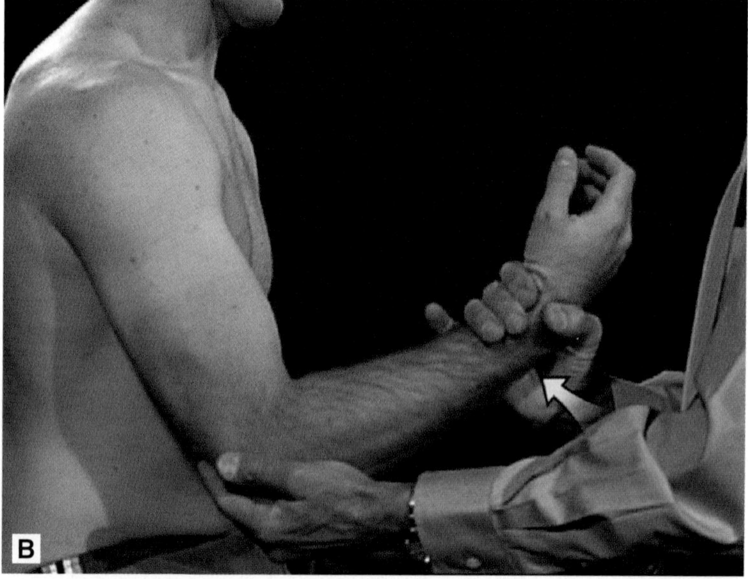

Fig. 6–23

Assess interosseus muscle (C8) strength by asking the patient to spread their fingers while you use your thumb and middle fingers to compress the patient's index and fifth finger together, attempting to overcome finger abduction (Fig. 6–24A, B).

With each muscle group, note any weakness and compare side to side. *(During strength testing, the patient should be comfortable and as pain free as possible. Reassurance and gentleness on the part of the examiner will help the patient perform with maximal effort.)*

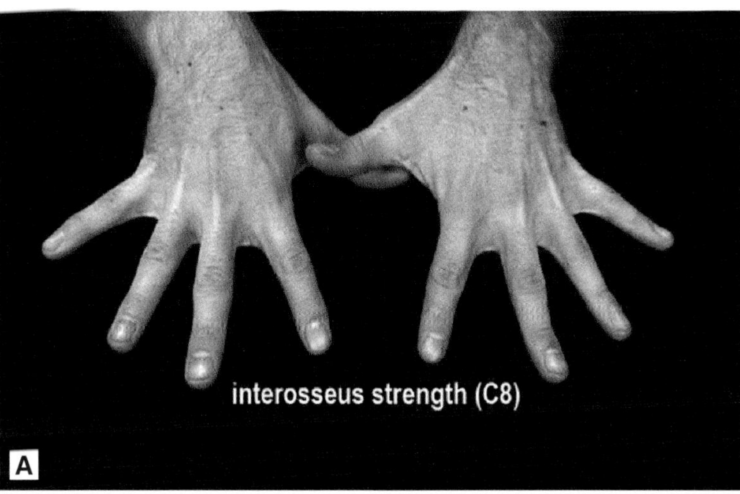

Fig. 6–24

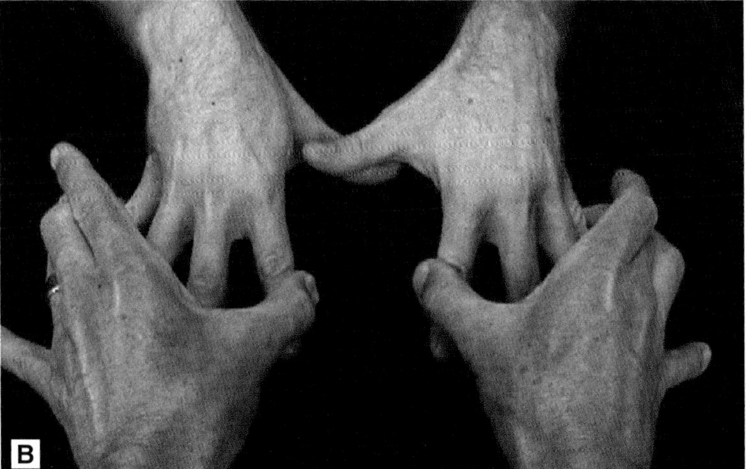

Fig. 6–24

Now check sensation to light touch and/or pin prick over the lateral deltoid (C5), thumb and index finger (C6), middle finger (C7), and ring and little fingers (C8) (Fig. 6–25A through D). Compare side to side.

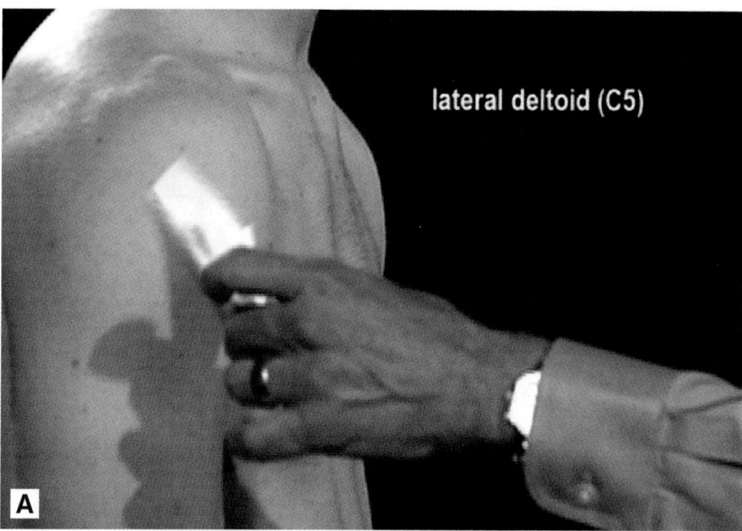

Fig. 6–25

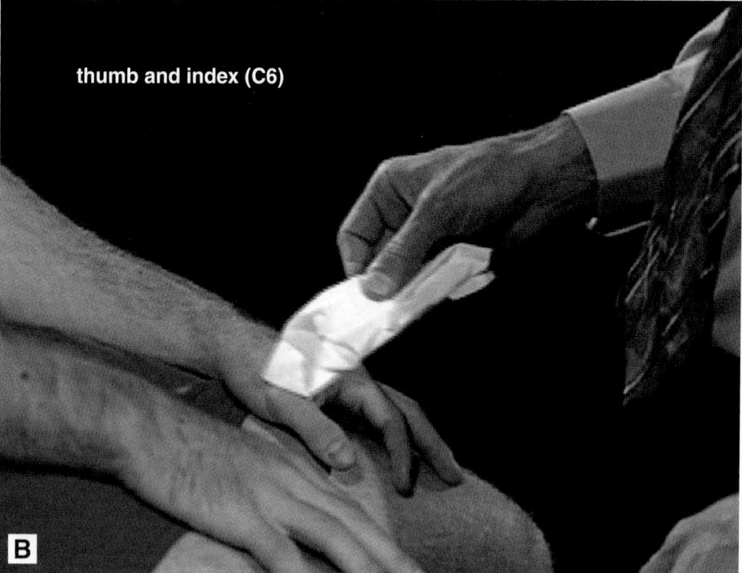

Fig. 6–25

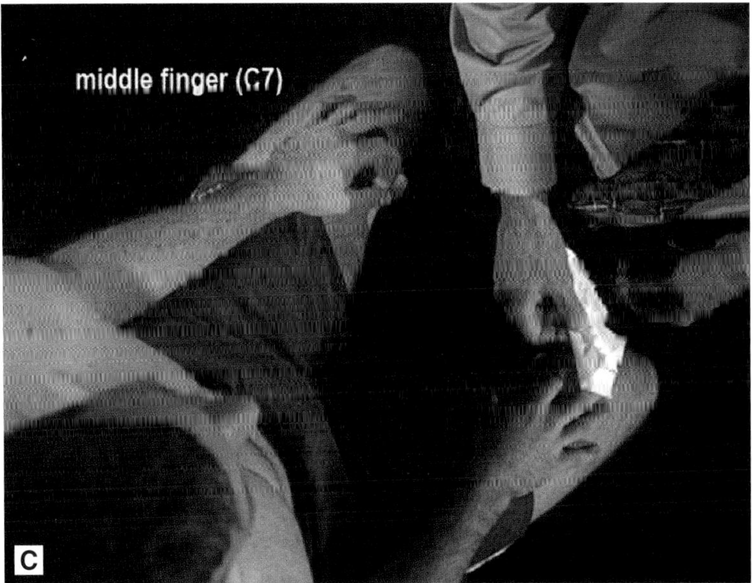

Fig. 6–25

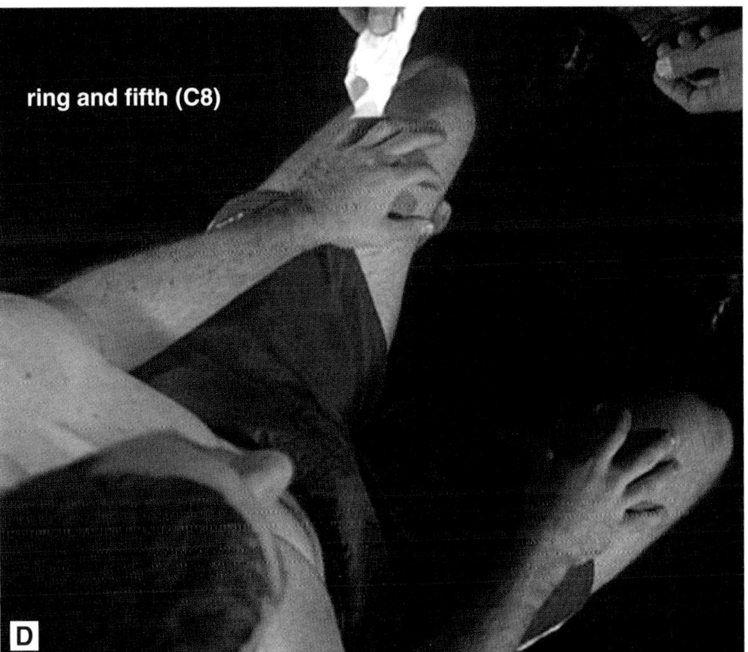

Fig. 6–25

Further confirmation of suspected cervical nerve root irritation may be obtained by performing the Spurling maneuver. Rotate the patient's head toward the painful side and move the neck into extension. Note any radicular pain. Now, add a firm but gentle compressive force to the skull, using one hand to push down on the occiput (narrowing the ipsilateral neuroforamen) (Fig. 6–26A). Reproduction of pain in a radicular pattern suggests nerve root irritation (Fig. 6–26B).

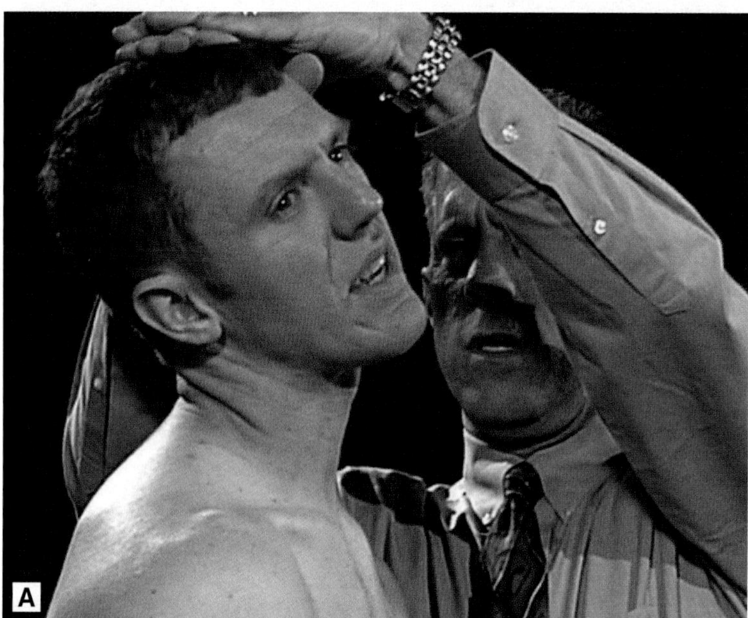

Fig. 6–26

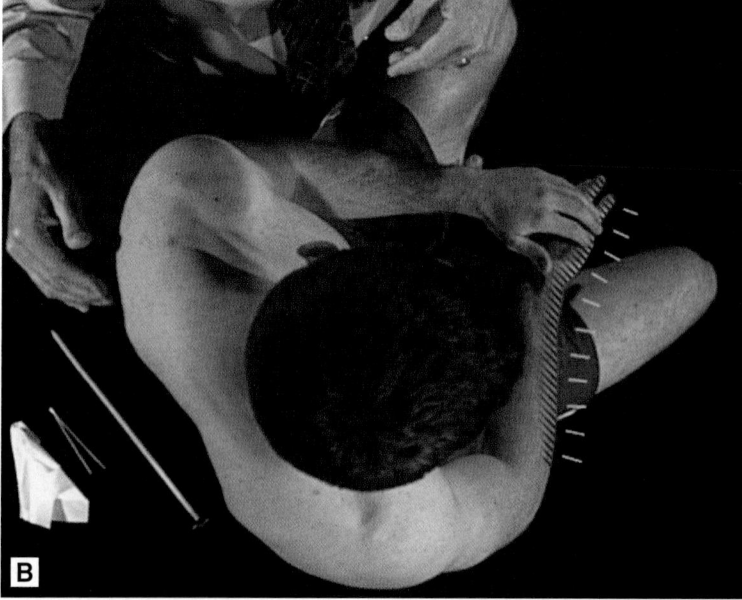

Fig. 6–26

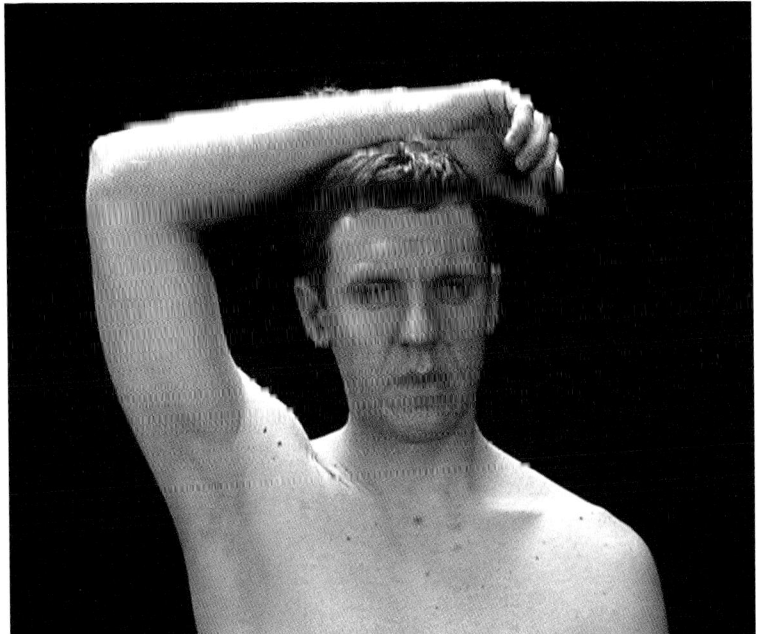

Fig. 6–27

An additional, potentially helpful clinical sign in evaluating possible cervical radiculopathy is the "abduction relief sign." Ask the patient to place the wrist or forearm of the affected extremity on the vertex of the skull (Fig. 6–27). Substantial improvement or relief of upper extremity pain with this maneuver suggests nerve root irritation as the underlying problem.

During your assessment of strength and sensation, note any nonphysiologic "breakaway" weakness or nondermatomal patterns of altered sensation. Additionally, note any signs of significant overreaction as manifest by inappropriate guarding, rubbing, grimacing, or sighing. This response pattern is frequently a clinically important indicator of accompanying psychological distress.

Special Testing

Suspected Myelopathy If cervical myelopathy is suspected, check for the presence of pathologic reflexes, possibly indicating an upper motor neuron lesion. Check for the presence of the Hoffman sign, by supporting the patient's forearm with your nondominant hand and laying the patient's middle finger over the radial aspect of the middle finger of your dominant hand (Fig. 6–28A). Place your thumb on the patient's third fingernail (Fig. 6–28B). Apply a sudden downward force to the fingernail, sliding your thumb off the end of the finger, "flicking" the tip of the finger rapidly and repeatedly. Note any sudden (involuntary) flexion of the patient's thumb and index finger immediately following each "flick" of the middle finger. This flexion response is analogous to the Babinski sign in the lower extremities and suggests possible cervical myelopathy (but is not nearly as specific as the Babinski sign) (Fig. 6–29).

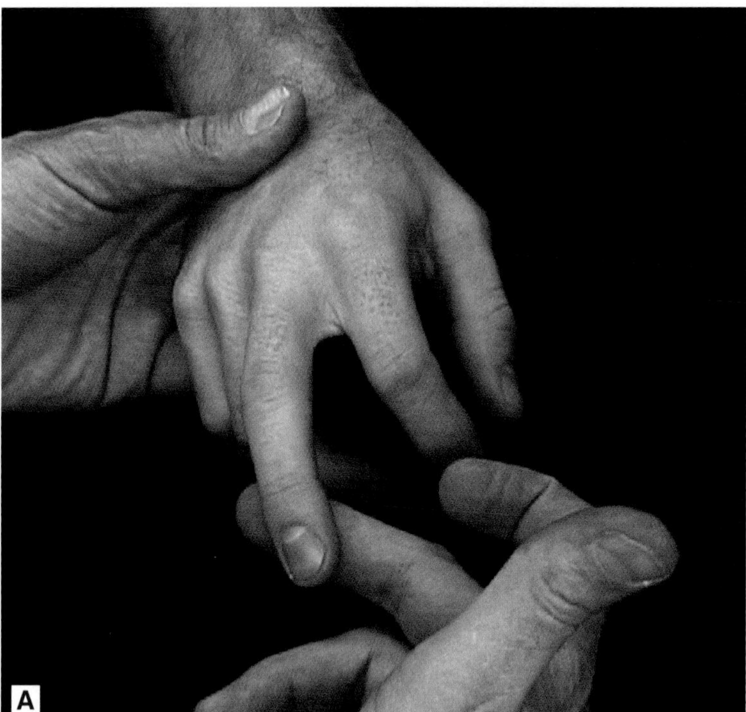

Fig. 6–28

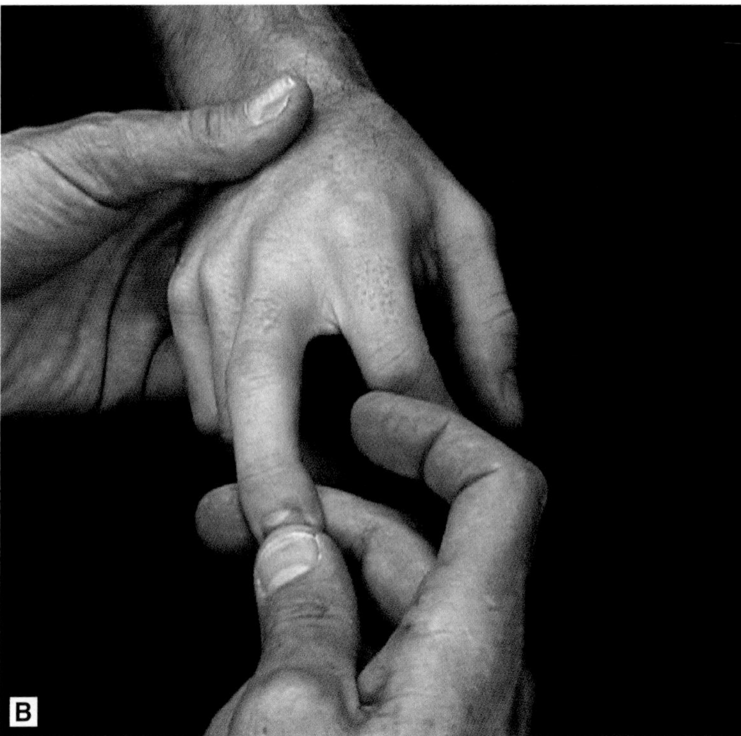

Fig. 6–28

Hoffman Sign
• analogous to Babinski
• not reliable as
isolated finding

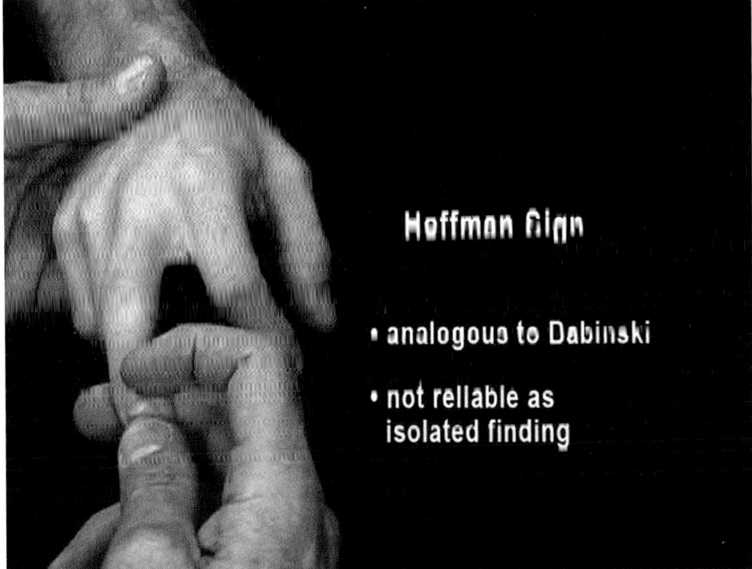

Fig. 6–29

Next, check the knee and ankle reflexes and note any hyperreflexia. Check for ankle clonus. With the foot and ankle relaxed, rapidly and forcefully dorsiflex the foot with your dominant hand. Note any sustained, rhythmical (involuntary) beats of plantar flexion (Fig. 6–30). Two or more beats of clonus are pathologic and suggest an upper motor neuron lesion.

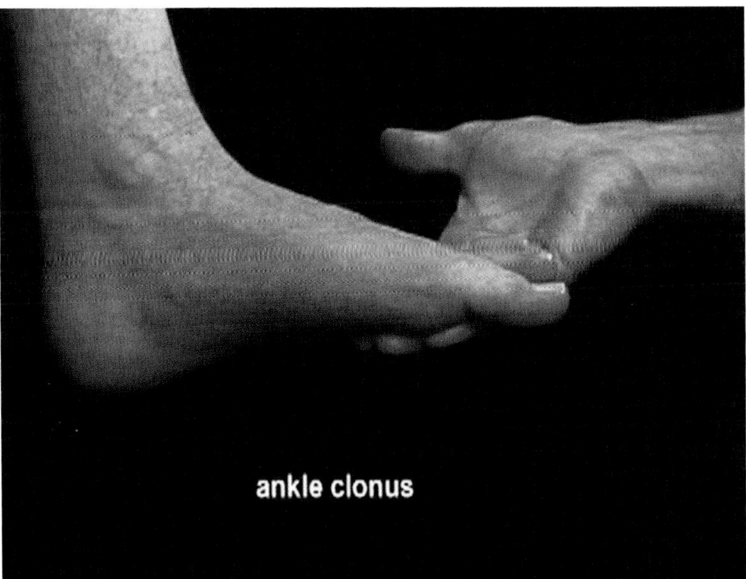

Fig. 6–30

Next, check the plantar reflexes. After explaining what you are about to do to the patient, use the handle of a reflex hammer (or the tip of a retracted ballpoint pen) to firmly stroke the lateral sole from the heel to forefoot (Fig. 6–31A, B). Look for an extensor plantar response, an upgoing great toe and spreading of toes 2 through 5. This finding, the Babinski sign, strongly suggests an upper motor neuron lesion (Fig. 6–32).

Lastly, observe the patient's gait for any abnormality (broad base, unsteadiness, etc) (Fig. 6–33).

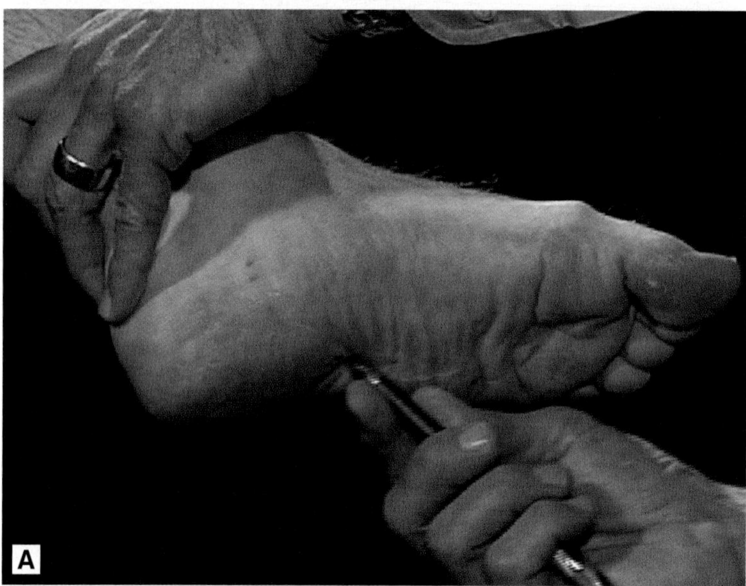

Fig. 6–31

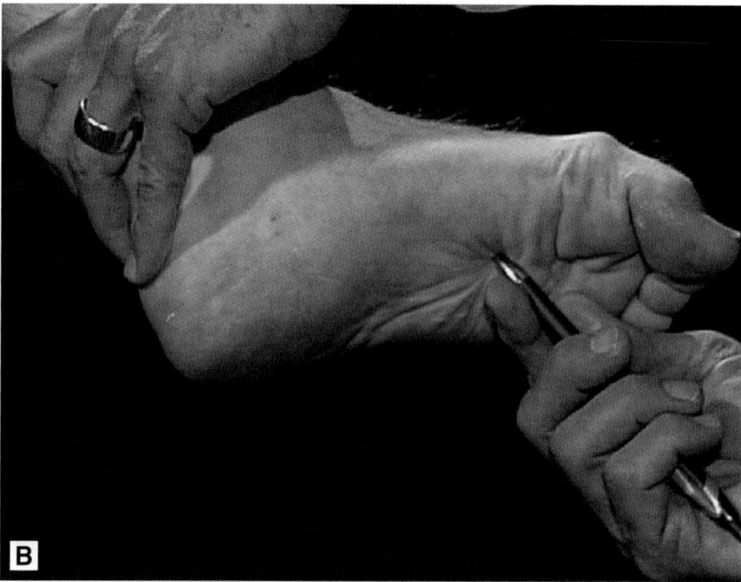

Fig. 6–31

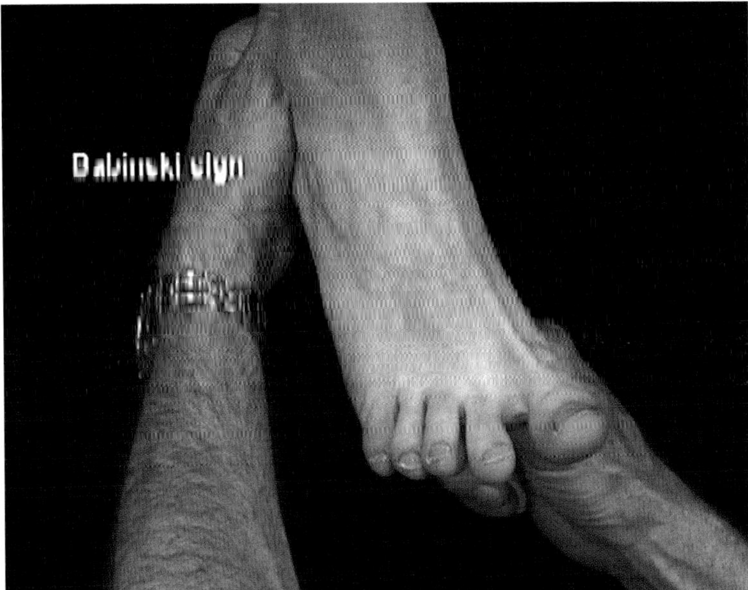

Fig. 6–32

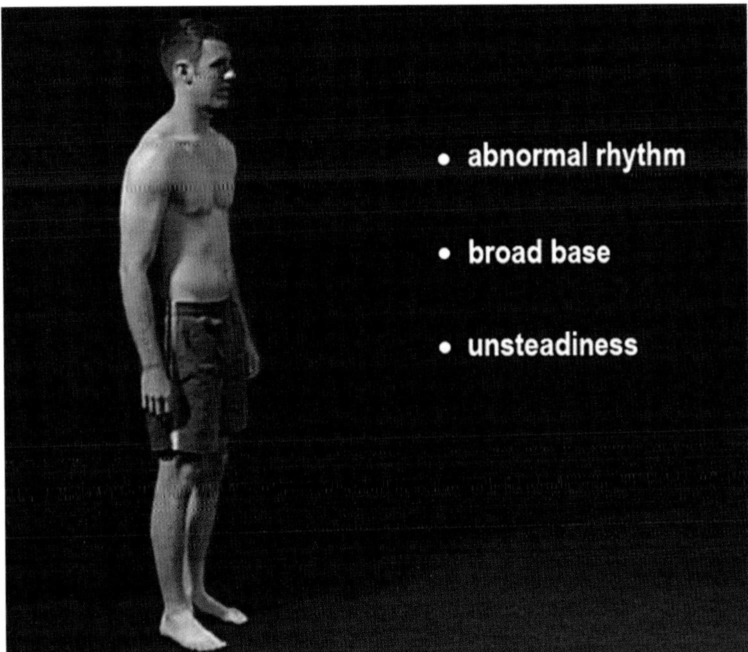

Fig. 6–33

Special Testing

Suspected Referred Visceral Pain In patients with neck pain and a surprisingly normal musculoskeletal examination, it may be appropriate to suspect possible referred visceral pain. Additional history should be obtained and pulmonary, cardiac, and GI examinations should be performed.

RMSE OF THE NECK
Practice Checklist

Basic Examination

Observation

____Observe posture, movement, and behaviors (throughout history and PE)

Inspection

Patient sitting

____Note resting posture and alignment

____Inspect skin (anteriorly and posteriorly)

Palpation

____Palpate occiput/inion and spinous processes (base of skull to upper T spine)

____Identify discrete myofascial trigger points or fibromyalgia tender points (suboccipital muscle insertions; mid to upper trapezius, supraspinatus and medial scapular borders, and others)

Range of Motion

____C spine flexion

____C spine extension

____C spine rotation, R and L

____C spine lateral flexion (lateral bending), R and L

Special Testing: *Suspected Shoulder Pathology (Neck and Proximal Arm Pain)*

____Screening *or* regional examination of shoulder(s)

Special Testing: *Suspected Nerve Root Irritation (Neck and Upper Limb Pain)*

____Biceps reflexes (C5)

____Brachioradialis reflexes (C6)

____Triceps reflexes (C7)

____Deltoid muscle strength, abduction (C5)

____Biceps muscle strength, resisted elbow flexion (C6)

____Triceps muscle strength, resisted elbow extension (C7)

____Interosseous muscle strength, resisted finger abduction (C8)

____Sensation over lateral deltoid (C5)

____Sensation at thumb and index (C6)

____Sensation at middle finger (C7)

____Sensation at ring and little finger (C8)

____Spurling sign: reproduction of radicular pain by applying gentle/firm pressure to occiput during combined rotation and extension to the affected side

____Abduction relief sign: relief of radicular pain with placing distal forearm/wrist of affected upper extremity on occiput

Special Testing: *Suspected Myelopathy*

____Hoffman sign: with hand relaxed, flick tip of middle finger; note involuntary flexion of thumb and index finger together

____Knee and ankle reflexes; note hyperreflexia

Patient sitting or lying

Ankle clonus: with foot and ankle relaxed, rapidly and forcefully dorsiflex the foot

____Babinski sign: firmly stroke the lateral sole from the heel to forefoot; note extension of great toe and spreading of digits

Patient standing

____Gait: note broad base or unsteadiness

Special Testing: *Suspected Referred Visceral Pain*

____Pulmonary, cardiac, and gastrointestinal examinations

COMMON NECK PROBLEMS

- Acute uncomplicated neck pain
- Whiplash injury
- Cervical degenerative spondylosis
- Cervical radiculopathy

Acute Uncomplicated Neck Pain Acute neck pain is a common, usually self-limited disorder. Patients may experience pain from sharp to aching in quality, posterior or lateral in distribution, in a territory from the occiput to T1. There is frequently associated pain in the interscapular or shoulder regions, but no radiation to the upper limb. Pain may occur following minor trauma, athletic injury, or prolonged periods of cervical flexion, extension, or rotation: at work, during reading, or overhead activities. Frequently, no clear precipitating event is evident, but inquiry should be made regarding occupational, recreational, or personal habits: computer and telephone use (computers, keyboards, head position, use of headsets), as well as lifting and carrying (packages, car seats) and asymmetric loads (heavy handbags, book bags). A brief inquiry about sleep positions and pillow use may be helpful in delineating additional contributing factors.

Examination often reveals reduced range of movements, diffuse tenderness, and spasm over the cervical spine particularly from C4 to T1. Whether pain originates in muscles, ligaments, disks, facet joints, or other structures is frequently unclear. However, given the often self-limited and benign course of acute neck pain, it is usually not clinically relevant. Efforts should be directed at pain control, restoration of function, and return to normal activities while avoiding unnecessary (and frequently misleading) imaging studies.

Whiplash Injury Whiplash is only a mechanism of injury of the cervical spine (not a specific clinical diagnosis), which most frequently occurs secondary to motor vehicle accidents or athletic injury. Acceleration and deceleration forces may result in injury to intervertebral disks, apophyseal joints, and paraspinal soft tissues. Patients may experience both posterior and anterior cervical discomfort with referral to shoulders or the interscapular region (similar to mechanical neck pain).

Physical examination frequently reveals diffuse tenderness, spasm, and a reduced range of movement, particularly of the lower cervical spine, usually without radicular symptoms or signs. The severity of initial symptoms and impairment of cervical range of motion are important prognostic indicators. In patients with functional limitations only, efforts should be directed at pain relief and early resumption of activity and preventing long-term disability. Patients with radiculopathy, spinal fracture, or dislocation should be referred for orthopedic assessment.

Cervical Degenerative Spondylosis Degenerative changes of the vertebral bodies, secondary to cervical degenerative disk disease, and uncovertebral and facet joint osteoarthritis are referred to as cervical spondylosis. This commonly occurs in older individuals related to the loss of the integrity of the intervertebral disk, secondary osteoarthritic changes in the uncovertebral and apophyseal joints, and hypertrophy and redundancy of the ligamentum flavum. Symptoms, when present, may involve local neck pain, sometimes with referral to the shoulders or scapulae. Stiffness and crepitus on motion, positional pain, and sleep difficulty may also be present. Physical examination may reveal tenderness, muscle spasm, and reduced cervical range of movements. Efforts should be directed at pain control, restoration of function, and return to normal activities. (*It is important to note that the finding of degenerative changes on imaging studies has* not *been shown to be associated with neck pain.*)

Cervical Radiculopathy Neck pain combined with neurogenic pain referred to the upper extremity strongly suggests cervical nerve root irritation. Far less common than uncomplicated idiopathic neck pain, cervical radiculopathy usually results from disk herniation, facet joint hypertrophy, and/or uncovertebral osteophytes causing mechanical irritation of the nerve root and its dural attachment as it enters the neuroforamen. Physical examination may reveal variable tenderness, paravertebral muscle spasm, and reduced range of movement of the cervical spine. Neurologic testing may reveal diminished reflexes, strength, or sensation in the affected root distribution. In addition to pain control, individuals with neck pain and neurologic findings may require more advanced imaging studies.

Less Common Neck Problems

- Cervical myelopathy
- Rheumatoid arthritis and spondylarthritis
- Malignancy
- Infection
- Referred visceral disease
- Chronic neck pain

Cervical Myelopathy Acute or chronic neck or thoracic pain may be accompanied by a progressive loss of neurologic function due to cord compression (myelopathy). Both the spinal pain itself and the symptoms of myelopathy may be quite subtle. Clinical suspicion is usually generated by a thoughtful history and physical examination. Changes in bladder or bowel habits, impotence, gait unsteadiness, and incoordination are important signs of myelopathy. Physical examination should include assessment for hyperreflexia, pathologic reflexes, and a possible sensory level. If clinical findings suggest possible myelopathy, both plain x-rays and advanced imaging studies (MRI) are indicated.

Rheumatoid Arthritis and Spondylarthritis Spinal disease of the neck secondary to inflammatory arthritis is nearly always due to rheumatoid arthritis (RA) of the cervical spine or a spondyloarthropathy (eg, ankylosing spondylitis, psoriatic spondylitis, or spondylitis of inflammatory bowel disease) involving the cervical and thoracolumbar spines.

Rheumatoid spinal involvement is confined to the neck and tends to occur late in the course of erosive disease. Inflammatory synovitis can cause progressive laxity of the ligaments between C1 and C2 (resulting in atlantoaxial instability), and/or lower cervical intervertebral instability (resulting in subaxial subluxation). Despite the seriousness of this process, there may be little or no pain with significant RA of the neck.

Symptoms of spondylitis involving the neck may also be subtle, but are more commonly associated with morning stiffness, pain, and loss of ROM than seen in RA.

Malignancy Spinal pain due to metastases or primary tumors, has a number of characteristic features usually seen in combination: age older than 50; a prior history of malignancy; unexplained weight loss; severe, unrelenting spinal pain, worse at night and with recumbency; and poor response to analgesics. Physical examination should be complete, including appropriate neurologic testing. If clinical findings suggest possible malignancy, imaging studies are indicated.

Infection Spinal infections, including vertebral osteomyelitis, septic diskitis, or spinal epidural abscess, may present with acute, subacute, or chronic spinal pain. Important predisposing factors include an immunocompromised status, corticosteroid use, diabetes mellitus, recent or current skin or urinary tract infections, and intravenous drug use. Clinical features may include fever, night sweats, and unexplained weight loss. Physical examination may reveal focal spinal tenderness in addition to muscle spasm. If clinical findings suggest possible spinal infection, imaging studies are indicated.

Referred Visceral Disease Although relatively uncommon, a variety of visceral disorders can refer pain to the spine. Pulmonary, pleural, cardiac, and pericardial diseases may present with neck and shoulder pain. Gastrointestinal (GI), pancreatic, genitourinary (GU), and atherosclerotic vascular diseases may present with thoracic, flank, and low back pain. Inquiring about a significant pulmonary, cardiac, GI, GU, or vascular history may provide important clues clarifying the patient's "spinal" complaints.

Chronic Neck Pain Neck pain persisting beyond 3 months despite conservative management (unassociated with an underlying systemic disease) develops in a minority of patients and represents a significant clinical problem. Important additional historical features may relate to the patient's age, work and home, and personal and psychosocial history. Occupational risk factors associated with chronic neck pain include physical stresses involved in manual labor, mental stress in both manual and office workers, as well as job-related stress due to lack of autonomy, lack of variation in workload, and lack of cooperation among workers. Pending litigation or disability determinations, marriage and family stress, drug or alcohol problems, and a history of anxiety, depression, or somatization may be important contributing factors. These "yellow flags" of chronic neck pain identify patients at higher risk for persistent, disabling symptoms and should point management efforts toward earlier referral to multidisciplinary specialized centers.

7

The Regional Musculoskeletal Examination of the Low Back

INTRODUCTION

The *regional musculoskeletal examination* (RMSE) of the **low back** is designed to build on the sequences and techniques taught in the SMSE and GMSE. It is intended to provide a comprehensive assessment of structure and function combined with special testing to permit you to evaluate common important musculoskeletal problems of the low back seen in an ambulatory setting. The skills involved require practice and careful attention to technique. However, they can be learned and mastered on normal individuals.

CLINICAL UTILITY

The RMSE of the low back is clinically useful as the initial examination in individuals whose history clearly suggests an acute or chronic low back problem: back-predominant spinal pain or lower extremity–predominant pain (possible lumbosacral nerve root irritation) or associated systemic or visceral disease. With practice, a systematic, efficient RMSE of the low back can be performed in ~4 to 5 minutes.

Furthermore, the RMSE of the low back provides the foundation for learning additional, more refined diagnostic techniques through your later exposure to orthopedic surgeons, rheumatologists, physiatrists, physical therapists, and others specifically involved in the diagnosis and treatment of back problems.

OBJECTIVES

This instructional program will enable you to identify essential anatomical features, functional relationships, and common pathologic conditions involving the low back. Essential content includes

- Observation of posture, gait, and movement
- Inspection, palpation, and range of motion of the lumbosacral spine
- Examination of the hip
- Evaluation for possible nerve root irritation
- Evaluation for important signs of psychological distress
- Evaluation for sacroiliitis/spondylarthritis
- Consideration of systemic or visceral disease.

Most importantly, this program will prepare you to perform an organized, integrated, and clinically useful regional examination of the low back.

ESSENTIAL CONCEPTS

Structural and Functional Anatomy The spinal column is composed of four balanced curves: the cervical lordosis, thoracic kyphosis, lumbar lordosis, and coccygeal kyphosis (Fig. 7–1). The compensatory nature of these balanced curves allows the normal resting erect posture to be maintained with minimal muscular effort.

The vertebrae have important common features: an anterior element, the weight-bearing vertebral body; and posterior elements, the neural arch and facet joints (Fig. 7–2A, B).

The intervertebral disks are shock-absorbing cushions between vertebral bodies which distribute weight over the surface of the vertebral end plates. They convert vertical loads into horizontal thrusts which are absorbed by the elastic mechanism of the disks. Concentric crossing layers of tough fibrous tissue, the annulus fibrosis, make up the outer circumference of the intervertebral disk, enclosing a central, gelatinous core, the nucleus pulposus (Fig. 7–3A through C).

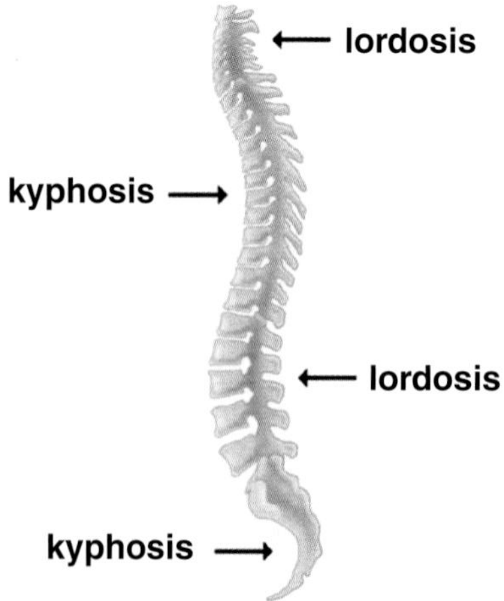

Fig. 7–1. (Modified with permission from Lawry GV, Kreder HJ, Hawker G, Jerome D. Fam's Musculoskeletal Examination and Joint Injection Techniques, 2nd ed. Mosby/Elsevier, 2010, p. 104.)

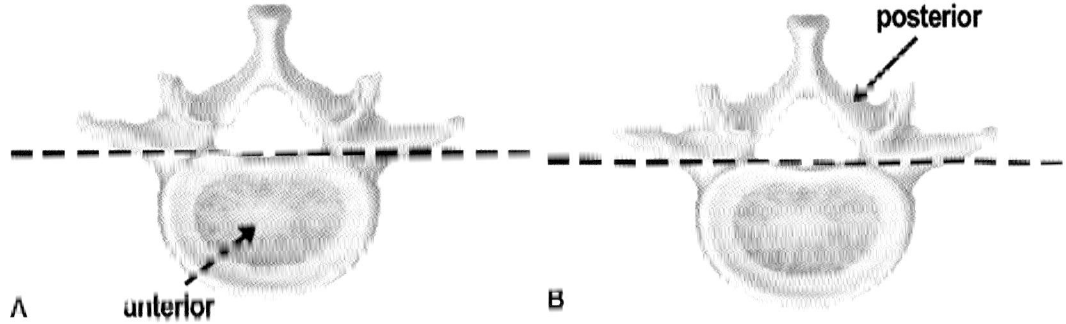

Fig. 7–2. (Modified with permission from Lawry GV, Kreder HJ, Hawker G, Jerome D. Fam's Musculoskeletal Examination and Joint Injection Techniques, 2nd ed. Mosby/Elsevier, 2010, p. 104.)

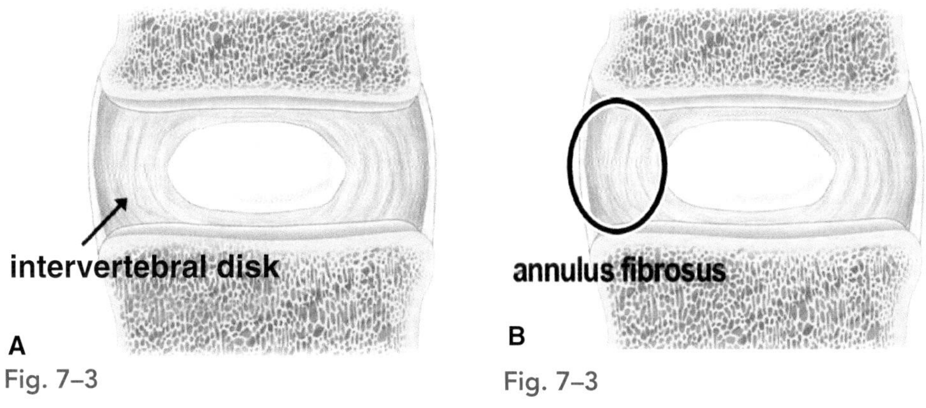

Fig. 7–3

Fig. 7–3

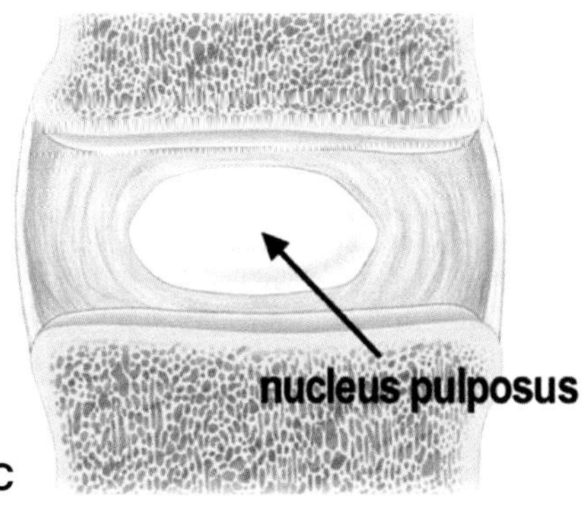

Fig. 7–3. (Modified with permission from Lawry GV, Kreder HJ, Hawker G, Jerome D. Fam's Musculoskeletal Examination and Joint Injection Techniques, 2nd ed. Mosby/Elsevier, 2010, p. 106.)

Posterior to the vertebral body is the neural arch. It is made up of two pedicles attached to the vertebral body and two laminae which fuse in the midline to form the posteriorly projecting spinous process and give rise (at the junction of the pedicle and lamina on each side) to the laterally directed transverse processes (Fig. 7–4A through D).

In addition to these bony projections, superior articular processes and inferior articular processes project from the junction of the pedicles and laminae forming the facet (apophyseal) joints (Fig. 7–5A through C) on each side. These "stacking joints" glide on one another during lateral movement of the spine and prevent sliding of one vertebra on another during flexion and extension.

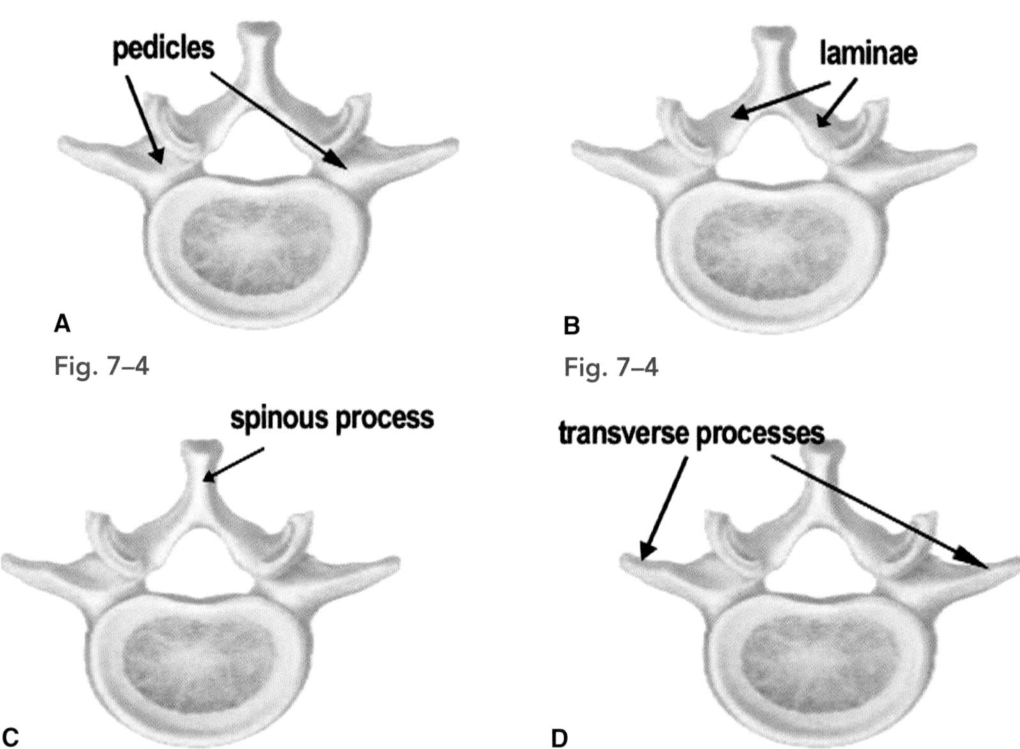

Fig. 7–4. (Modified with permission from Lawry GV, Kreder HJ, Hawker G, Jerome D. Fam's Musculoskeletal Examination and Joint Injection Techniques, 2nd ed. Mosby/Elsevier, 2010, p. 104.)

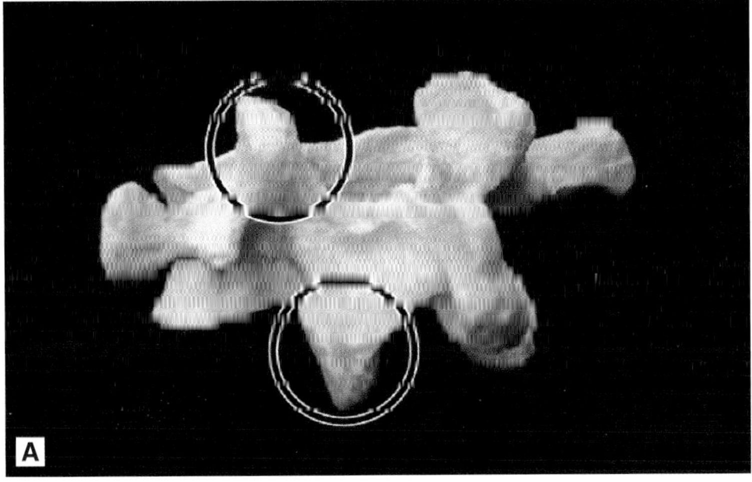

Fig. 7–5

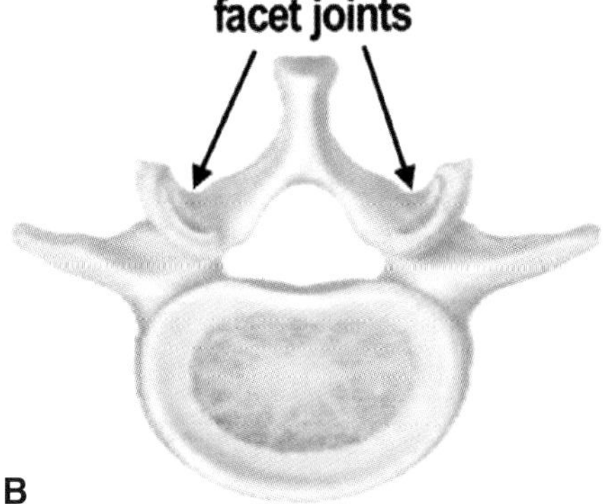

Fig. 7–5

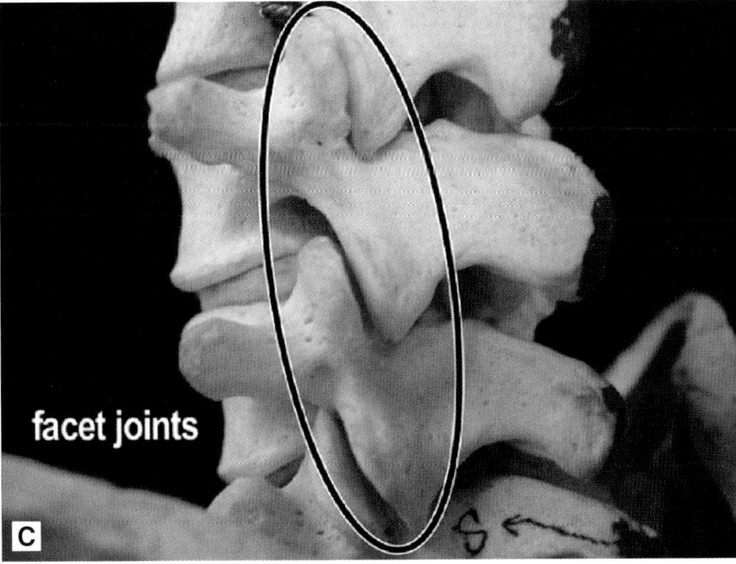

Fig. 7–5. (Part B modified with permission from Lawry GV, Kreder HJ, Hawker G, Jerome D. Fam's Musculoskeletal Examination and Joint Injection Techniques, 2nd ed. Mosby/Elsevier, 2010, p. 104.)

Two primary ligaments stabilize the anterior elements of the spinal column. The anterior longitudinal ligament is a broad, strong, fibrous band that runs from the occiput to the sacrum, where it anchors the anterior vertebral surfaces and intervertebral disks, preventing excessive extension of the spine (Fig. 7–6A). The posterior longitudinal ligament also runs the length of the spinal column but is a weaker and narrower band, broadening where it attaches posteriorly to the intervertebral disk (Fig. 7–6B).

Multiple ligaments also stabilize the posterior elements of the spine. The ligamentum flavum interconnects the vertebral laminae (the posterior roof of the spinal canal) and interspinous and supraspinous ligaments interconnect the spinous processes (Fig. 7–6C, D). These interconnecting ligaments partially limit forward and lateral flexion of the spine.

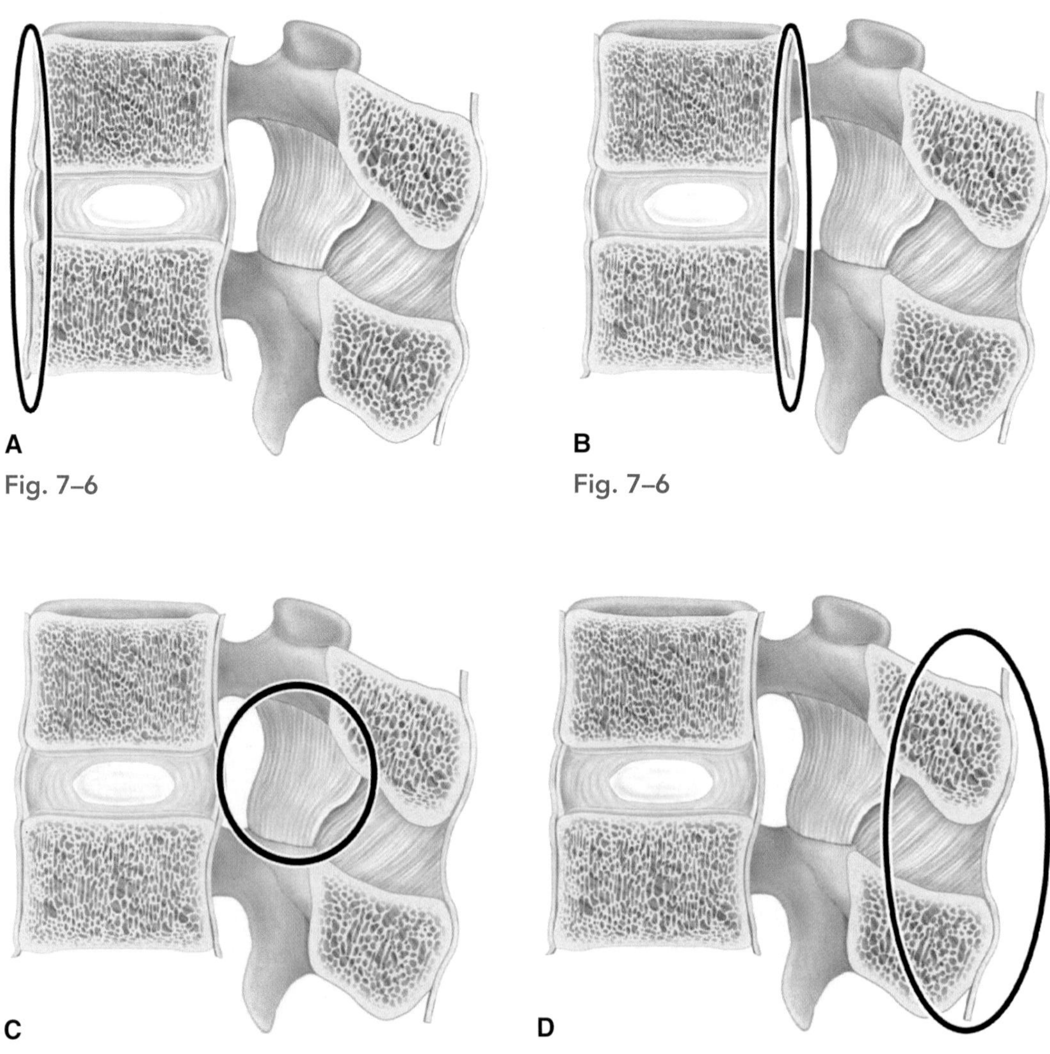

Fig. 7–6. (Modified with permission from Lawry GV, Kreder HJ, Hawker G, Jerome D. Fam's Musculoskeletal Examination and Joint Injection Techniques, 2nd ed. Mosby/Elsevier, 2010, p. 106.)

The larger cross-sectional area of the lumbar vertebral end plates facilitates load bearing by the intervertebral disks (Fig. 7–7A). Larger surface area of lumbar facet joints (apophyseal joints) provides increased torsional and sheer stability to these spinal segments, limiting rotation but allowing side bending (Fig. 7–7B). These features combine to allow the lumbar spine a significant range of motion, including flexion, extension, lateral bending, and rotation.

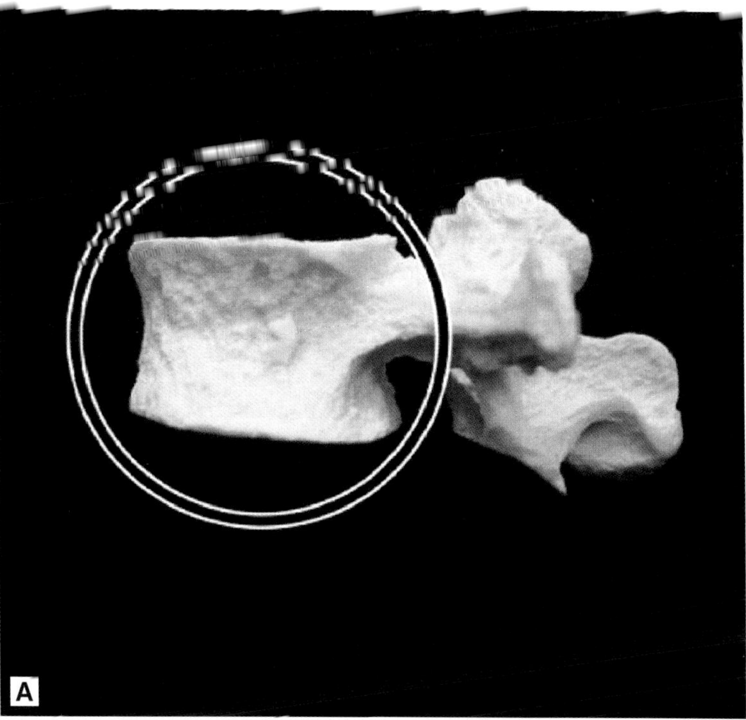

Fig. 7–7

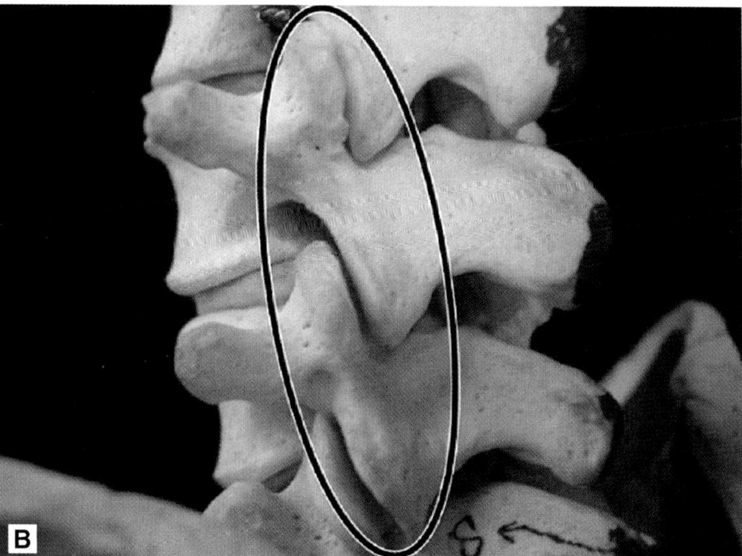

Fig. 7–7

The wedge-shaped sacrum provides the interior anchor for the spinal column where it articulates with the posterior bony pelvis at the sacroiliac (SI) joints on each side (Fig. 7–8A, B). The sacroiliac joints are irregular, narrow articulations that join the spinal column to the pelvis on each side and lend stability to the posterior pelvic circle. The SI joints are both synovial and fibrous joints, which permit little or no movement (Fig. 7–9). The **coccyx** consists of four small fused vertebrae at the inferior end of the spinal column (Fig. 7–10).

Clinical History The patient's history is the essential first step in all musculoskeletal diagnosis and directs the focus of an appropriate physical examination. The musculoskeletal physical examination is used to confirm or refute diagnostic hypotheses generated by a thoughtful history. Appropriate

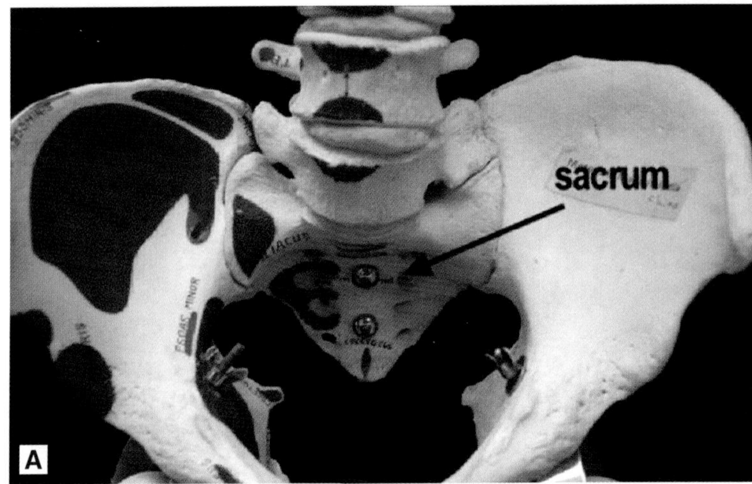

Fig. 7–8

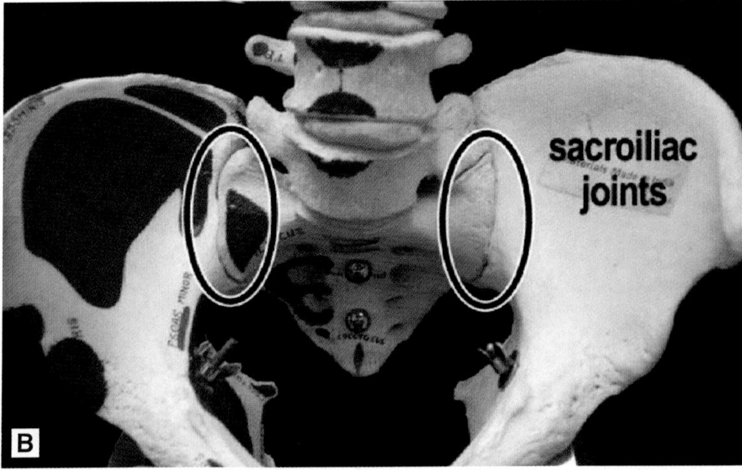

Fig. 7–8

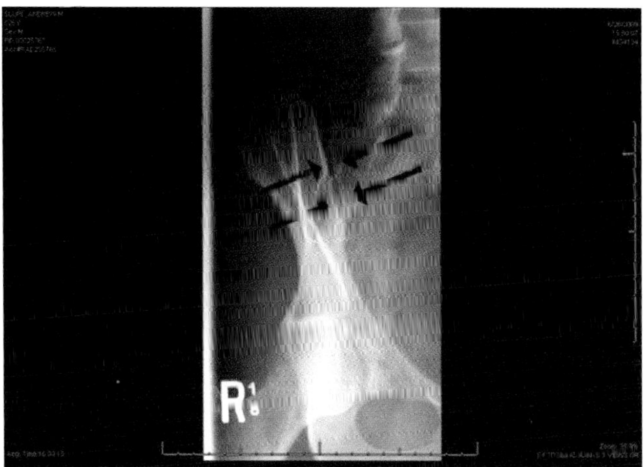

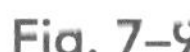

Fig. 7–9

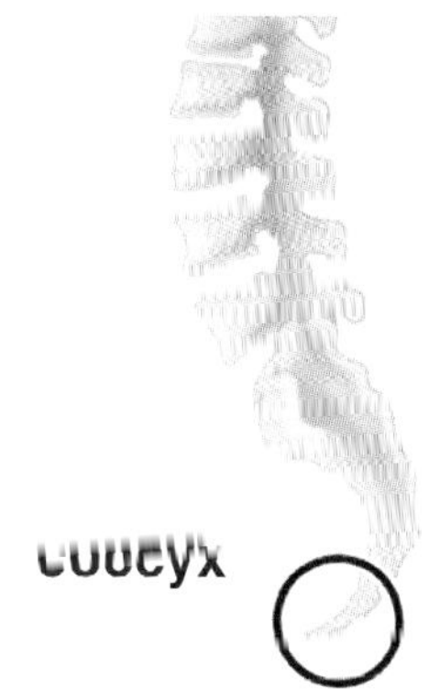

Fig. 7–10. (Modified with permission from Lawry GV, Kreder HJ, Hawker G, Jerome D. Fam's Musculoskeletal Examination and Joint Injection Techniques, 2nd ed. Mosby/Elsevier, 2010, p. 104.)

evaluation of low back pain requires a careful delineation of pain characteristics and associated features. A helpful mnemonic to characterize low back pain is **OPQRSTU** where **O** = Onset, **P** = Precipitating and ameliorating factors, **Q** = Quality, **R** = Radiation, **S** = Severity, **T** = Timing, and **U** = Urinary symptoms.

Evaluation of low back pain centers on answering four important questions:

Is there evidence of major trauma or injury?

Is there evidence of neurologic compromise requiring surgical consultation?

Is there an underlying serious systemic disease?

Is there social or psychological distress that may amplify, prolong, or complicate the pain?

Major etiologic categories of diagnosis in patients presenting with low back pain include mechanical, systemic, and visceral disease.

Mechanical factors: The vast majority of primary care visits for back pain are for uncomplicated, idiopathic, mechanical low back pain (back-predominant spinal pain). A fraction of patients present with mechanical low back pain complicated by neurologic features of sciatica or pseudoclaudication (lower extremity–predominant pain). In addition, low back pain may occasionally be secondary to spinal fractures: traumatic (younger individuals) or osteoporotic (older individuals).

Systemic diseases: Low back pain is uncommonly associated with systemic problems, including neoplastic diseases, (metastatic malignancy and primary tumors), infectious diseases (osteomyelitis, diskitis, and abscess formation), and inflammatory spondylarthritis (ankylosing spondylitis and spondylarthropathies).

Visceral diseases: Low back pain is uncommonly associated with gastrointestinal disease (peptic ulcer, gall bladder, and pancreatic diseases), genitourinary and gynecologic disorders (renal stones, renal infection, endometriosis, chronic pelvic inflammatory disease, and prostatitis), and arteriosclerotic vascular disease (abdominal aortic aneurism).

Most low back pain is attributed to muscle and/or ligamentous strain, facet joint arthritis, intervertebral disk herniation, or other miscellaneous causes. However, despite advances in imaging and neurodiagnosis, the etiology of most acute and chronic low back pain is complex and frequently poorly understood.

The thrust of a brief, focused history should inquire about risk factors pointing to fracture, malignancy, infection, underlying visceral or systemic disease, or the need for urgent surgical consultation. The musculoskeletal physical examination of the low back should be focused and used to confirm or refute diagnostic hypotheses generated by a focused, but thoughtful history.

Acute uncomplicated idiopathic neck and low back pain accounts for the vast majority of spinal pain seen in clinical practice. A focused clinical history and physical examination is important, and in the absence of serious underlying conditions, a diagnosis of acute nonspecific neck or low back pain can be made. A definitive anatomic diagnosis cannot be made in as many as 85% of patients presenting with acute neck or low back pain, but up to two-thirds of such patients have resolution of their symptoms in 4 to 8 weeks.

Fortified by this information, the clinician is able to direct subsequent management efforts at reassurance and resumption of normal functional activity rather than extensive and expensive (and frequently misleading) imaging studies.

THE EXAMINATION, OVERVIEW

Observe the patient's posture, movement, and behaviors throughout the history and different components of the physical examination.

Begin by observing the patient's gait. Note any uneven rhythm or asymmetry. Ask the patient to walk on heels and toes. Note any weakness or asymmetry. Observe the resting posture and alignment. Note any asymmetry or deformity. Inspect for the normal thoracic kyphosis and lumbar lordosis. Inspect the skin.

Next, assess skin tenderness to light touch and/or skin rolling over the lumbosacral region. Note the reaction pattern. Palpate the spinous processes from the mid-thoracic spine to the sacrum. Note any focal tenderness.

Observe lumbar flexion by instructing the patient to bend forward at the waist. Assess lumbar extension by having the patient bend backward. Assess lumbar lateral flexion (lateral bending) by asking the patient to bend to the right and to the left. Simulate lumbar spinal rotation by passively rotating the pelvis while keeping the shoulders and hips in the same plane or simulate axial loading by applying light pressure to the top of the skull. Note the reaction pattern.

Next, assess for the Trendelenburg sign on the right and left sides. Now, ask the patient to lie down.

Palpate for trochanteric bursitis (lateral trochanter). Next, palpate the insertion site of the gluteus medius tendon (posterior/superior trochanter) and the mid gluteus.

Assess hip flexion by grasping the heel and moving the thigh up toward the chest. Return the hip to 90° of flexion while holding the knee at 90° of flexion. Now, move the ankle medially to assess hip external rotation (ER) and move the ankle laterally to assess hip internal rotation (IR).

If indicated by the patient's history or from observations during the basic examination, perform special testing for possible nerve root irritation.

With the patient lying down, perform a supine straight leg raise on both the symptomatic and non-symptomatic sides. Estimate the angle at pain onset. Next, ask the patient to sit up. Check the knee and ankle reflexes. Assess strength by testing combined foot inversion and ankle dorsiflexion, great toe dorsiflexion, and foot eversion.

Next, assess a distracted, seated straight leg raise by "testing quadriceps strength" by bringing the knee into full extension and asking the patient to resist downward force applied to the shin. Note reaction pattern (as knee is brought into full extension).

Check sensation of the medial foot and ankle, and dorsum of the foot, and lateral foot and ankle.

If cauda equina syndrome is suspected, check perianal sensation, anal reflex, and sphincter tone.

If indicated by the patient's history or from observations during the basic examination, complete your assessment by specifically noting the presence or absence of Waddell's behavioral signs.

If indicated by the patient's history or from observations during the basic examination, perform special testing for possible sacroiliitis or inflammatory spondyloarthropathy.

Ask the patient to stand. Palpate each sacroiliac joint. Note any tenderness. Then, measure lumbosacral spinal mobility by performing a "modified Schober test." With the patient lying down, stress the sacroiliac joints by performing the FABER (hip **f**lexion, **ab**duction, and **e**xternal **r**otation) maneuver. Note any SI region pain. Next, apply simultaneous downward compression to the iliac crests. Note any SI region pain. If a spondyloarthropathy is clinically indicated from the patient's history and physical examination up to this point, also record spondylitis-specific measurements.

If indicated by the patient's history or from observations during the basic examination, perform special testing for possible visceral or vascular disease.

With the patient lying down, perform a careful abdominal examination and check for an abdominal aortic aneurysm. Check lower extremity pulses and perfusion. Perform a pelvic examination or male GU examination and digital rectal examination.

THE EXAMINATION, COMPONENT PARTS

Observation Gentleness and reassurance during the physical examination will establish a bond of trust and allow the patient to relax and give their best effort during each component of the examination. Observation of movement and pain-related behaviors during the history and physical examination is important and provides an opportunity to observe function and range of motion at a time when the patient is unaware that such observations are being made. Discrepancies may become apparent between the level of pain and function observed during the history and subsequent physical examination, providing important clues regarding the patient's level of perceived distress.

The patient should be comfortable yet appropriately undressed. This usually includes undershorts with or without a gown for men and underwear with a gown for women. Adjusting the gown whenever necessary to permit adequate visualization is very important.

Inspection Observe the patient's gait. Check for any limp or uneven rhythm. Note the swing and stance phases and any abnormal swaying of the trunk. Ask the patient to localize any pain during ambulation. Observe heel and toe walking. Note any asymmetry or weakness (Fig. 7–11A, B).

Next, observe standing posture and alignment. Note any asymmetry or deformity. Inspect the skin and note any scars from prior surgery or significant injury. Check for lipomas, neurofibromas, pigmented spots, or hairy patches in the lumbosacral region (sometimes associated with congenital

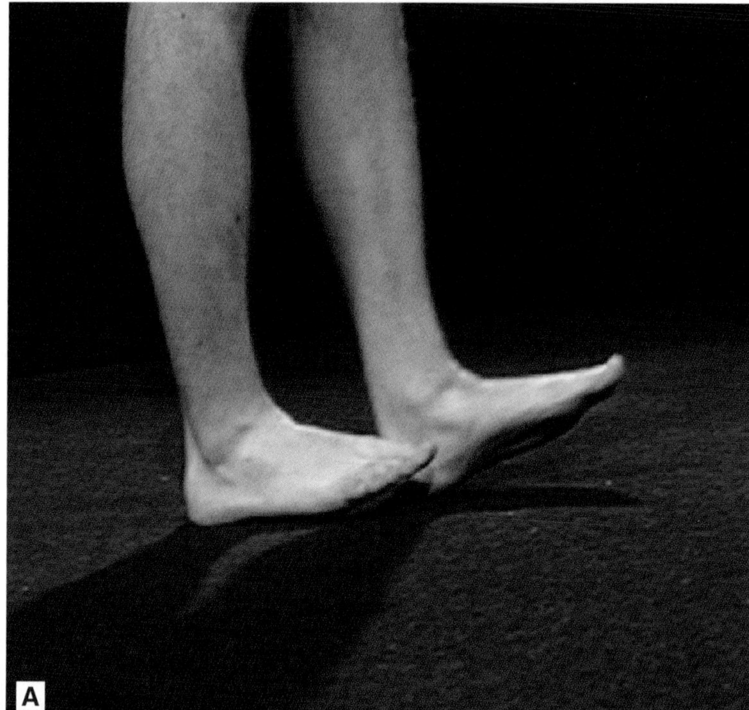

Fig. 7–11

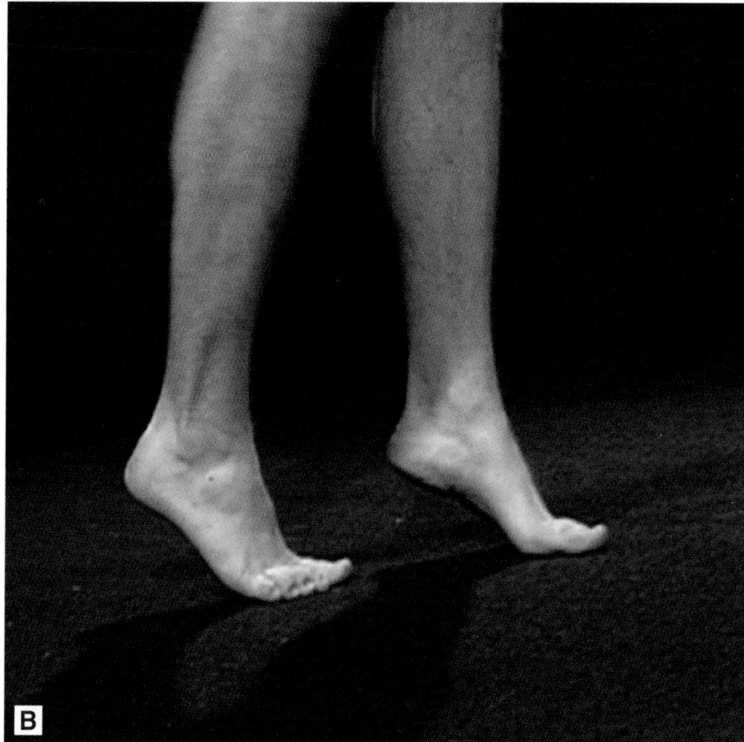

Fig. 7–11

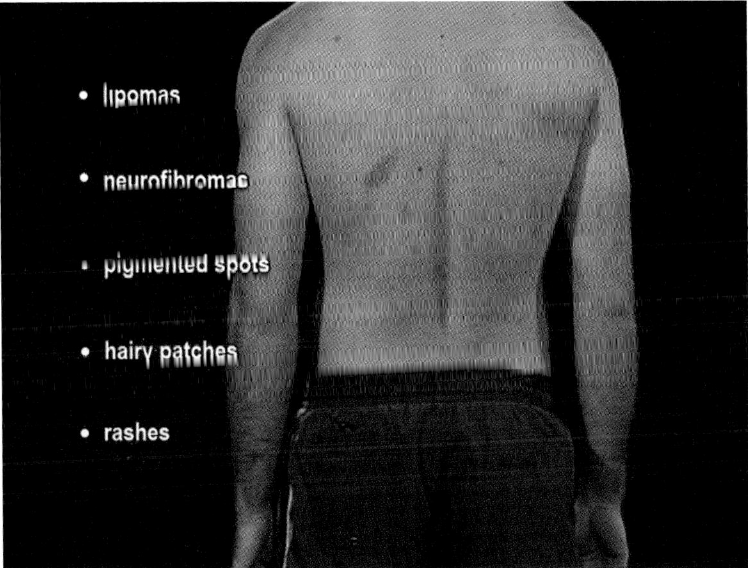

Fig. 7–12

structural abnormalities of the LS spine). Note any rashes (particularly vesicles characteristic of herpes zoster) (Fig. 7–12).

Palpation Lightly stroke or roll the skin on both sides of the lumbosacral spine. Note the patient's response. Widespread sensitivity of the superficial soft tissues over the lumbar region (excluding prior scars) may be a sign of significant psychological distress (Fig. 7–13A). Beginning in the upper thoracic

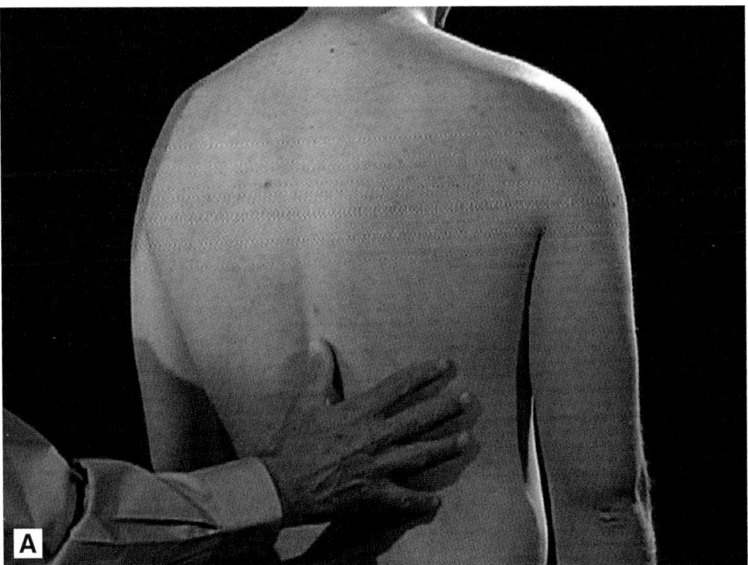

Fig. 7–13

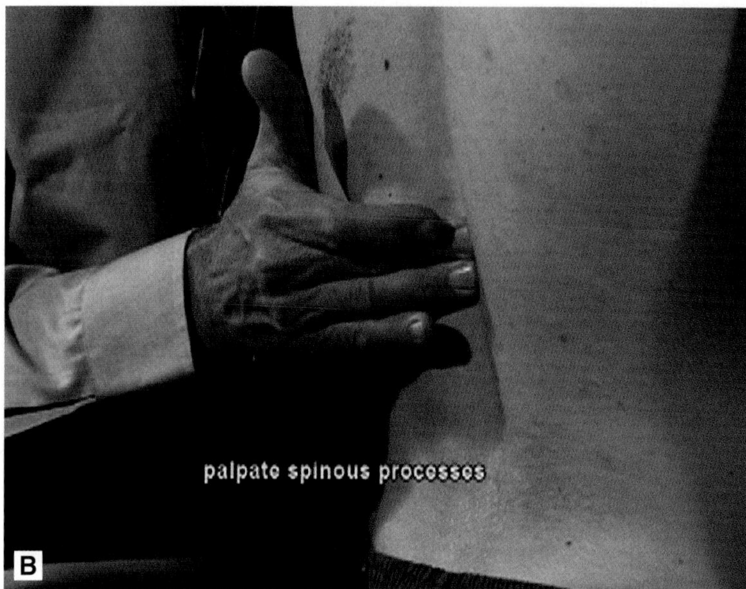

Fig. 7–13

spine and proceeding inferiorly to the sacrum, palpate the spinous processes (Fig. 7–13B). If clinically indicated, palpation may be facilitated with the patient lying prone.

Focal, midline tenderness may be seen with spinal (compression) fractures, metastatic malignancy, or spinal infection. *The significance of such tenderness depends heavily on the historical context* (Fig. 7–14). Bony tenderness felt over a wide area, not localized to one structure and often extending from the thoracic spine to the sacrum or pelvis, may be an important indicator of psychological distress (Fig. 7–15).

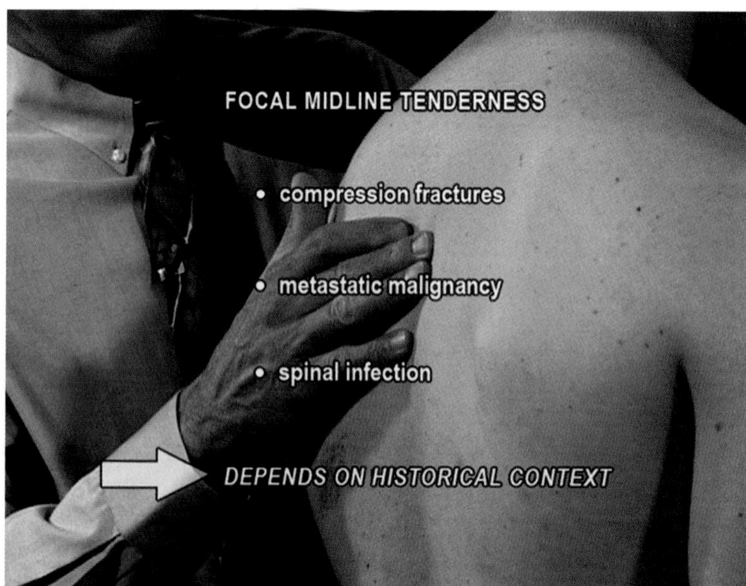

Fig. 7–14

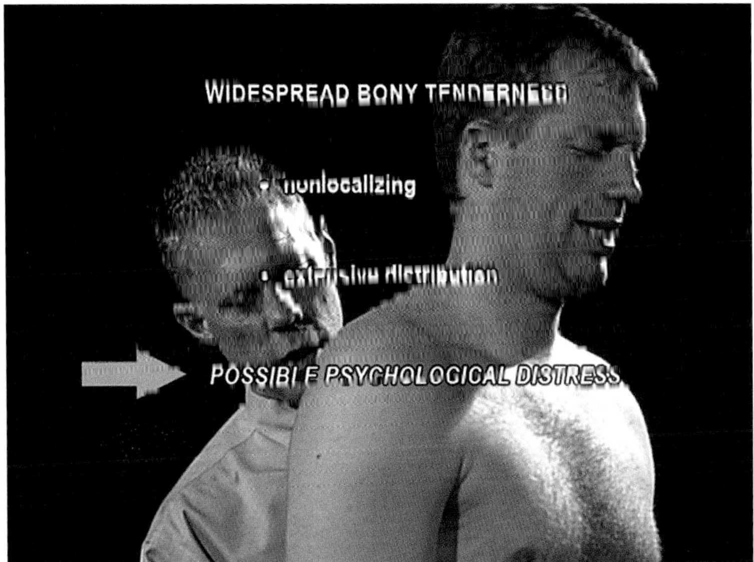

Fig. 7–15

Range of Motion Next, observe lumbosacral range of motion. Assess lumbar flexion by instructing the patient to bend forward at the waist and attempt to touch the toes. Normal lumbar flexion should involve progressive reversal of the lumbar curvature from lumbar lordosis in the standing position (Fig. 7–16A) to flattening of the lordosis in midflexion and to flattening or even slight lumbar kyphosis at the end of full flexion (Fig. 7–16B).

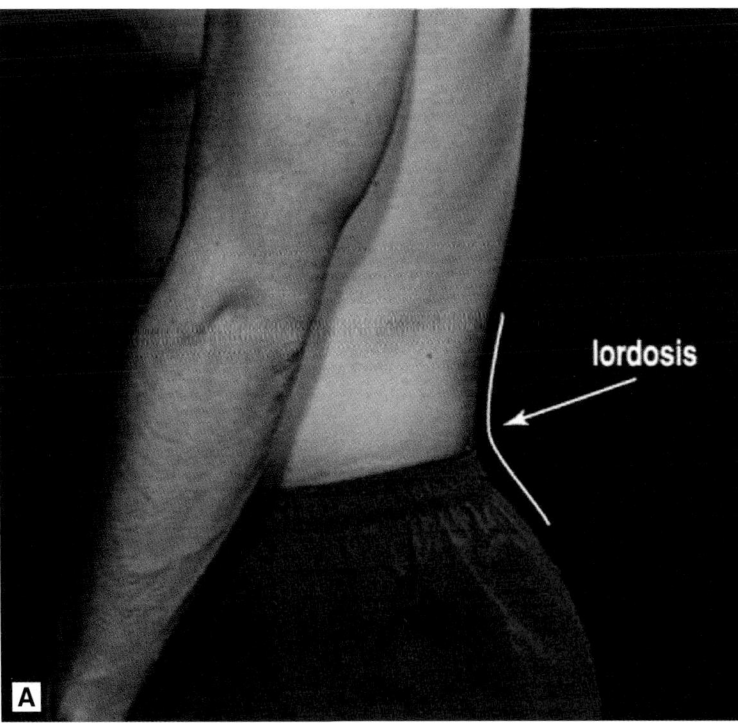

Fig. 7–16

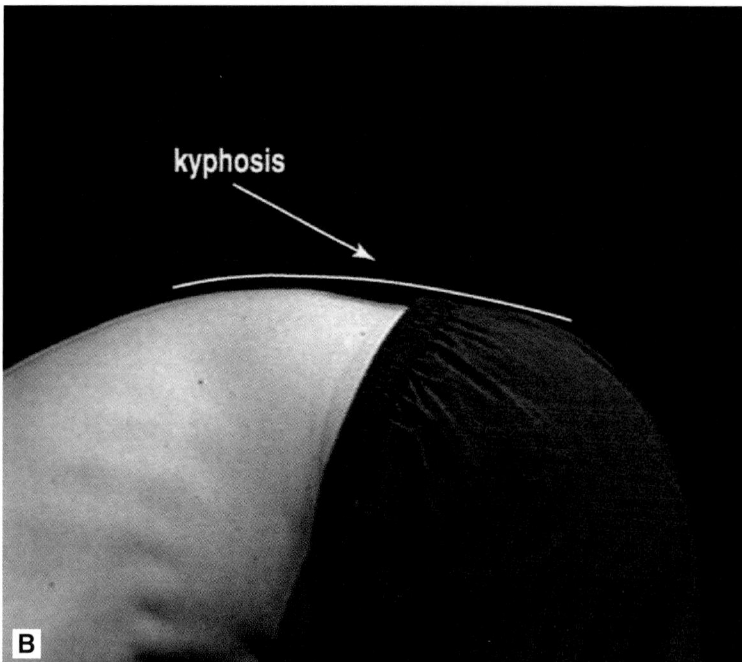

Fig. 7–16

Observing the patient from behind in lumbar flexion (Fig. 7–17A) also allows you to inspect for evidence of scoliosis by noting any asymmetry or prominence of the posterior rib cage on either side (caused by the significant rotatory component of scoliosis usually present in the thoracic spine) (Fig. 7–17B).

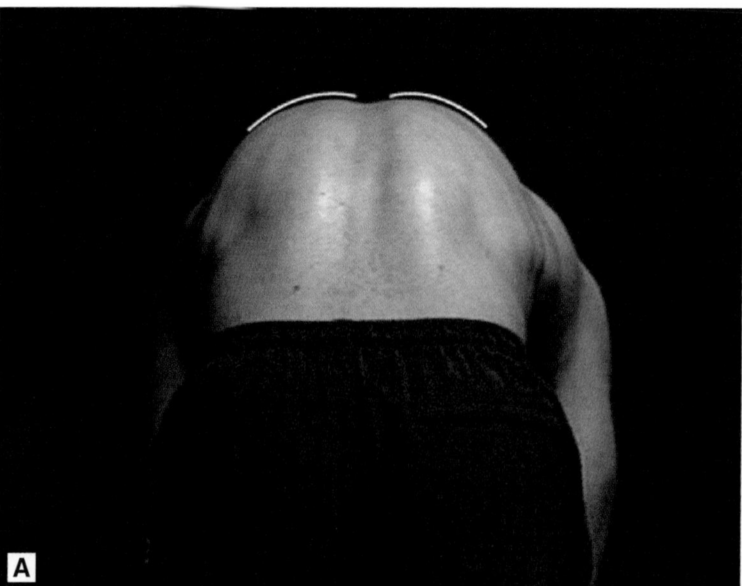

Fig. 7–17

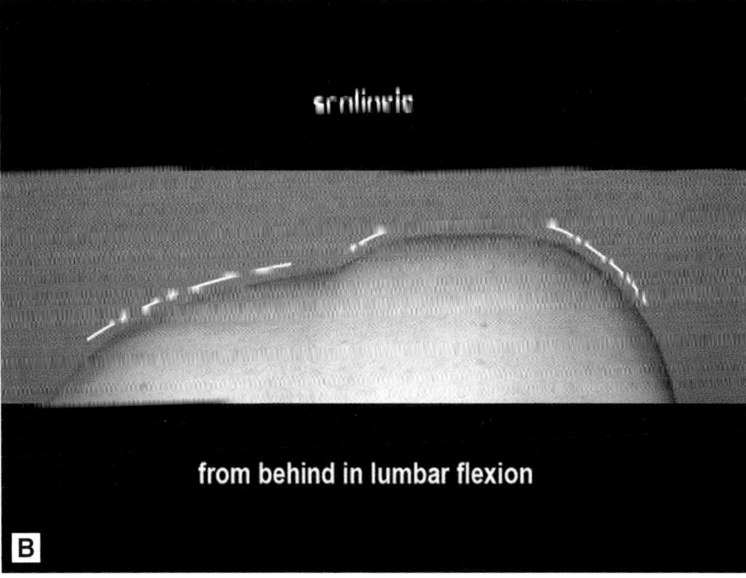

Fig. 7–17

Next, assess lumbosacral extension by asking the patient to bend backward. Simultaneously supporting the low back with one hand and one shoulder with the other hand provides stability and permits you to help the patient into full extension (Fig. 7–18).

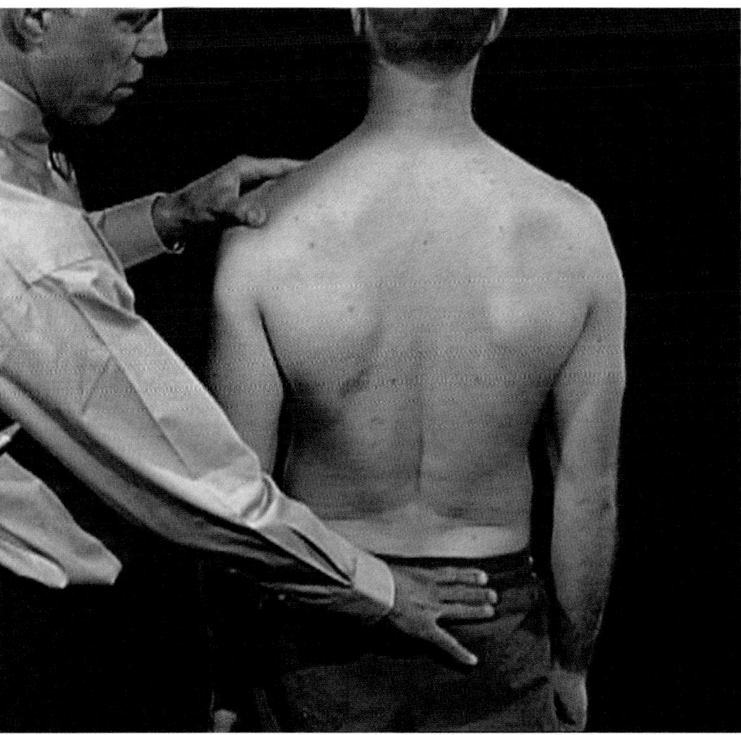

Fig. 7–18

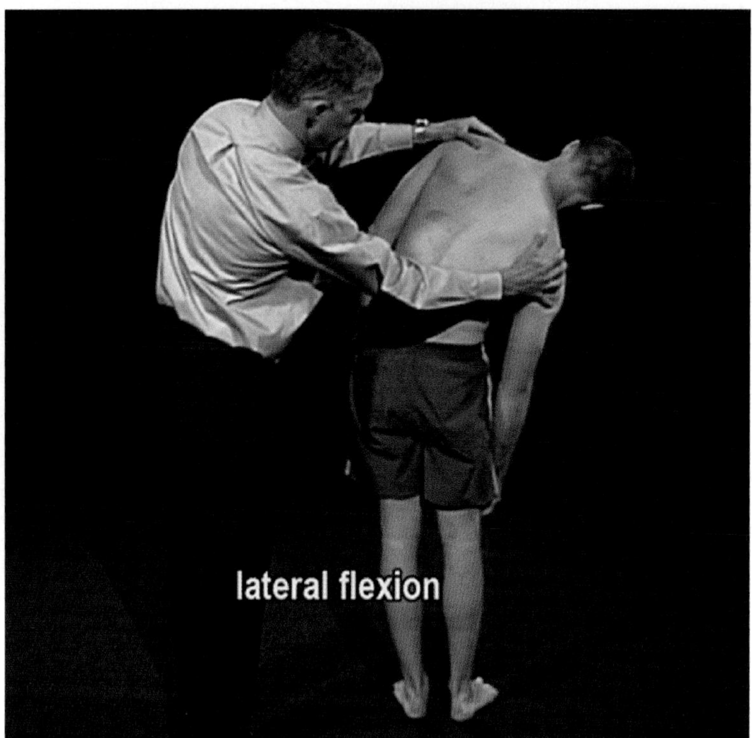

Fig. 7–19

Assess lumbar lateral flexion (lateral bending) by asking the patient to bend to the right and to the left (Fig. 7–19). Place your hands on both shoulders and, if necessary, provide gentle pressure to help the patient into lateral flexion. Assess the patient's response. Note any abnormalities of flexion, extension, and lateral bending. Most importantly, note whether these motions are painful and the location and radiation of the pain (Fig. 7–20).

Screening for Waddell Categories

Simulation Testing Next, assess simulated spinal rotation. Have the patient stand relaxed, with the feet nearly together and the arms at the side. Hold the distal forearms against each trochanter and gently rotate the pelvis ~10° to 15° to the right and to the left. This should permit the shoulders and hips to passively rotate in the same plane (without lumbar spinal rotation) and should not aggravate low back pain (Fig. 7–21). Note the response.

If appropriate, check for low back pain in response to axial loading. Explain to the patient that you are "going to apply gentle pressure over the top of the head to check for any aggravation of low back pain." Apply gentle, light pressure (~5 lb of force, sufficient to blanch your fingernails) to the top of the skull (Fig. 7–22). Light pressure to the skull of a standing patient should not significantly increase low back symptoms. *Neck pain in response to this maneuver may occur and should be discounted.* Note the response.

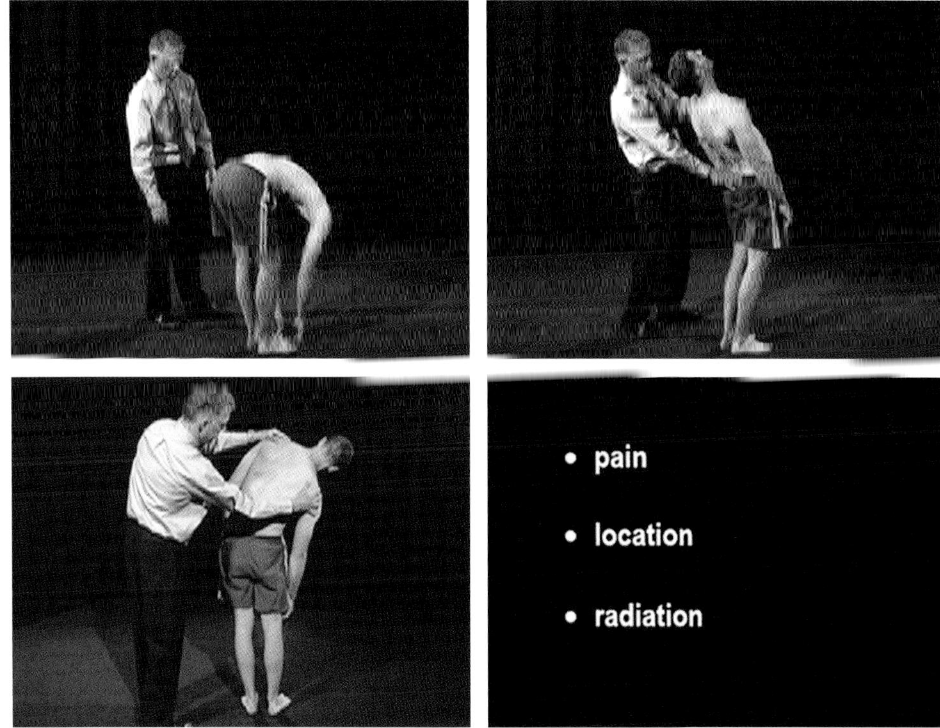

Fig. 7–20

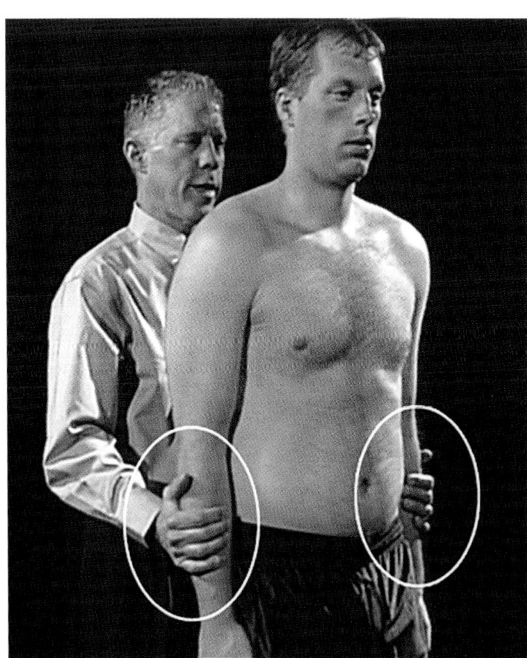

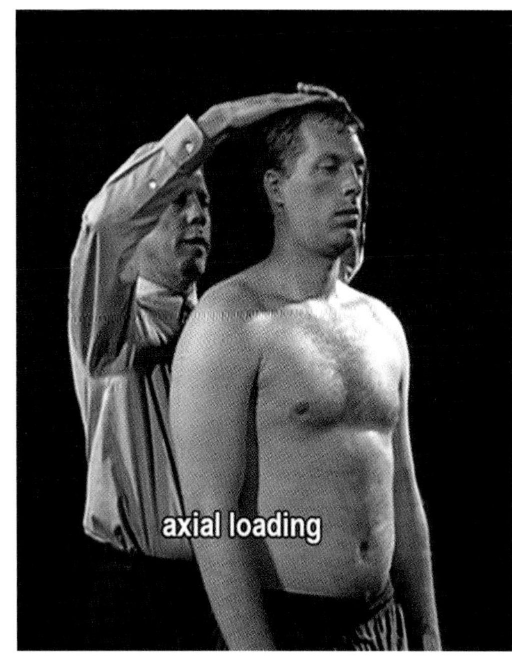

Fig. 7–21

Fig. 7–22

Hip Examination Since symptoms of "low back pain" may originate from the pelvis as well as the lumbosacral spine, it is important to include an examination of the hips in patients presenting with low back complaints. In addition, patients with low back problems frequently complain of "hip pain" when referring to symptoms at the LS junction and/or buttocks (Fig. 7–23). Hence, a careful assessment of both the spine and hips is essential.

With the patient still standing, observe the pelvis from behind and identify the level of the iliac crests (Fig. 7–24A, B). Ask the patient to stand on one foot. Note whether the iliac crests remain level or whether the pelvis drops on the side opposite the standing leg (Fig. 7–25A, B). This pelvic "droop" is referred to as the Trendelenburg sign and is a sensitive indicator of intrinsic hip disease and/or muscle weakness on the weight-bearing side. The Trendelenburg sign is also considered positive if the patient has to lean toward the weight-bearing side to keep the hip from dropping. Repeat this test with the opposite leg.

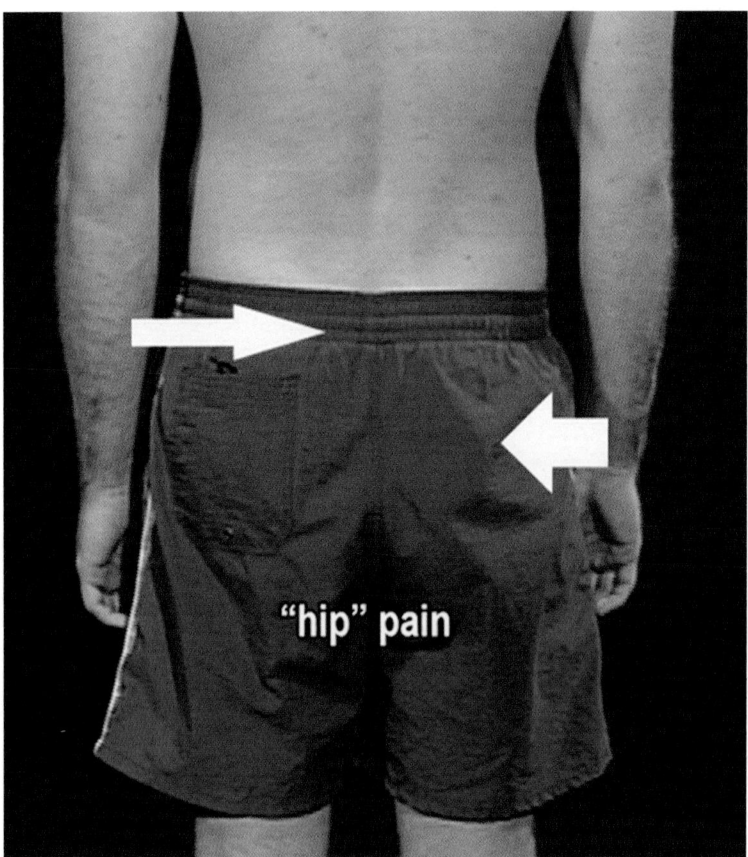

Fig. 7–23

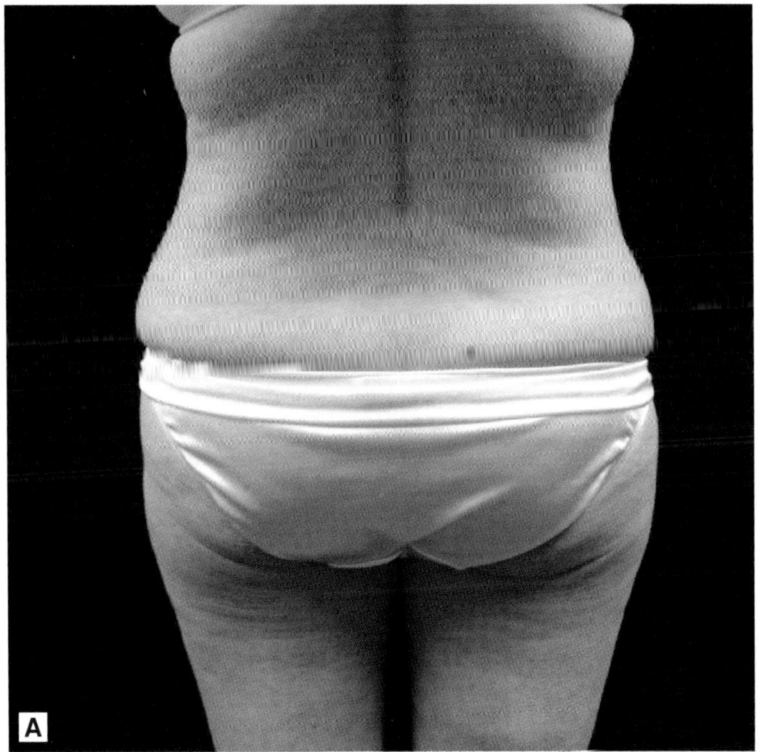
Fig. 7–24

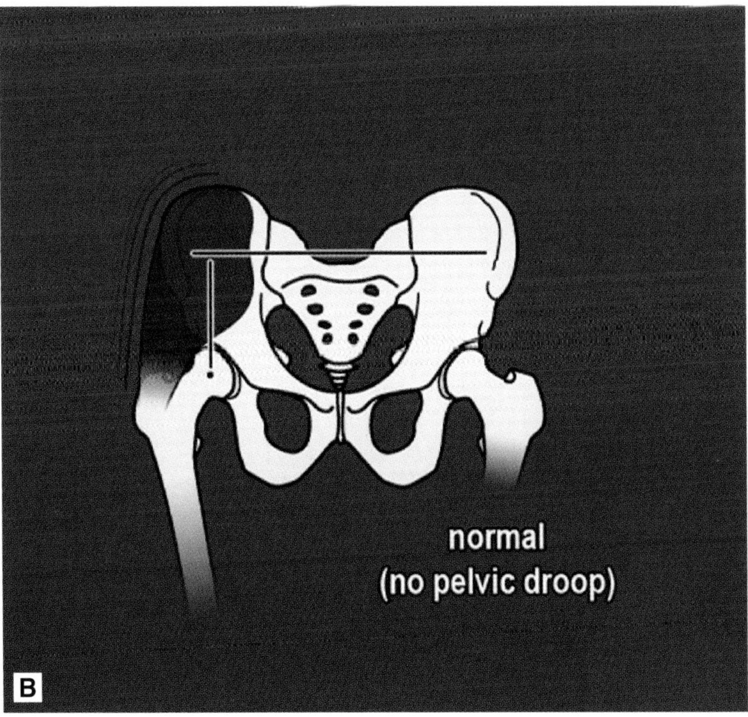

Fig. 7–24

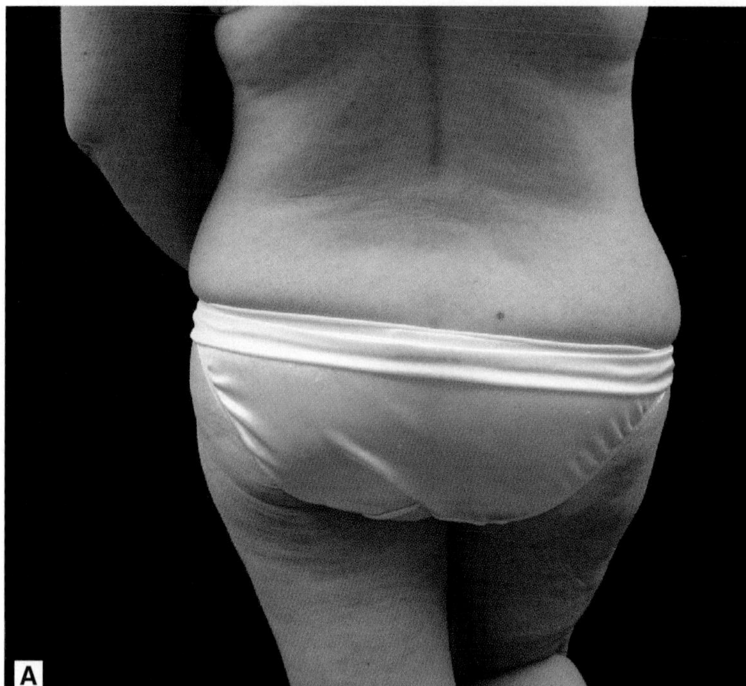

Fig. 7–25

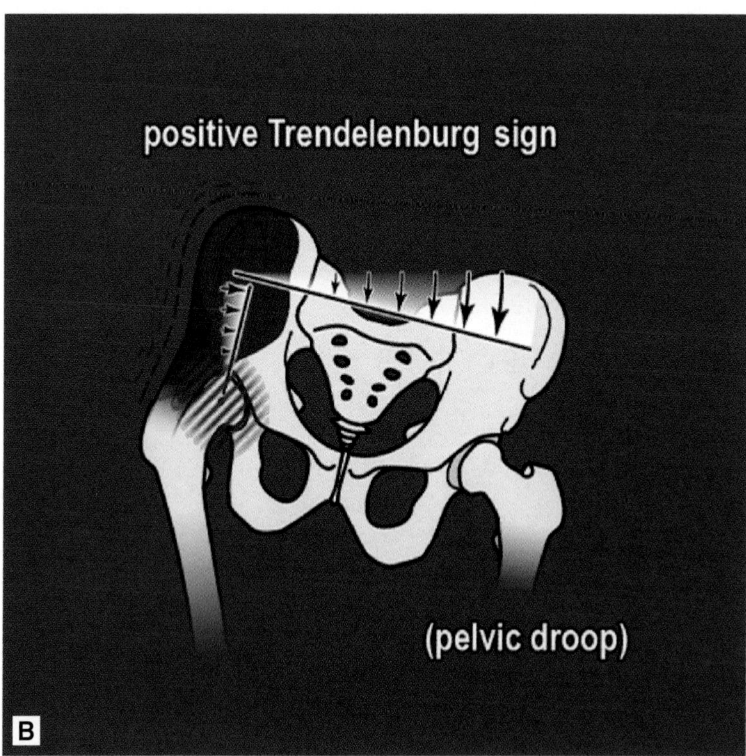

Fig. 7–25

Now ask the patient to lie supine and bring the hips into moderate flexion (with the feet still on the examination table). While standing on the patient's right side, place your thumbs on the superior anterior iliac spines on each side. Your remaining fingers, directed posteriorly toward the table, now lie over each greater trochanter. Check for possible trochanteric bursitis by applying firm pressure to the lateral region of each trochanter. Note any tenderness (Fig. 7-26A).

Next, slide your fingers posteriorly and superiorly on the trochanter to the region of the insertion of the gluteus medius tendon. Apply firm pressure to this area at the posterior aspect of the top of the trochanter. Note any tenderness, suggesting gluteus medius tendinitis (Fig. 7-26B). (*The trochanteric syndrome may include tenderness at the trochanteric bursa and/or the gluteus medius insertion.*)

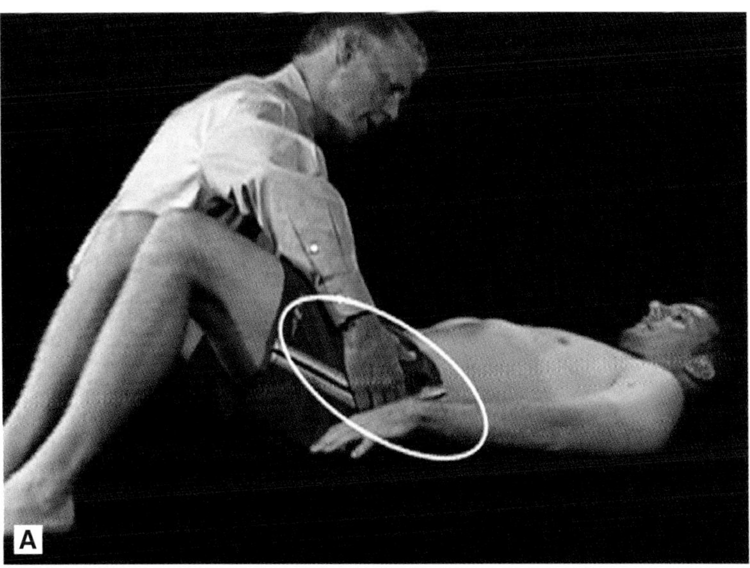

Fig. 7–26

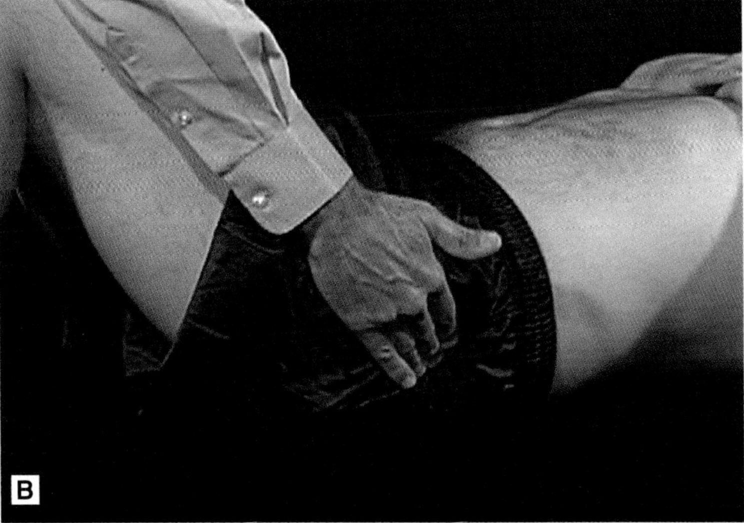

Fig. 7–26

Next, check hip range of motion. Assess hip flexion by moving the thigh up toward the thorax. Normal hip flexion brings the anterior thigh nearly to the chest. Return the hip and knee to 90° of flexion. Keeping the thigh perpendicular and the shin parallel to the examination table while testing hip rotation permits easy visualization of the arcs of movement. Moving the ankle medially assesses hip external rotation (Fig. 7–27A). Moving the ankle laterally assesses hip internal rotation (Fig. 7–27B). Apply firm but gentle pressure to adequately assess range of motion. Note any pain. Watch the patient's face while you perform hip rotation. A change in facial expression may be your first indication that hip range of motion is painful.

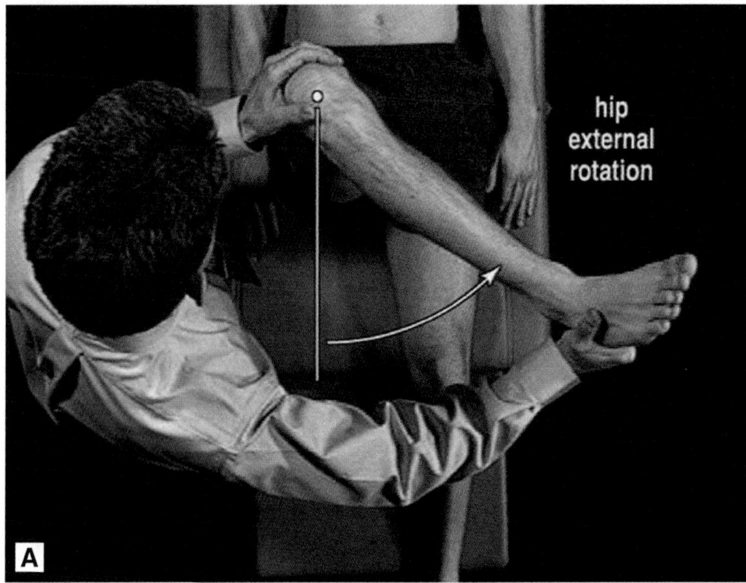

Fig. 7–27

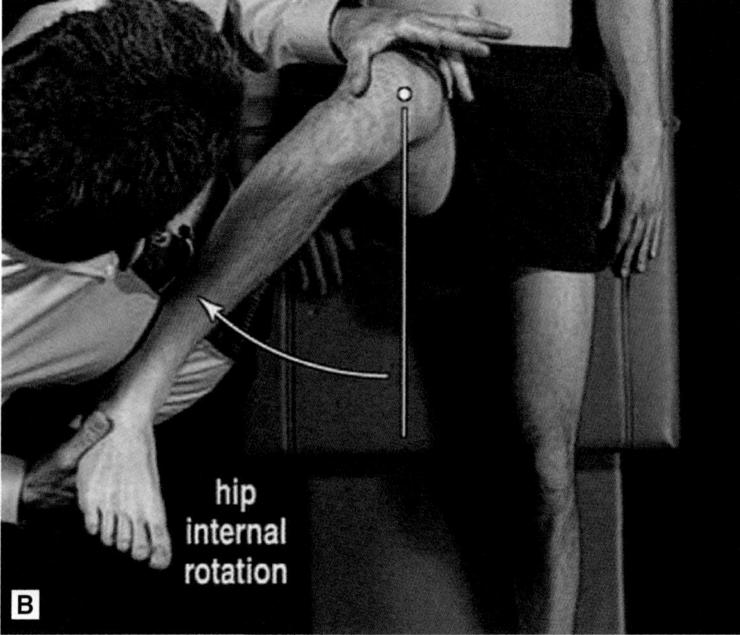

Fig. 7–27

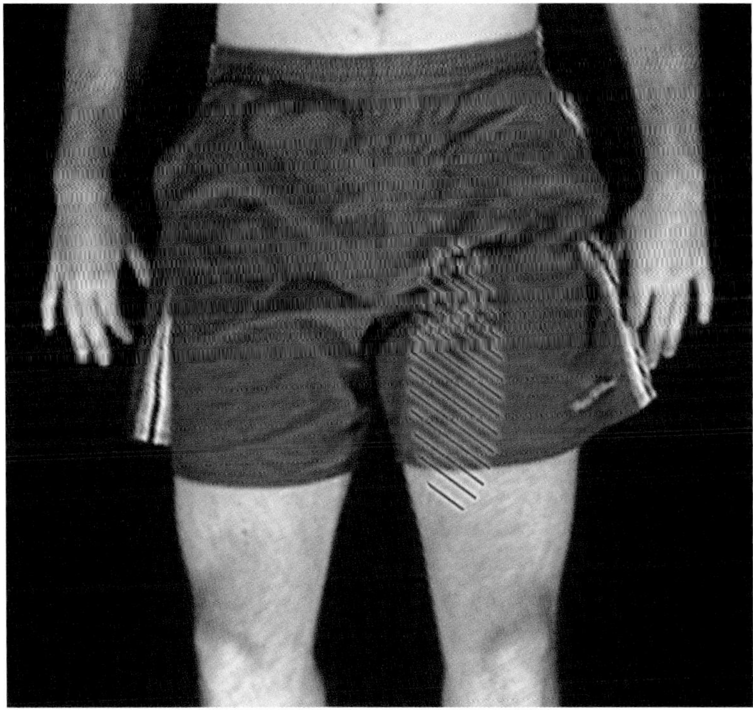

Fig. 7–28

Pain originating from the hip joint itself is usually felt in the groin or medial thigh (Fig. 7–28). (*Note: In patients with total hip replacements, be cautious in assessing hip range of motion; flexion, adduction, and internal rotation may dislocate the femoral component.*) (Fig. 7–29).

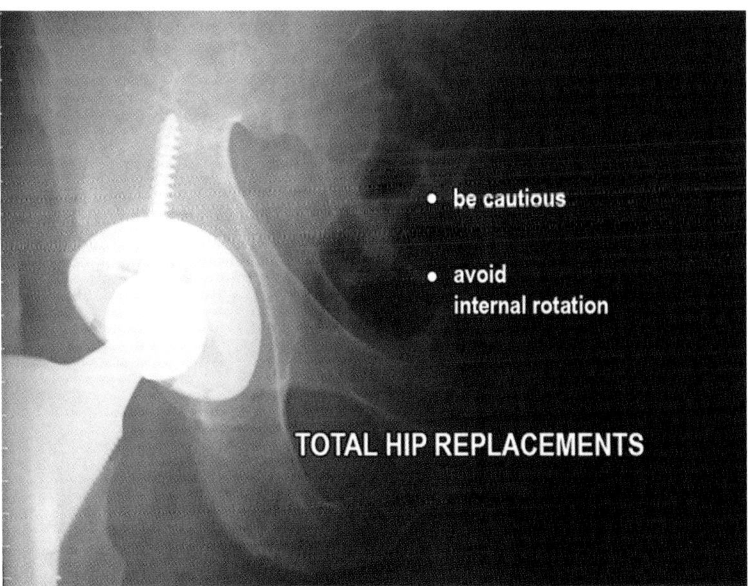

Fig. 7–29

It is important to recognize that the leg becomes a powerful lever arm at the end of hip rotation. In particular, application of appropriate pressure to assess the end of internal rotation causes the ipsilateral hemipelvis to rotate upward in a cephalad direction, jamming the facet joints in the lower lumbosacral spine on that side (Fig. 7–30A). The patient may report "hip pain" with this maneuver. Ask the patient to point to where he feels the discomfort (Fig. 7–30B). Pain from the lower lumbosacral facet joints is usually felt posteriorly on the same side at the level of the belt line (suggesting its origin from the LS spine and not the hip).

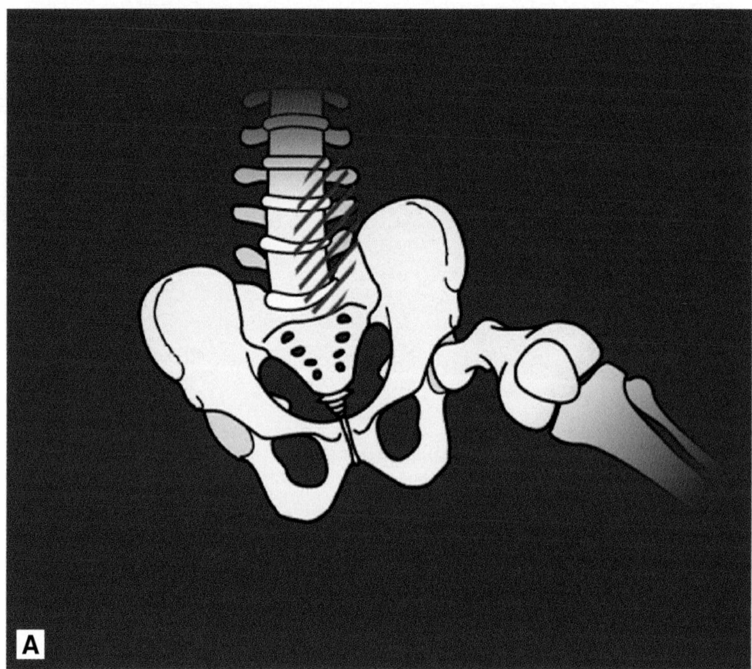

Fig. 7–30

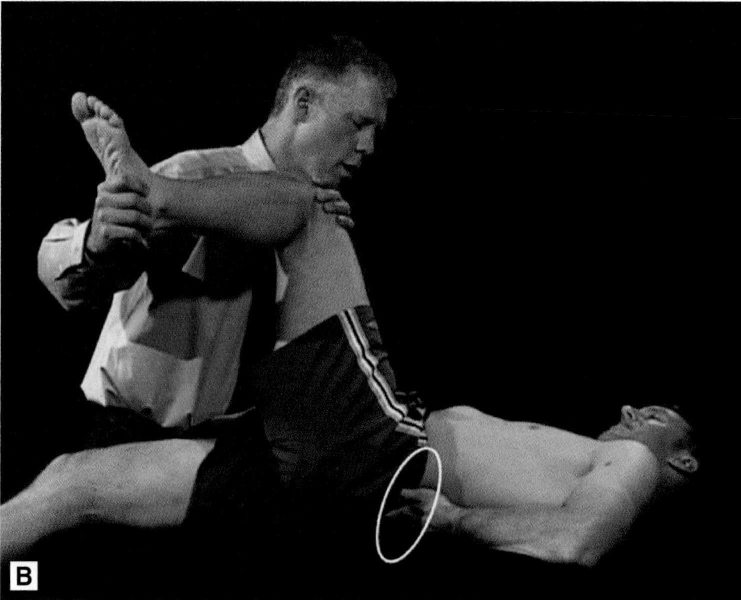

Fig. 7–30

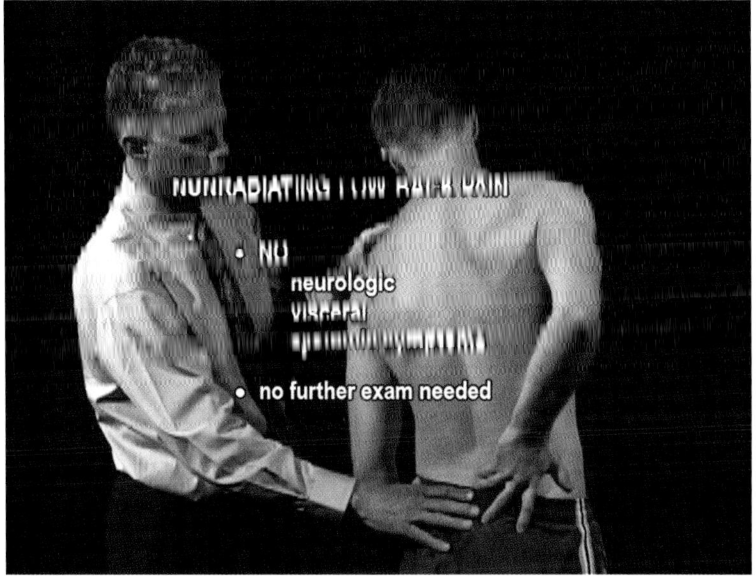

Fig. 7–31

In patients presenting with regional, nonradiating (back-predominant) pain with no historic features suggesting neurologic, visceral, or systemic disease, no further physical examination may be necessary (Fig. 7–31).

However, in individuals suspected of having nerve root irritation, significant psychological distress, possible visceral disease, sacroiliitis, or spondyloarthropathy, additional assessment is indicated.

Special Testing

Suspected Nerve Root Irritation If lumbosacral radiculopathy is suspected, ask the patient to lie supine. Place the patient's heel in the palm of your hand with the knee fully extended and the leg relaxed. Gently and progressively lift the heel off the table until the patient experiences pain. The straight leg raise results in tension on the L5 and S1 nerve roots, especially between 30° and 70° of leg elevation (Fig. 7–32).

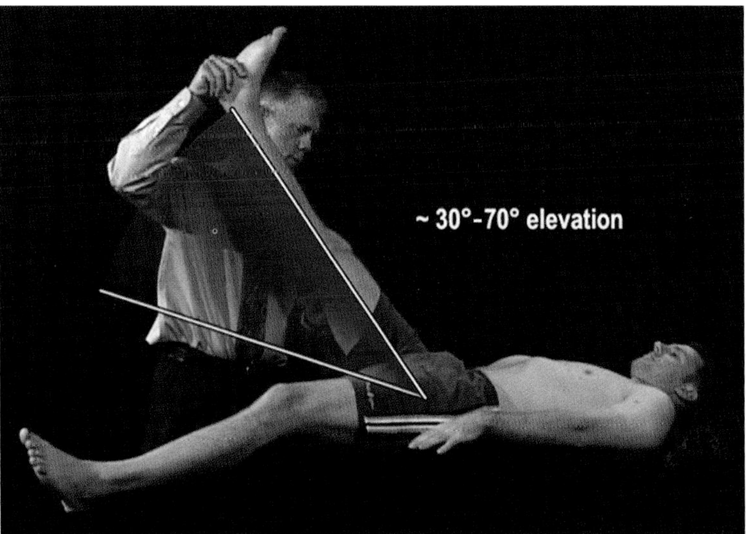

Fig. 7–32

The development of "tightness" in the hamstrings during straight leg raising does not constitute a positive test (Fig. 7–33A). Note whether the patient's discomfort is localized to the back or posterior thigh (negative straight leg raise) (Fig. 7–33B) or whether pain radiates below the knee (positive straight leg raise)

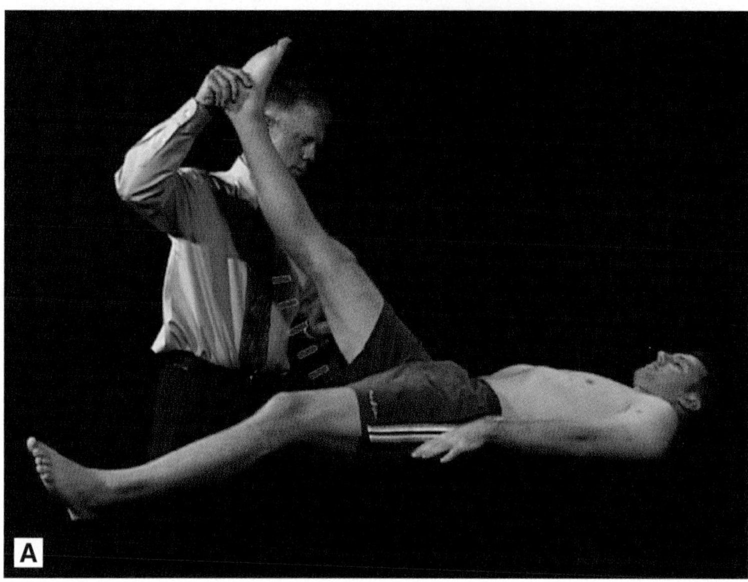

Fig. 7–33

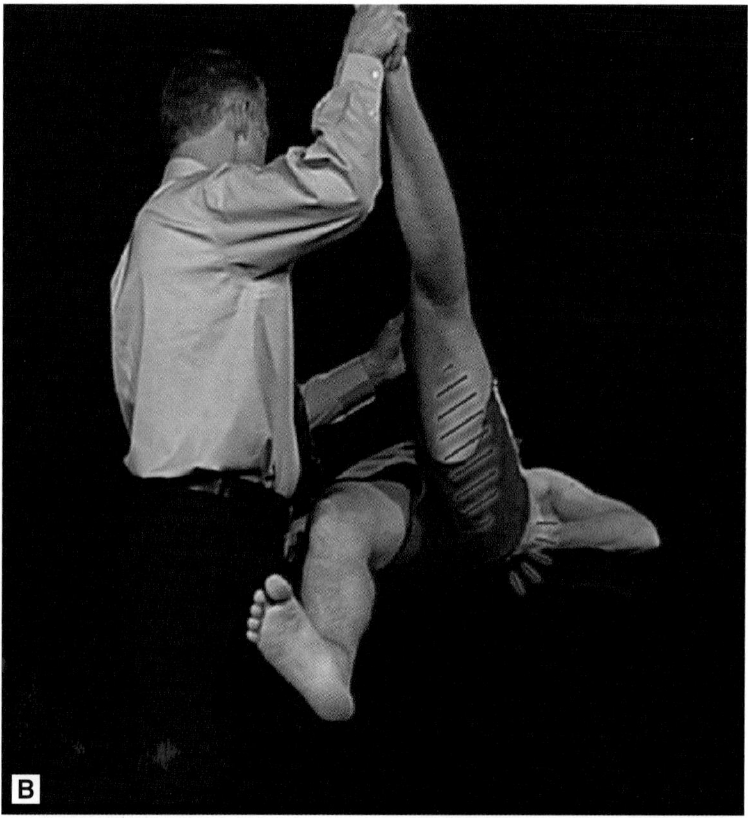

Fig. 7–33

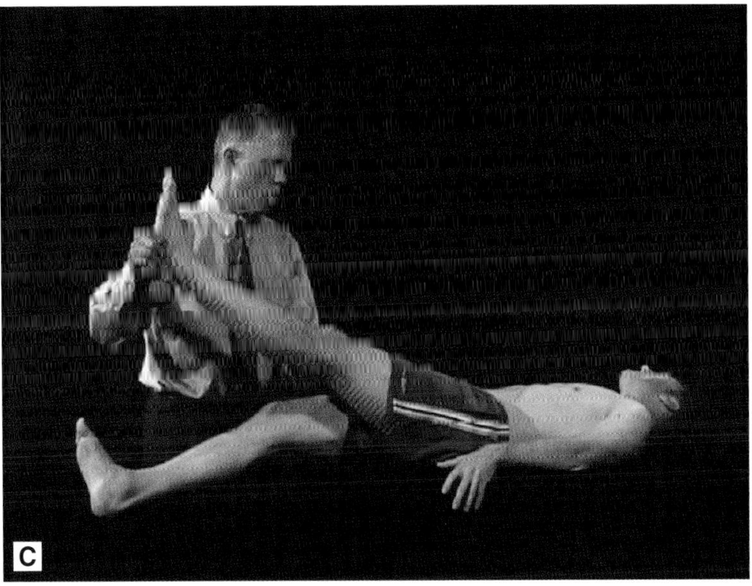

Fig. 7–33

(Fig. 7–33C). Note the location of pain and estimate the angle at pain onset. Now, repeat the straight leg raise on the opposite side. Estimate and record the angle at pain onset, if any.

Assessing the straight leg raise in both the symptomatic and nonsymptomatic sides allows you to check for a so-called "crossed straight leg raising sign." A positive crossed straight leg raise is defined as the reproduction of sciatic pain in the symptomatic leg when passive straight leg raising is performed on the opposite (asymptomatic) leg (Fig. 7–34). A positive straight leg raise on the symptomatic side is moderately sensitive but nonspecific for disk herniation. A positive "crossed straight leg raise," although uncommon, is highly specific for disk herniation.

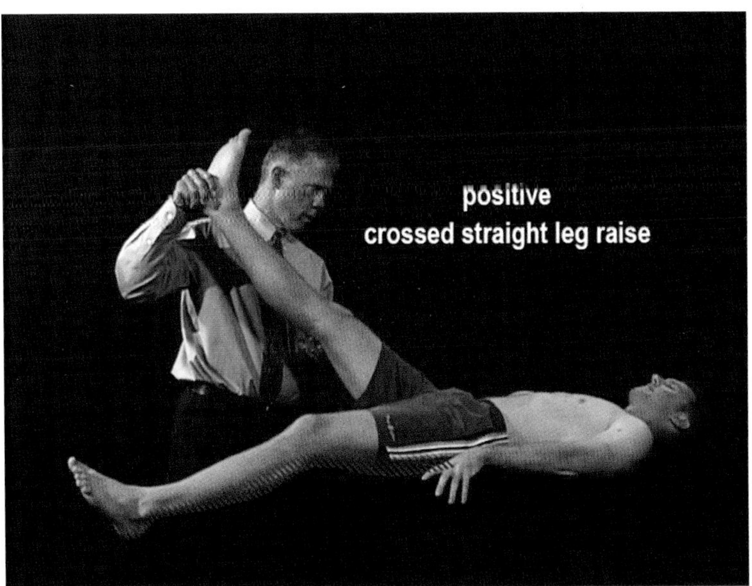

Fig. 7–34

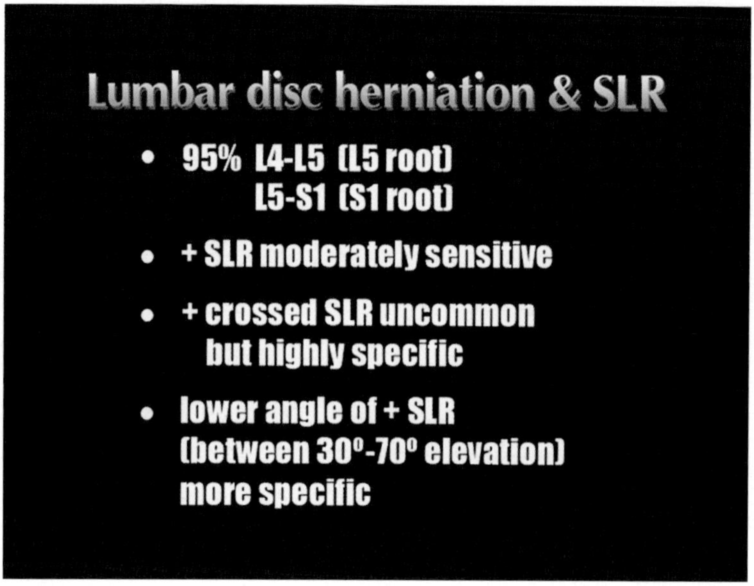

Lumbar disc herniation & SLR

- 95% L4-L5 (L5 root)
  L5-S1 (S1 root)
- + SLR moderately sensitive
- + crossed SLR uncommon but highly specific
- lower angle of + SLR (between 30°-70° elevation) more specific

Fig. 7–35

The lower the angle of elevation required to produce a positive straight leg raise (in the arc 30°-70°), the greater the likelihood of significant disk herniation (Fig. 7–35).

Now ask the patient to sit up. Assess the patellar reflex (L4) in response to rapid, forceful percussion of the patellar tendon midway between the tibial tuberosity and lower pole of the patella. Next, check the Achilles reflex (S1). With the patient relaxed, apply gentle but firm upward pressure to the sole of the foot at the level of the metatarsal heads, gently stretching the Achilles tendon until you feel firm resistance. Strike the tendon in its mid portion, at the level of the malleoli (Fig. 7–36). In addition to visual assessment, you can also assess the force of plantar flexion against your hand. Compare side to side.

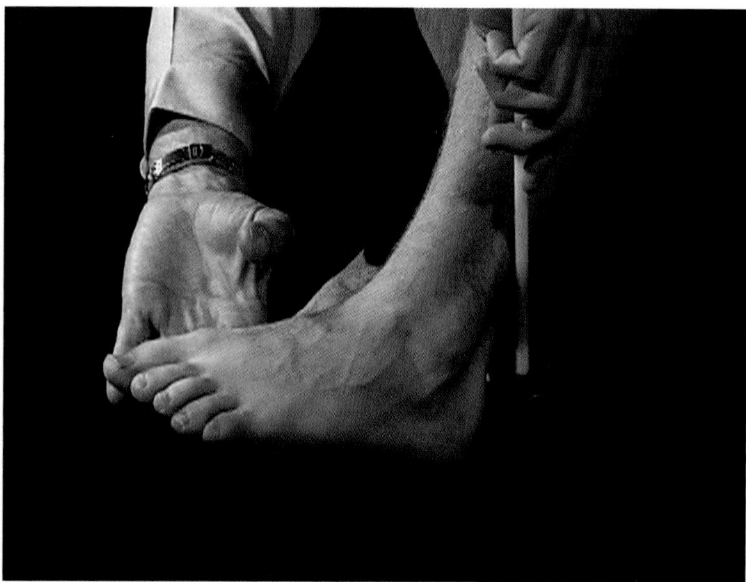

Fig. 7–36

Next, assess distal lower extremity strength. Check combined foot inversion and ankle dorsiflexion (L4) by asking the patient to twist the forefoot toward the inner aspect of the ankle and lift it up toward the head (Fig. 7–37A). Ask the patient to hold it in that position while you apply downward force on the medial aspect of the forefoot. Note any weakness.

Assess great toe dorsiflexion (L5) by asking the patient to raise the big toe up toward the head and hold it in that position. Apply downward force with two fingers. Note any weakness (Fig. 7–37B).

Check combined foot eversion and dorsiflexion (S1) by asking the patient to twist the forefoot toward the outer aspect of the ankle and lift the foot up toward the head. Ask the patient to hold it in that

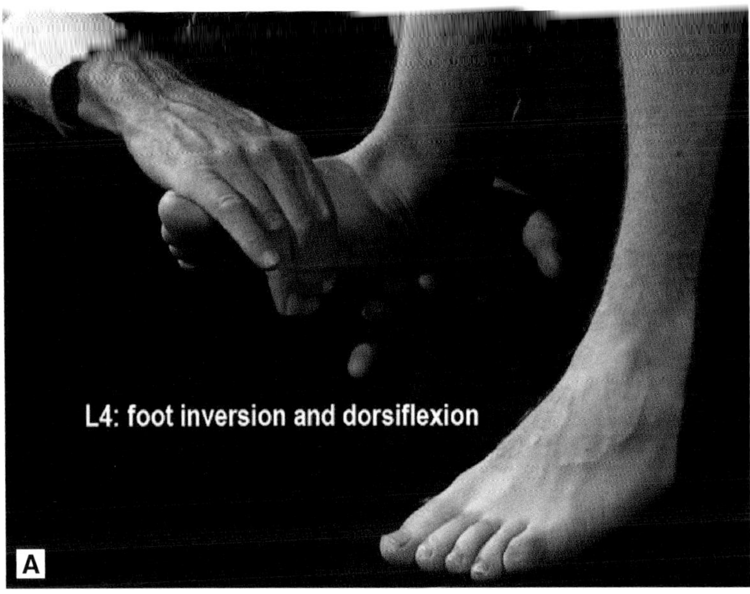

Fig. 7–37

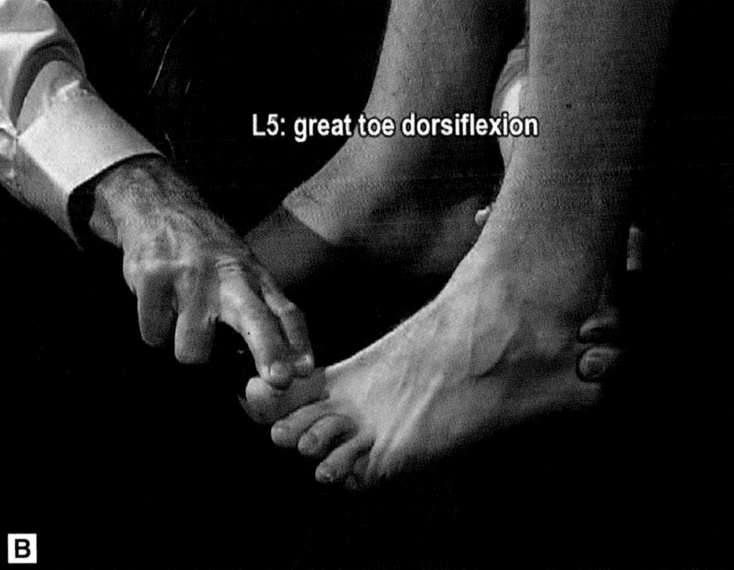

Fig. 7–37

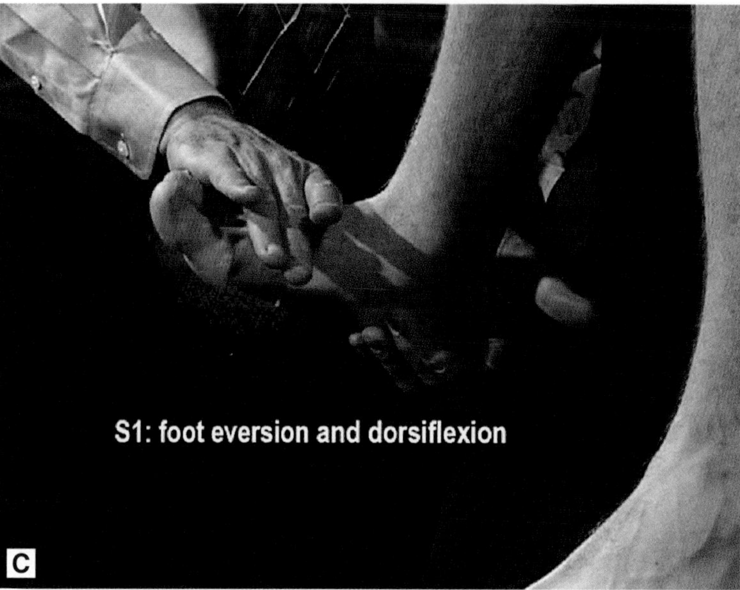

Fig. 7–37

position while you apply downward force to the lateral aspect of the forefoot. Note any weakness and compare side to side (Fig. 7–37C).

If possible S1 root weakness is detected, you can further assess ankle plantar flexor strength by having the patient stand and repetitively rise on the toes of one foot while supporting their arms against the wall. Observing 10 toe raises on each side may provide a more dynamic assessment of S1 strength than toe walking alone (Fig. 7–38).

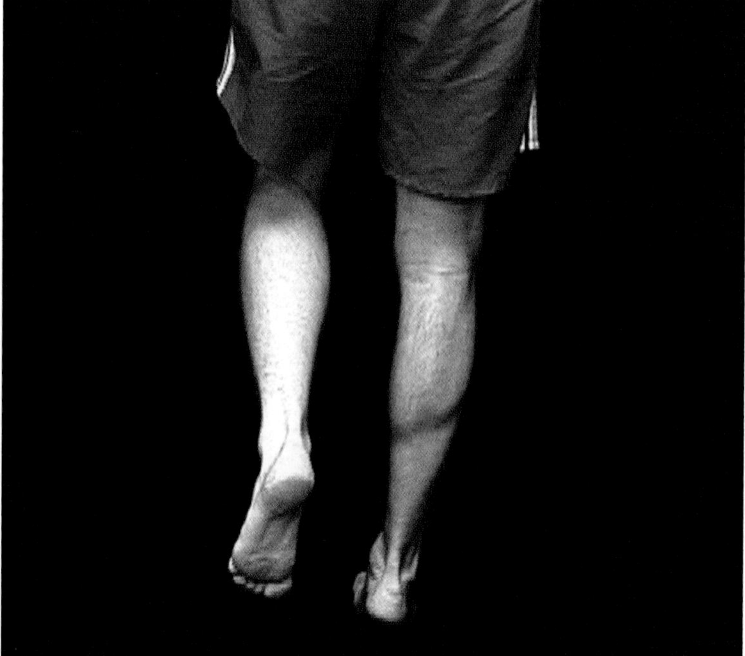

Fig. 7–38

Note any generalized "giving way" or so called "breakaway" weakness not explainable on a neurologic basis. Such findings may indicate psychological distress.

Next, assess a distracted straight leg raise in the seated position by telling the patient that you want to "check thigh muscle (quadriceps) strength." Palpate the distal quadriceps muscles with one hand and grasp the patient's heel in the palm of your other. Slowly elevate the shin from vertical to horizontal. Note whether this maneuver results in back pain, hamstring tightness, or radiating pain below the knee. As you gently extend the knee, estimate the angle at pain onset and the maximum tolerated angle of knee extension. Patients with no significant nerve root irritation will experience no pain (Fig. 7–39). If the seated straight leg raise is unexpectedly negative, complete the "distraction" and assess resisted quadriceps strength by attempting to flex the knee against the patient's resistance. Patient's with true sciatica secondary to disk herniation will often lean backward during the seated straight leg raise, in an effort to reduce the angle of leg elevation and nerve root irritation (Fig. 7–40). This response is called the "flip sign," named after the patient's tendency to suddenly "flip" backward to relieve nerve root tension.

Note whether there is a marked difference (>40° to 45°) between straight leg raising performed in the supine and sitting positions. A marked improvement during the seated straight leg raise compared with the supine straight leg raise may suggest an important component of psychological distress.

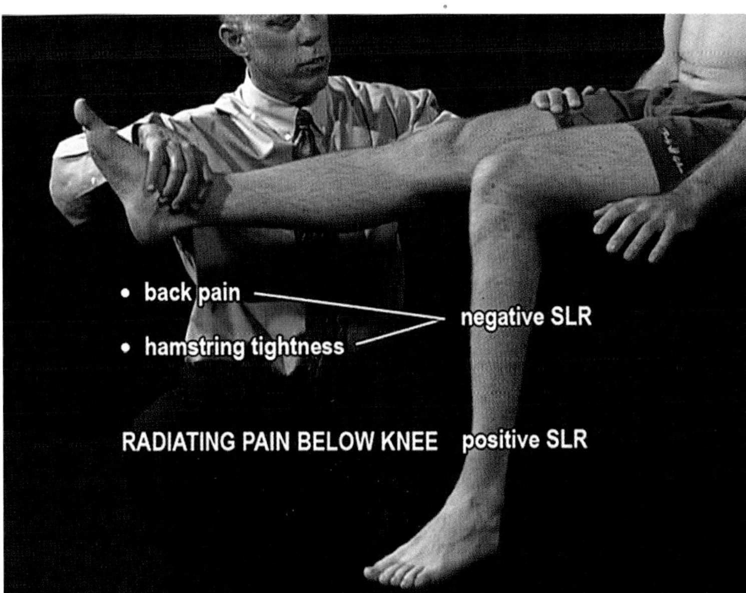

Fig. 7–39

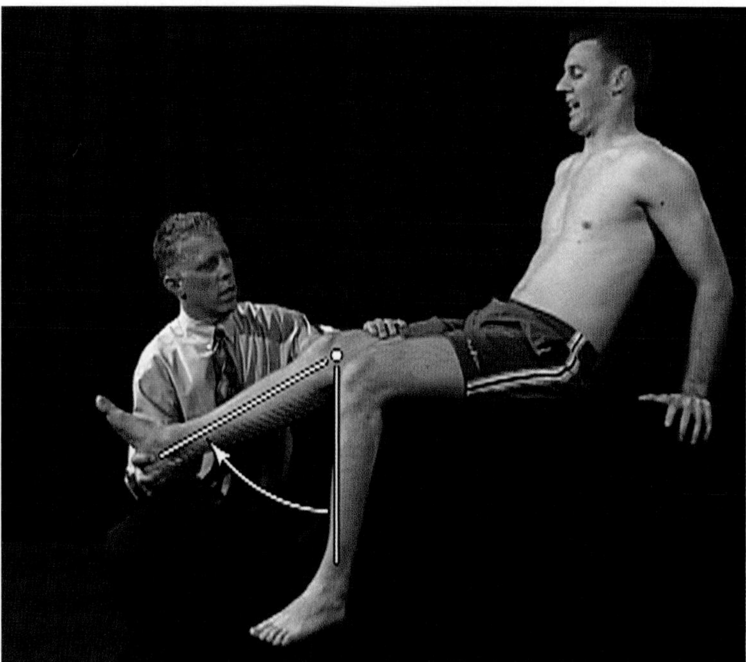

Fig. 7–40

Now, assess the sensation of the medial foot and ankle (L4), the dorsum of the foot (L5), and the lateral foot and ankle (S1) to light touch and/or pin prick. (Fig. 7–41A through C) Compare side to side.

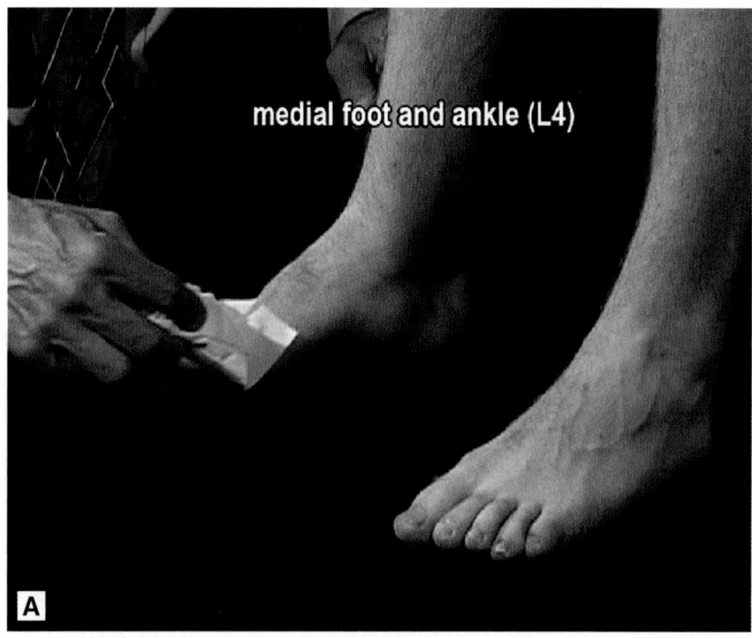

Fig. 7–41

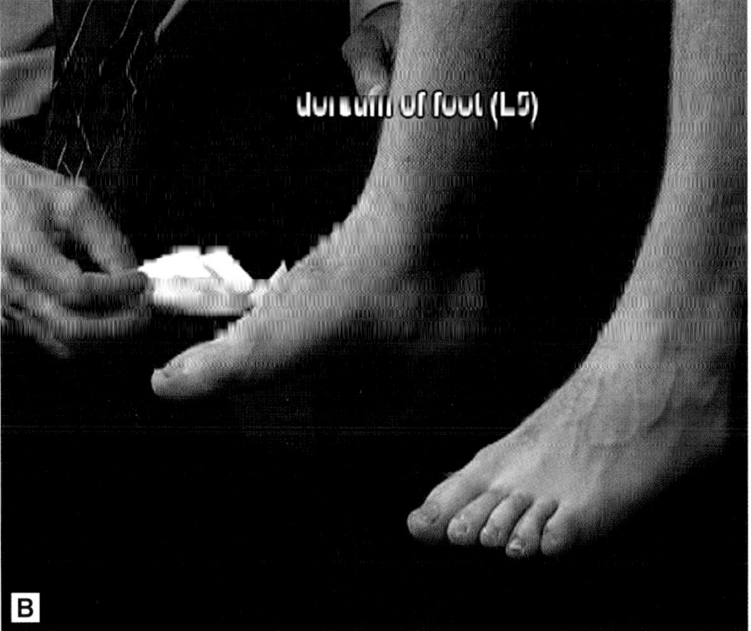

Fig. 7–41

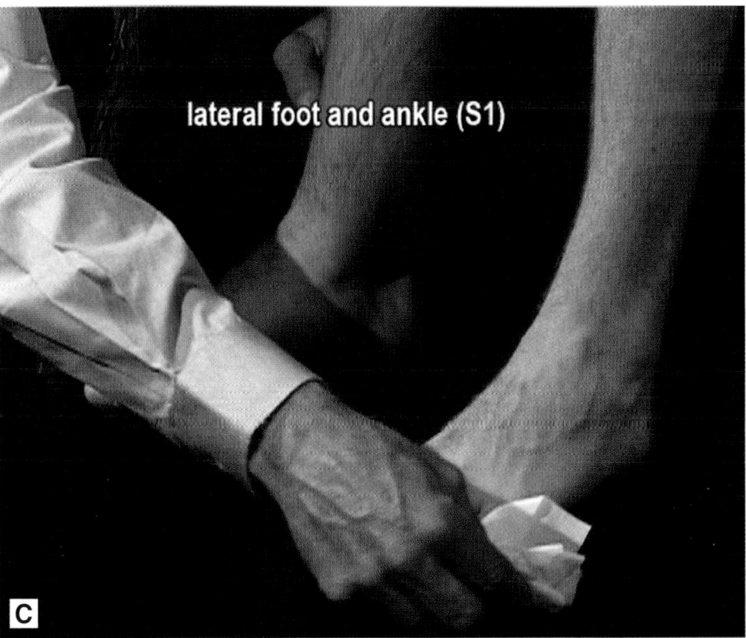

Fig. 7–41

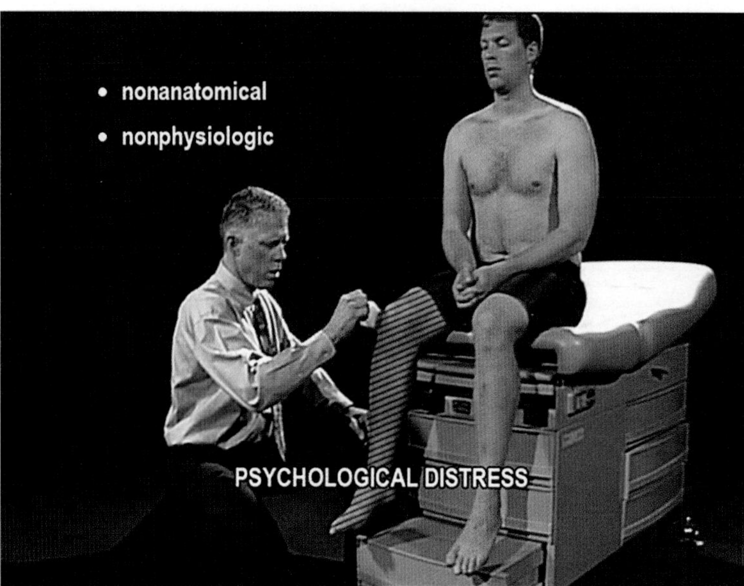

Fig. 7–42

Note any regional sensory alterations that are not explainable on a neuroanatomic basis (eg, decreased sensation of an entire limb). The finding of nonanatomical, nonphysiologic motor or sensory disturbances may also indicate psychological distress (Fig. 7–42).

Patients with a history and physical examination suggesting possible cauda equina syndrome should have additional testing: check perianal sensation, the anal reflex (so-called "anal wink"), and digital rectal examination to assess sphincter tone.

Suspected Psychological Distress: Waddell Categories Your history and physical examination provide important opportunities to observe movement and pain-related behaviors. If the accumulating clinical findings during the "basic" examination suggest possible psychological contributions to the patient's back pain, perform the examination components you would to evaluate "suspected nerve root irritation." This will permit you to more deliberately assess for the presence of Waddell's behavioral signs. The Waddell signs were developed as a clinical assessment tool to help clinicians recognize important features of psychological distress and illness behaviors complicating low back pain.

These signs are grouped into five categories of response:

- **Nonorganic tenderness:** superficial or nonanatomic tenderness
- **Simulation tests:** axial loading or simulated rotation
- **Distraction tests:** discrepant straight leg raising
- **Regional disturbances:** "giving way" weakness or nondermatomal sensory disturbances
- **Overreaction**

The presence of significant superficial or nonanatomical tenderness (Fig. 7–43A); back pain in response to simulated axial loading or pelvic rotation (Fig. 7–43B); marked differences in response to supine and seated straight leg raising (Fig. 7–43C); nonphysiologic regional disturbances in motor or sensory function (Fig. 7–43D); and the presence of significant overreaction manifested by inappropriate guarding, limping, bracing, rubbing, grimacing, or sighing during the examination (Fig. 7–43E) are important clinical signs and should not be ignored.

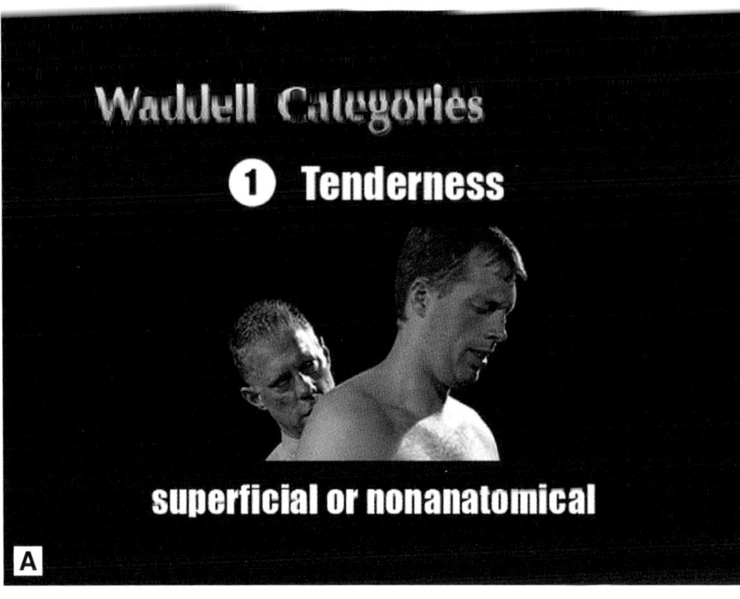

Fig. 7–43

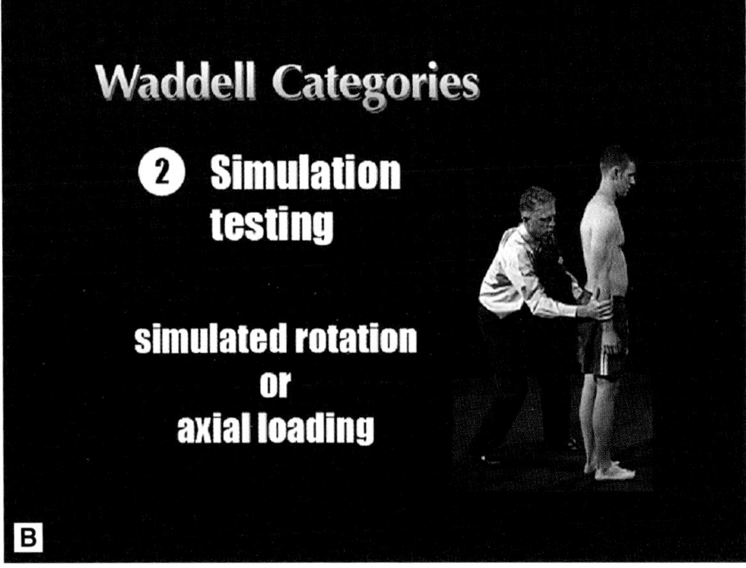

Fig. 7–43

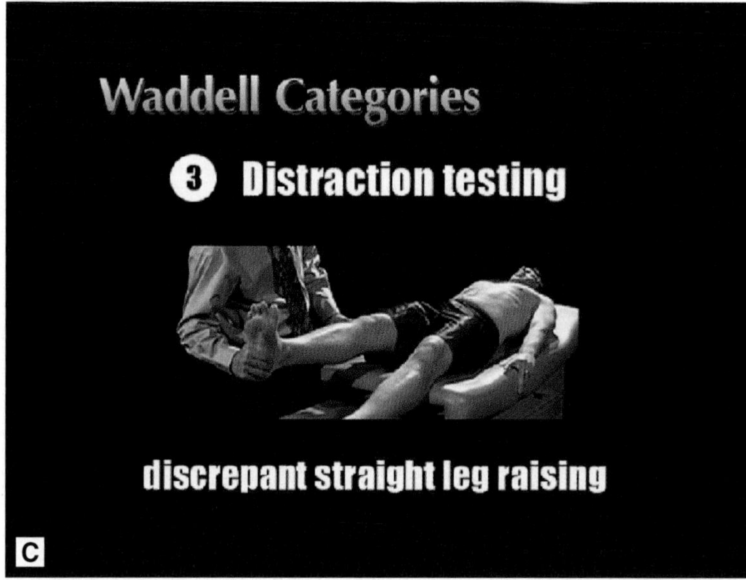

Fig. 7–43

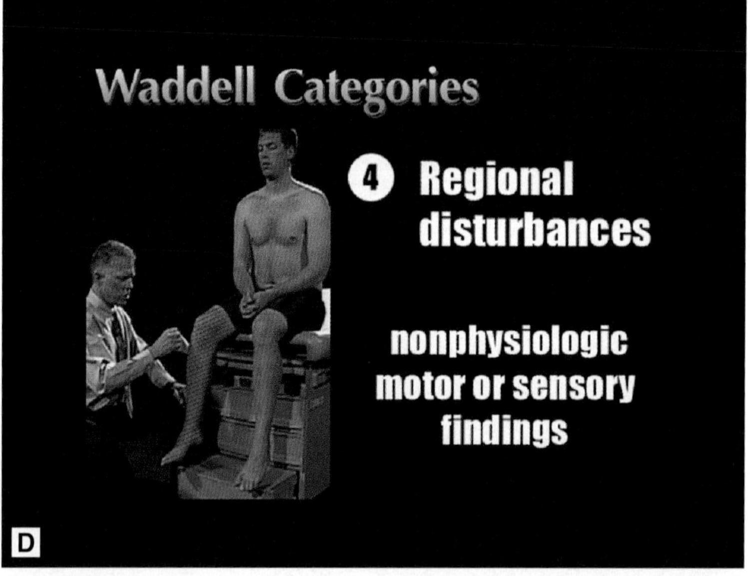

Fig. 7–43

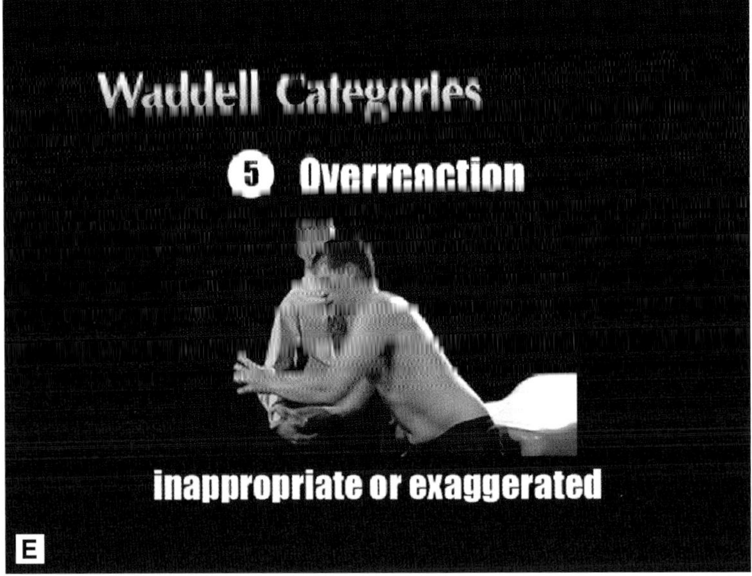

Fig. 7–43

The assessment of the Waddell categories can be readily integrated into a rapid, organized, and sequential examination of the low back. The presence of signs in three or more Waddell categories may indicate significant psychological distress complicating the patient's low back pain.

Overinterpretation of behavioral signs must be avoided. Isolated behavioral signs should not be considered clinically significant. Furthermore, the presence of behavioral signs does not rule out an anatomic problem.

Properly understood, the presence of signs in three or more Waddell categories "simply shows the health care provider that abnormal illness behavior may be present as a coping strategy and that other learned cognitive and behavioral patterns and psychological influences may need to be addressed to improve treatment outcome" (Waddell). The Waddell behavioral signs (also referred to as "nonorganic physical signs in low back pain") can be very useful in clarifying your clinical assessment. These "yellow flags" highlight important distinctions enabling the examiner to identify and clarify both the physical and nonorganic elements of the clinical presentation. With this information, your management strategy can be focused on appropriate interventions: physical treatment can be directed toward physical pathology and proper attention can be directed toward identifying (and hopefully modifying) important psychosocial factors, which may tend to perpetuate pain and disability.

Suspected Sacroiliitis and Spondylitis If the patient's age (<40) and clinical history suggest possible inflammatory low back pain, a more focused assessment of the sacroiliac joints and spine is appropriate (Fig. 7–44).

With the patient standing, identify the sacral dimples at the lumbosacral junction. The sacroiliac joints lie beneath a line formed between the sacral dimples and the coccyx. Firmly palpate/percuss each sacroiliac joint (Fig. 7–45). Note any tenderness. (*Without a prior clinical suspicion of sacroiliitis, SI joint palpation/percussion is of very limited clinical value.*)

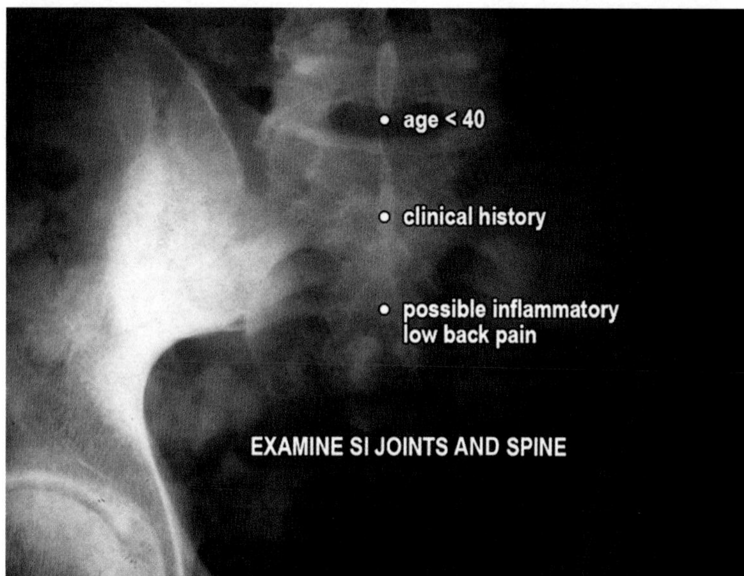

Fig. 7–44

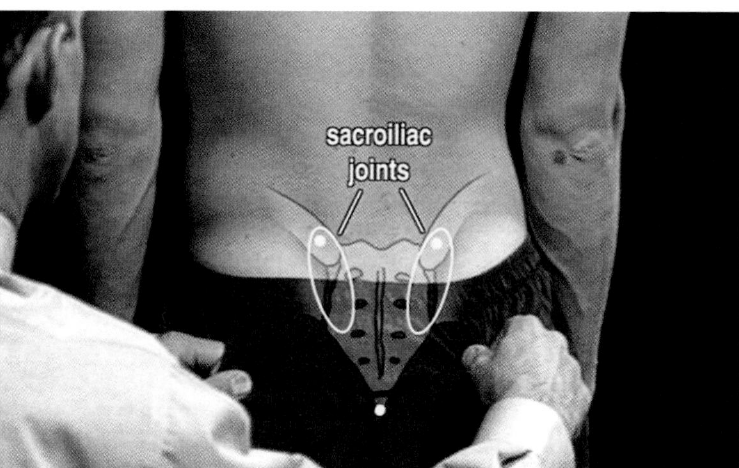

Fig. 7–45

Next, measure lumbosacral spinal mobility by checking a "modified Schober test." Locate the sacral dimples at the lumbosacral junction and draw a small line between them. With the spine in a resting neutral position, use a tape measure to mark a point 10 cm above and 5 cm below the lumbosacral junction (Fig. 7–46A, B). Now ask the patient to bend forward and attempt to touch the toes. Assess lumbosacral spinal mobility by measuring the distraction between the upper and lowest skin marks and record the distance between them at the end of full flexion: Schober 15 cm to ____ cm (Fig. 7–46C). (Normal distraction with LS flexion is >5 cm.)

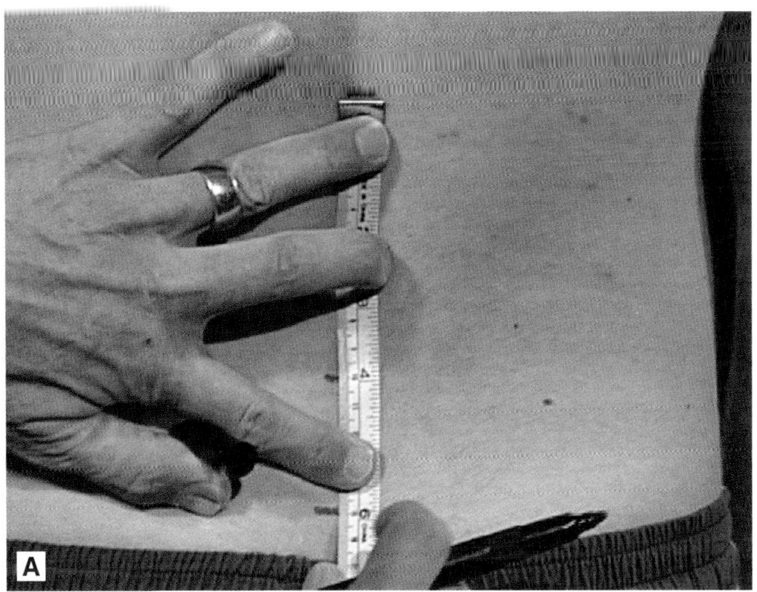

Fig. 7–46

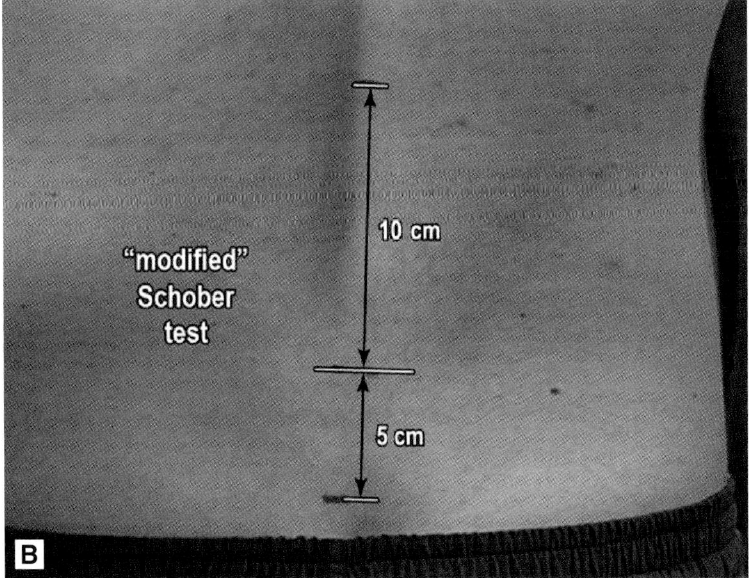

Fig. 7–46

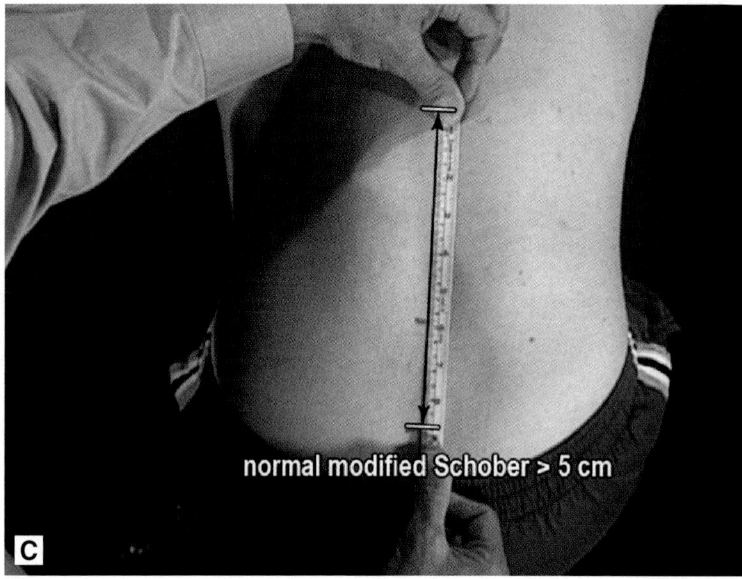

Fig. 7–46

Next, ask the patient to lie supine. Bring the hip and knee into flexion when you cross one leg over the opposite leg and rest the patient's lateral malleolus on the opposite distal thigh ("crossing the legs"). Now, gently but firmly apply pressure to the medial aspect of the flexed knee, pushing it toward the examination table. This maneuver is called the FABER test and refers to the position of the hip in **F**lexion, **AB**duction, and **E**xternal **R**otation, stressing the ipsilateral sacroiliac joint (Fig. 7–47A). A "positive

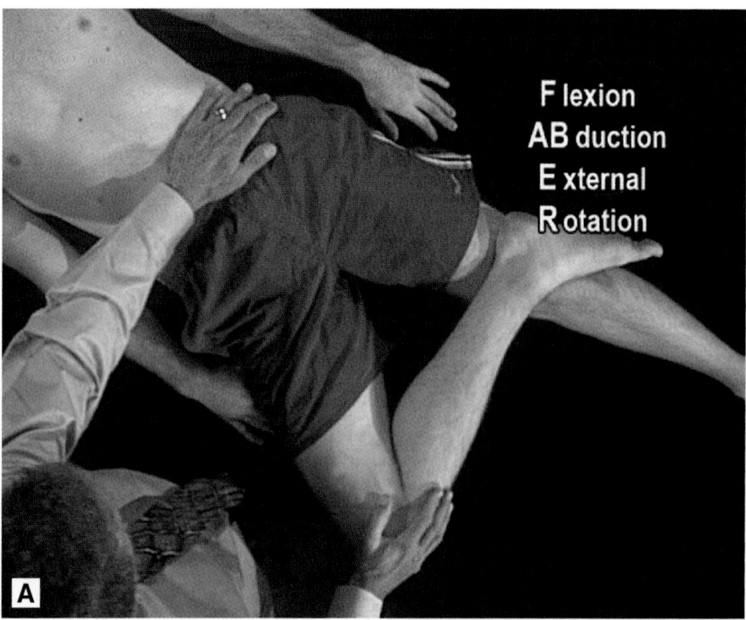

Fig. 7–47

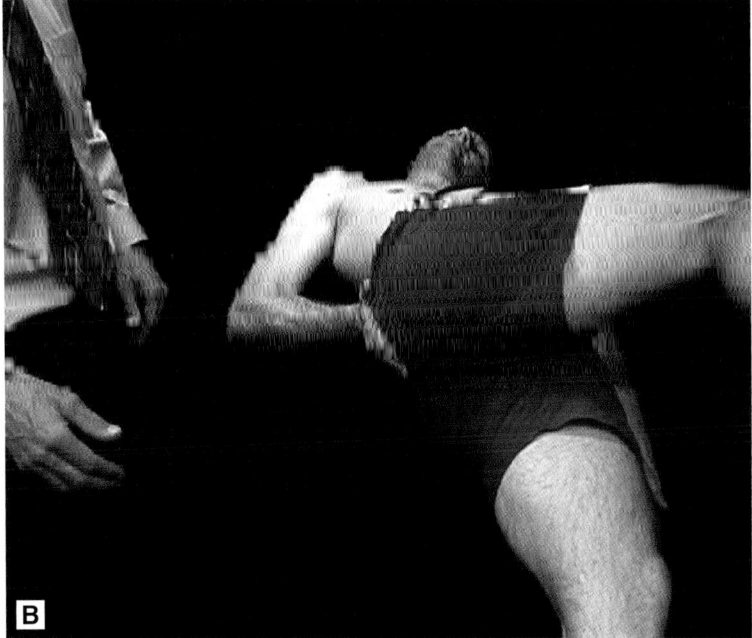

Fig. 7–47

FABER test" requires reproduction of sacroiliac pain on the same side, felt in the upper inner buttock region (Fig. 7–47B) (rather than lumbosacral junction, trochanter, or groin). This test may be difficult to interpret in patients with intrinsic hip disease (who may feel discomfort in the groin or gluteal region rather than the SI joint). Perform the FABER maneuver on the opposite side and compare.

Next, gently but progressively press downward on both superior anterior iliac spines, driving the iliac wings posteriorly toward the examination table (Fig. 7–48A). This maneuver stresses both sacroiliac joints

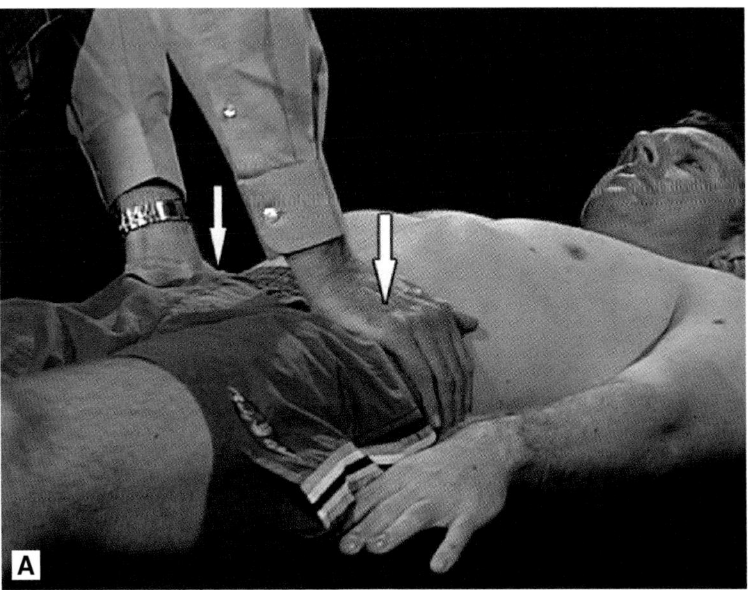

Fig. 7–48

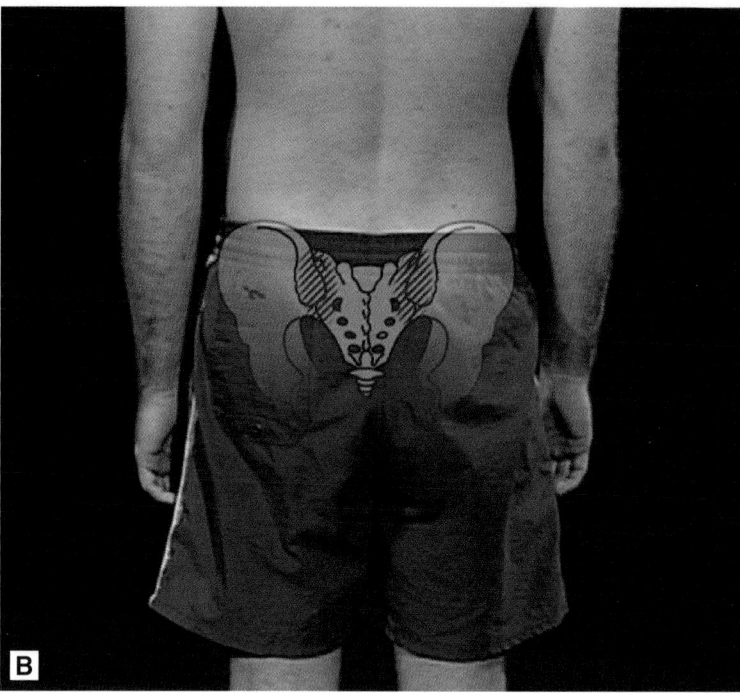

Fig. 7–48

and a "positive compression test" requires reproduction of the patient's pain localized to the sacroiliac joint on one or both sides (Fig. 7–48B) (induction of discomfort in other regions is not considered a positive test).

In patients whose history and examination confirms the suspicion of a spondyloarthropathy, make several additional spondylitis-specific measurements (Fig. 7–49).

Ask the patient to stand. Perform and record the modified Schober test (see Fig. 7-46C).

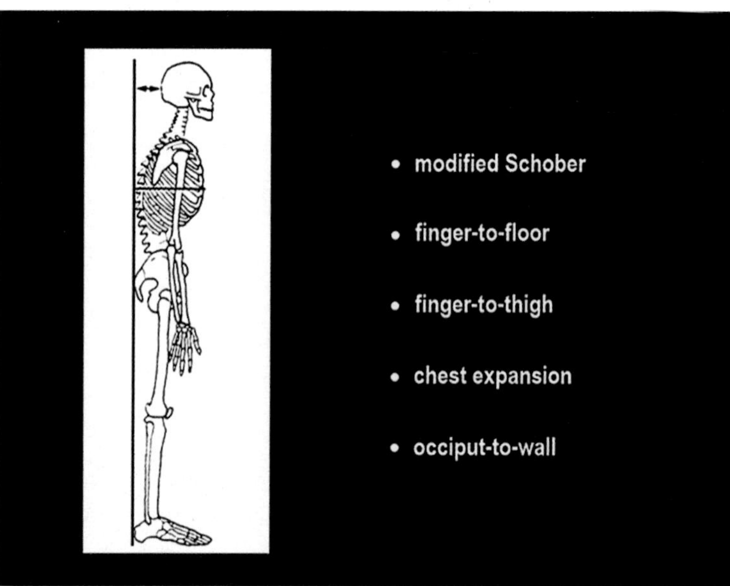

Fig. 7–49

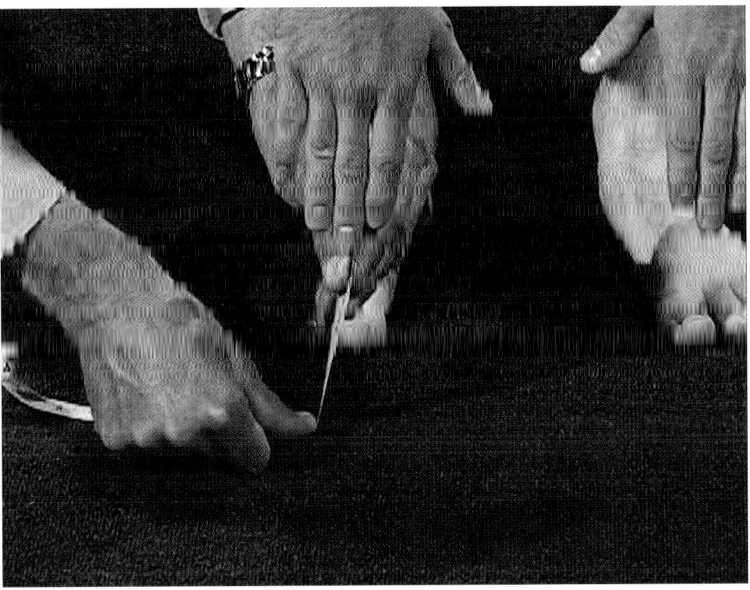

Fig. 7–50

Check the patient's "finger to floor" distance. With the patient in full forward flexion, measure the distance from the patient's third fingertip and to the floor (Fig. 7–50).

Next, check the "finger to thigh distraction" by asking the patient to stand fully upright against the wall with their arms at the side. Mark each thigh at the level of the third fingertip. Then, ask the patient to bend to one side as far as they can (maximum lateral flexion). Mark the leg at this point and measure the total distraction. Repeat on the opposite side (Fig. 7–51).

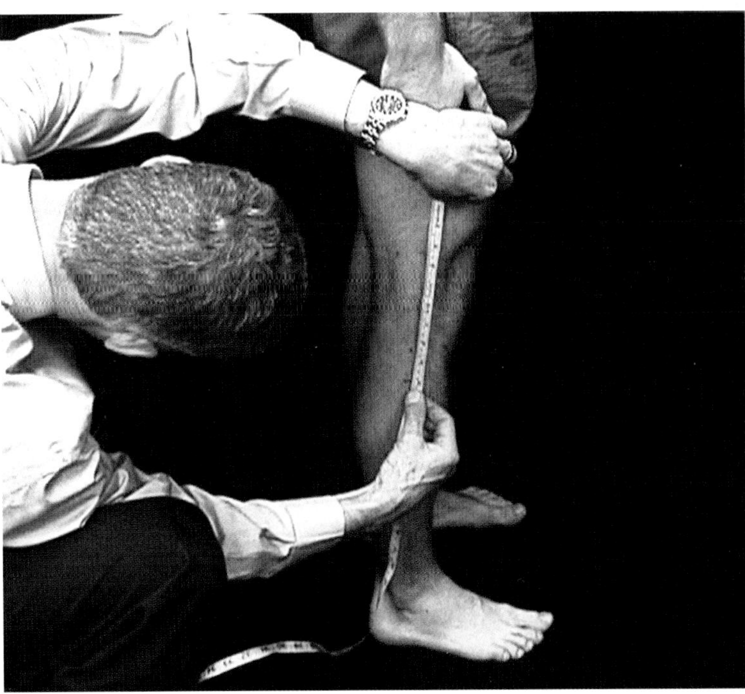

Fig. 7–51

Next, check chest expansion by placing the tape measure at the fourth intercostal space, approximately at the level of the nipples (Fig. 7–52A). Measure the difference in chest circumference at the end of full expiration and full inspiration. (Fig. 7–52B).

Lastly, ask the patient to stand with their heels, buttocks, and scapulae against the wall. With the neck maximally extended, measure the distance from the occiput to the wall (normal occiput to wall = 0 cm, since the occiput should touch the wall) (Fig. 7–53). Record the values in centimeters for each of these measurements. (*An alternative measurement is the tragus-to-wall measurement, also recorded in centimeters.*)

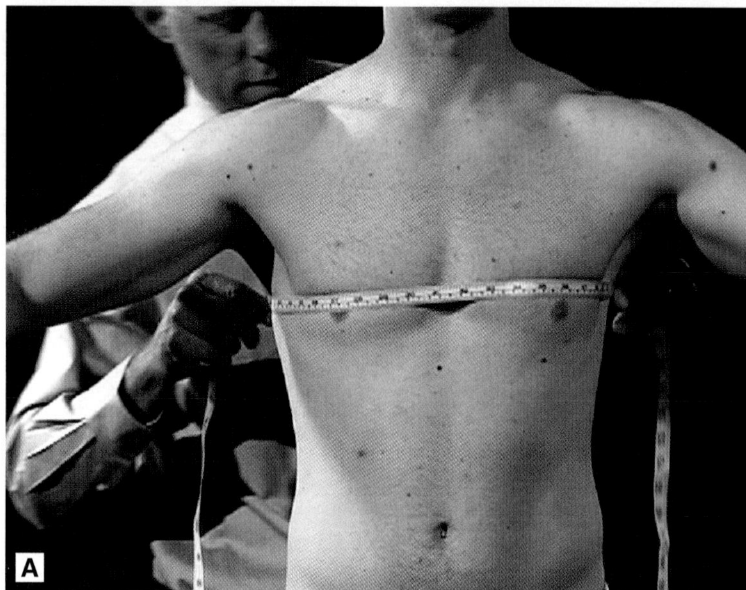

Fig. 7–52

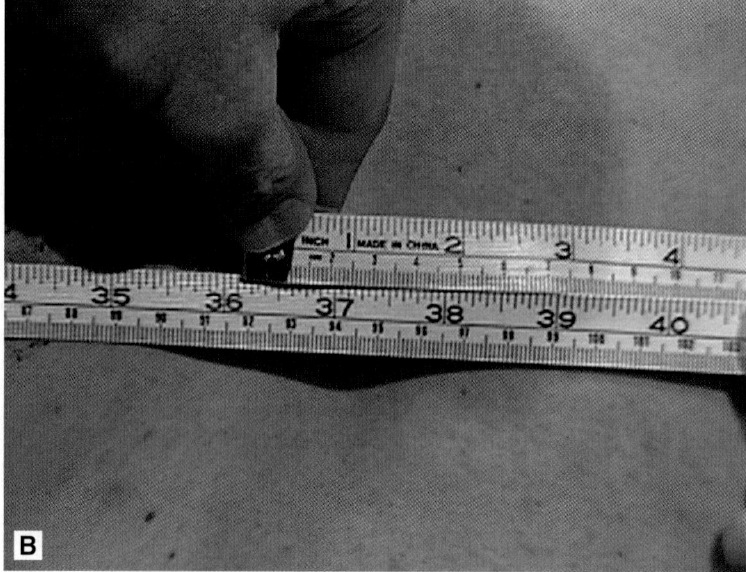

Fig. 7–52

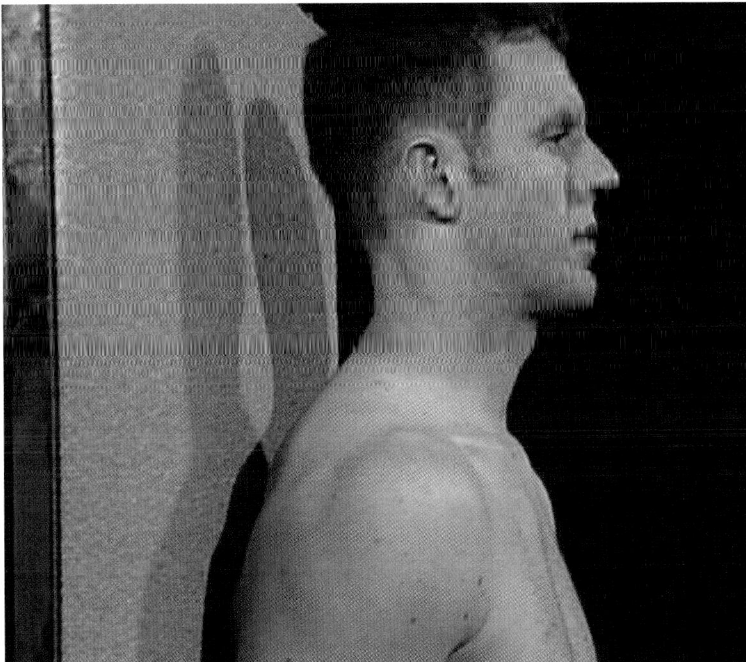

Fig. 7–53

Suspected Visceral or Vascular Disease If the patient's age, clinical symptoms, and associated problems suggest gastrointestinal, genitourinary, gynecologic, or vascular problems, additional focused examinations of these organ systems may be appropriate.

RMSE OF THE LOW BACK I

Practice Checklist

Basic Examination

Observation

Patient standing

____Observe posture, movement, and behaviors (throughout Hx and PE)*

Inspection

____ Observe gait

____ Observe heel and toe walking

____ Observe resting posture, alignment, and curvature

____Inspect skin

Palpation

____Assess skin tenderness to light touch or "skin rolling"*

____Palpate spinous processes (mid T to sacrum)

Range of Motion

____LS flexion

____LS extension

____LS lateral bending

____Simulated rotation (pelvis) or axial loading (head)*

Hips

____Trendelenburg test, R and L

Patient lying

____Palpate trochanteric bursa (lateral trochanter)

____Palpate gluteus medius insertion (superior/posterior trochanter)

____Hip flexion

____Hip external rotation

____Hip internal rotation

---

*Waddell signs in three or more of five categories during observation, basic examination, and special testing suggest possible psychological distress.

RMSE OF THE LOW BACK II

Special Testing: *Suspected Nerve Root Irritation*

Patient lying

Straight Leg Raising

Straight leg raising (R and L legs; estimate angle at pain onset)

Patient sitting

Reflexes

Patellar reflexes (L4)

Achilles reflexes (S1)

Muscle Strength*

_____Foot inversion and ankle dorsiflexion (L4)

_____Great toe dorsiflexion (L5)

_____Foot eversion (S1)

_____"Quadriceps strength" (distracted SLR in sitting position)

Sensation*

_____Medial foot and ankle (L4)

_____Dorsum of foot (L5)

_____Lateral foot and ankle (S1)

_____*(Perianal sensation, anal reflex, and sphincter tone [cauda equina syndrome])*

Special Testing: *Suspected Psychological Distress**

Waddell Categories

_____Superficial tenderness *or* nonanatomic tenderness

_____Simulated rotation *or* axial loading

_____Discrepant straight leg raises

_____"Giving way" weakness *or* nondermatologic sensory disturbances

_____Overreaction

---

*Waddell signs in three or more of five categories during observation, basic examination, and special testing suggest possible psychological distress.

RMSE OF THE LOW BACK III
Practice Checklist

Special Testing: *Suspected Sacroiliitis/Spondyloarthropathy*

Sacroiliac Joints

Patient standing

____Palpate/percuss SI joints for tenderness (upper inner buttocks)

____Modified Schober test of LS spinal mobility: 15 cm to ___cm

Patient lying

____ FABER test (hip flexion, abduction, and external rotation)

____ Iliac compression (on superior anterior iliac spines)

Special Testing: *Spondylitis Measurement Set*

Lumbosacral, Thoracic, and Cervical Spines

Patient standing

____Modified Schober test of LS spinal mobility: 15 cm to ___cm

____Finger-to-floor distance in maximal forward flexion: ___cm

____Middle finger-to-lateral thigh distraction in maximal lateral flexion: R =___cm; L =___cm

____Chest expansion measured at level of fourth intercostal space: ___cm

____Occiput-to-wall distance: ___cm

Special Testing: *Suspected Visceral or Vascular Disease*

Patient lying

____Perform abdominal examination

____Check for AAA and lower extremity pulse examination

Patient lying or standing

____Pelvic or male GU examination

____Rectal examination

COMMON LOW BACK PROBLEMS

- Acute uncomplicated low back pain
- Lumbosacral radiculopathy
- Degenerative spondylosis
- Degenerative lumbar spinal stenosis
- Chronic low back pain/chronic pain syndrome
- Spinal fractures
- Osteoporotic compression fractures

Acute Uncomplicated Low Back Pain Acute low back pain is a common, usually self-limited, but frequently recurrent problem. It is often precipitated by lifting or bending and can be felt in the lumbar spine, lumbosacral junction, buttock, and posterior thighs without radiation below the knees. Physical examination reveals diffuse lumbar spinal tenderness, muscle spasm, and diminished ROM, without radicular symptoms or signs. Whether the pain originates in the paraspinal muscles, ligaments, disks (annular tears), facet joints, or other structures is not clear and is usually not clinically relevant. Up to 85% of patients may return to normal activities within 1 month; however, recurrence may occur in up to 40% of patients within 6 months. Efforts should be directed at pain control, restoration of function, and return to normal activities.

Lumbosacral Radiculopathy Low back pain combined with neurogenic lower extremity pain (sciatica) strongly suggests lumbosacral nerve root irritation. Pain may be abrupt or gradual in onset and typically radiates from the buttock to the posterior or posterolateral thigh to the ankle or foot. There may be accompanying lower extremity numbness, tingling, or weakness. The knee flexed position, either supine or side-lying, often affords relief. Physical examination is remarkable for abnormal posture (list to one side), variable lumbosacral tenderness and muscle spasm, and reduced lumbosacral ROM. Straight leg raising, indicating lumbosacral root irritation, may be positive. Neurologic testing may indicate diminished reflexes, strength, or sensation in the affected root distribution. Nearly 95% of lumbosacral disk herniations involve L4/L5 (L5 nerve root) and L5/S1 (S1 nerve root) levels. In addition to pain control, individuals with low back pain and neurologic findings may require more advanced imaging studies.

Although rare, acute severe low back pain with bilateral sciatica, saddle anesthesia, and recent onset urinary dysfunction (retention, frequency, overflow incontinence) strongly suggests a cauda equina syndrome and constitutes a surgical emergency.

Degenerative Spondylosis Degenerative changes in the vertebral bodies, secondary to lumbar degenerative disk disease and facet joint osteoarthritis are commonly referred to as lumbar spondylosis, and typically occur in older individuals. It is important to note that the finding of degenerative changes on imaging studies has *not* been shown to be associated with back pain.

Symptoms, when present, are most often chronic low back pain sometimes with radiation to the buttocks. The pain is mechanical in quality, typically aggravated with activity and relieved by rest. Relatively brief morning stiffness, positional pain, and sleep difficulties may also be present. Physical examination often reveals tenderness to palpation in the lower lumbosacral spine and sacroiliac region (nonspecific findings). Lumbosacral movements may be painful and limited, especially lateral flexion and extension. Efforts should be directed at pain control, weight reduction (if appropriate), restoration of function, and return to normal activities.

Degenerative Lumbar Spinal Stenosis Spinal stenosis is a relatively common, clinically important cause of neurogenic lower extremity pain in older individuals. Varying combinations of degenerative disk disease with loss of disk height resulting in diskovertebral instability with redundancy and hypertrophy of the ligamentum flavum lead to narrowing of the spinal canal with lateral recess or foraminal stenosis at multiple levels. The facet joints experience increased mechanical loading and subsequent osteoarthritic changes with osteophyte formation. The onset of symptoms is typically insidious, often with a history of low back pain. The principal symptom is pain with tingling or numbness in one or both legs (buttocks, posterior thighs, calves) with ambulation or spinal extension. Symptoms are relieved by sitting or spinal flexion. Freedom from symptoms during exercise in a flexed position (leaning on a grocery cart, walking uphill, or bicycling) helps differentiate degenerative spinal stenosis from vascular claudication. Physical findings may include posterior thigh pain after 30 seconds of spinal extension, a wide-based gait, and abnormal motor or sensory testing (diminished vibratory sense) with normal lower extremity pulses.

Chronic Low Back Pain/Chronic Pain Syndrome Low back pain persisting beyond 3 months despite conservative management develops in a minority of patients and represents a significant clinical problem. Important additional historical features may relate to the patient's work, home, personal, and psychosocial history. Occupational risk factors associated with chronic low back pain include physical stresses involved in manual labor, mental stress in both manual and office workers as well as job-related stress due to lack of autonomy, lack of variation in workload, and lack of cooperation among workers. Pending litigation or disability determinations; marriage and family stress; drug or alcohol problems; and a history of anxiety, depression, or somatization are important contributing factors.

These "yellow flags" of chronic low back pain identify patients at higher risk for persistent, disabling symptoms and should point management efforts toward earlier referral to multidisciplinary specialized centers.

Spinal Fractures The evaluation of spinal pain associated with major trauma, motor vehicle accidents, and athletic or work-site injuries primarily involves the identification of fracture or dislocation. The clinical setting and initial screening history should identify such patients and an appropriate orthopedic assessment can be initiated.

Acute thoracic or lumbar spine pain associated with lesser trauma or injury such as minor fall, twisting, or heavy lifting in an older individual raises the possibility of an osteoporotic fracture.

Osteoporotic Compression Fractures Osteoporotic compression fracture of a mid-to-lower thoracic vertebra is one of the common causes of acute thoracic spine pain in the elderly. Risk factors include advanced age, female sex, personal or family history of fracture, cigarette smoking, low body weight, estrogen or testosterone deficiency, and corticosteroid use. Acute, severe spine pain, especially when accompanied by radiation bilaterally around the rib cage, strongly suggests a compression fracture. Focal spinal tenderness to palpation or gentle percussion (in the absence of neurologic symptoms or signs of malignancy or infection) increases the likelihood of a possible compression fracture.

LESS COMMON BACK PROBLEMS

- Spondyloarthropathies/inflammatory spinal pain
- Diffuse idiopathic skeletal hyperostosis
- Malignancy
- Infection
- Visceral disease

Spondyloarthropathies/Inflammatory Spinal Pain Spinal involvement in the spondyloarthropathies may involve the low back, thoracic spine, or neck and tends to occur early in the course of the disease. Initial symptoms are frequently vague and often overlooked. Characteristic features of inflammatory back pain include age younger than 40, an insidious onset, significant morning stiffness, improvement in spinal pain with exercise and worsening with prolonged rest, and a duration of longer than 3 months. These features, while not specific, strongly suggest inflammatory back pain and are quite different from typical mechanical low back pain. The presence of SI joint pain and tenderness and limited spinal movements should prompt further investigation, most importantly an AP pelvis x-ray (Ferguson view) to check for radiographic sacroiliitis. More advanced imaging with MRI scanning may be appropriate if clinical suspicion is high and initial plain x-rays are unrevealing.

Diffuse Idiopathic Skeletal Hyperostosis Diffuse idiopathic skeletal hyperostosis (DISH) is rare before the age of 40 to 50 years, and its prevalence increases with age, reaching about 10% in those older than 65 years. It typically occurs in individuals with abdominal obesity and multiple features of the metabolic (insulin resistance) syndrome. DISH is characterized by widespread heterotopic new bone formation, especially involving the axial spine and peripheral entheses. It predominantly affects the thoracic spine with flowing ossification of the anterior longitudinal ligament (and frequently discovered as an incidental finding on lateral chest radiographs). Patients may be asymptomatic or may complain of axial spinal stiffness, often greater than pain. Physical examination may reveal decreased spinal range of movement in both the lumbosacral and cervical spines. The absence of radiographic sacroiliitis readily distinguishes DISH from ankylosing spondylitis.

Malignancy Spinal pain due to metastases or primary tumors has a number of characteristic features usually seen in combination: age older than 50; a prior history of malignancy; unexplained weight loss; severe, unrelenting spinal pain, worse at night and with recumbency; and poor response to analgesics. Physical examination should be complete, including appropriate neurologic testing. If clinical findings suggest possible malignancy, imaging studies are indicated.

Infection Spinal infections, including vertebral osteomyelitis, septic diskitis, or spinal epidural abscess, may present with acute, subacute, or chronic spinal pain. Important predisposing factors include an immunocompromised status, corticosteroid use, diabetes mellitus, recent or current skin or urinary tract infections, and intravenous drug use. Clinical features may include fever, night sweats, and unexplained weight loss. Physical examination may reveal focal spinal tenderness in addition to muscle spasm. If clinical findings suggest possible spinal infection, imaging studies are indicated.

Visceral Disease Although relatively uncommon, a variety of visceral disorders can refer pain to the spine. Pulmonary, pleural, cardiac, and pericardial diseases may present with neck and shoulder pain. Gastrointestinal, pancreatic, genitourinary, and atherosclerotic vascular diseases may present with thoracic, flank, and low back pain. Inquiring about a significant pulmonary, cardiac, GI, GU, or vascular history and risk factors may provide important clues clarifying the patient's "spinal" complaints.

Suggested References

Hoppenfeld S. *Physical Examination of the Spine and Extremities*. New York, NY: Appleton-Century-Crofts; 1976.

Klippel JH, Stone JH, Crofford LJ, White PH. *Primer on the Rheumatic Diseases*. 13th ed. New York, NY: Springer; 2008.

Lawry G, Kreder HJ, Hawker J, Jerome D. *Fam's Musculoskeletal Examination and Joint Injection Techniques*. 2nd ed. Philadelphia, PA: Mosby/Elsevier; 2010.

Letha YG, ed. *Essentials of Musculoskeletal Care*. 3rd ed. Rosement, IL: American Academy of Orthopedic Surgery; 2005.

Index

Page numbers referencing figures are followed by a *f* and page numbers referencing tables are followed by a *t*.

A

abduction, 7, 8*f*. *See also* Passive abduction
  GH joint, 122, 122*f*–123*f*
abduction relief sign, 195
  cervical radiculopathy, 215, 215*f*
AC joints. *See* acromioclavicular joints
Achilles tendon, 63, 64*f*
Achilles tendon reflex, 254, 254f
ACL. *See* anterior cruciate ligament
acromioclavicular (AC) joints
  abnormalities of, 109
  GH joint and, 90
  inspection of, 107, 107*f*
    for asymmetry, 45, 45*f*
    for swelling, 45, 45*f*
  joint line, 108, 109*f*
  localization of, 108, 108*f*
  pain, 109, 129
  palpation of, 107, 107*f*, 109*f*
  structural and functional anatomy, 88
acromion, 45, 45*f*, 89, 89*f*
  AC joint examination and, 107, 107*f*
  anatomy and, 100, 100*f*
acute trauma, neurovascular examination, timing of, 82
acute uncomplicated low back pain, 234, 274–275
acute uncomplicated neck pain, 221, 234
adduction, plane and direction of movement, 7, 8*f*
adhesive capsulitis (frozen shoulder), 122, 127, 129
anatomical position, 7, 8*f*
ankle
  clonus, 217, 217*f*
  dorsiflexion, 17, 17*f*

ankle (*Cont.*):
  examination, 17, 17*f*
    GMSE, 29, 62–64, 62*f*–64*f*
  neutral position, 17, 17*f*
  plantar flexion, 17, 17*f*
  reflexes, 217
ankle plantar flexor strength, S1 root weakness assessment, 256, 256*f*
ankle reflexes, 224–225
annulus fibrosus, 226, 227*f*
anserine bursa, 136, 136*f*, 177, 178*f*
anserine bursitis, 182
anserine bursitis/tendinitis, 177
anterior arch, 186, 187*f*
anterior cruciate ligament (ACL)
  anatomical relationships of, 132–133, 133*f*
  injury, 181
  intact, 160, 160*f*, 162, 164
  integrity assessment, 158, 158*f*, 159*f*
  orientation of, 134, 135*f*
  ruptured, 161*f*
  tight, 161*f*
anterior drawer test, 162, 163*f*
anterior instability testing, shoulder, 123, 125*f*
anterior longitudinal ligament, 230, 230*f*
apophyseal joints. *See* facet joints; lumbar facet joints
apprehension sign, 127
apprehension test, 125, 125*f*
arthritis, 86. *See also* osteoarthritis
  crystalline, 180
  glenohumeral, 119, 122, 127, 129
  of knee, 180
  psoriatic, 180
  rheumatoid, 180, 223

arthritis (*Cont.*):
  septic, 180
  sternoclavicular, 130
athletic preparticipation examination. *See* physical examination
atlantoaxial joint (C1-C2), 187
atlantooccipital joints, 185, 185*f*
atlas. *See* C1
axial loading, low back pain and, 242, 243*f*
axial spine, direction of motion and, 5
axis. *See* C2

B

Babinski sign, 196, 217*f*, 218, 219*f*
back pain. *See* low back pain
back problems
  common, 274–276
  less common, 276–277
ballotable patella. *See* patellar tap
biceps muscle, 98, 98*f*
  heads of, 98, 98*f*, 99*f*
  strength, 208–209, 209*f*
  tendon of, 100, 100*f*, 101*f*, 114–121, 115*f*
biceps tendonitis, 129
bicipital groove, 92, 92*f*
bulge sign of knee, 53, 53*f*, 56, 141, 146
bursal inflammation, 181

C

C spine
  extension, 18*f*
  flexion, 18*f*
  lateral bending, 9*f*
  rotation, 9*f*
C1 (atlas), 184, 184*f*, 185*f*
C1-C2. *See* atlantoaxial joint
C2 (axis), 186, 186*f*
calves, from behind, 18*f*

cervical degenerative spondylosis, 222
cervical lordosis, 18*f*, 196, 196*f*, 226, 226*f*. *See also* resting cervical lordosis
cervical myelopathy, 195, 222
cervical nerve root irritation, finger confirmation of, 214
cervical radiculopathy, 222
  abduction relief sign, 215, 215*f*
cervical spine
  inspection, 102, 104, 104f, 105*f*
    lateral flexion assessment, 104, 106*f*
    rotation assessment, 104, 105*f*
  referred pain, 130
chest expansion test, 268*f*, 270, 270*f*
chronic degenerative tears, 181
chronic low back pain, chronic pain syndrome and, 276
chronic neck pain, 223
chronic pain syndrome, chronic low back pain and, 276
clavicle, 107, 107*f*, 108
CMC joint. *See* first carpometacarpal joint
coccygeal kyphosis, 226, 226*f*
coccyx, anatomy of, 232, 233*f*
collateral ligament tear, 181
complete physical examination, SMSE and, 5
coracoid process, 89, 89*f*
crossed straight leg raising sign
  lumbar disk herniation, positive, 253, 253*f*, 254*f*
  positive, 253, 253*f*
cruciate ligament tear, 181
crystalline arthritis, 180

D

degenerative lumbar spinal stenosis, 275–276
degenerative spondylosis, 275
deltoid muscle strength, 208, 208*f*
diagnosis, accurate, 4
diffuse idiopathic skeletal hyperostosis (DISH), 277
diffuse musculoskeletal pain, 28
DIP joints. *See* distal interphalangeal joints
direction of motion, 5
DISH. *See* Diffuse idiopathic skeletal hyperostosis
distal interphalangeal joints (DIP joints), positions, 10, 10*f*, 31, 31*f*, 32–33, 32*f*–34*f*, 68
  abnormalities, 39
distal lower strength assessment, 255
distal vastus lateralis, 147, 147*f*

E

effusions. *See also* Moderate effusion patellar tap
  elbow, 43, 43*f*
  examination
    large, 60–61
    moderate, 58–59, 58*f*, 59*f*
    small, 53–57, 53*f*–57*f*
  fluid wave of knee, 53, 53*f*
  knee, 52, 145, 145*f*
    large, 146, 146*f*, 153–154, 153*f*–154*f*
    moderate, 151–152, 153*f*
    small, 146–150
  shoulder, 102, 103
elbow
  effusion, 43, 43*f*
  examination, 13, 13*f*, 42–45, 42*f*–44*f*
extensor plantar response, 218, 218*f*

F

FABER test, 266–267, 266*f*
facet joints (apophyseal joints), 192, 192*f*, 193*f*
  anatomy of, 228, 229*f*
feet, from behind, 18*f*
femur, 132, 132*f*
fibromyalgia, 28, 28*f*, 200, 200*f*
fibromyalgia tender points, 201*f*
  assessment, 74, 75*f*, 76–81, 76*f*–81*f*
fibula, 132, 132*f*
fifth finger, light touch sensation assessment, 212, 213*f*
finger
  extension assessment, 10
  flexion, 10–11, 11*f*, 31
finger joint, palpating, 68
finger-to-floor test, 268*f*, 269, 269*f*
finger-to-thigh distraction test, 268*f*, 269, 269*f*
first carpometacarpal joint (CMC joint), 38, 38*f*–39*f*
first metatarsal head, 69*f*
fist
  dorsal view, 11*f*
  maneuver for making, 11, 11*f*
  palmar view, 11*f*
flexion, 7, 8*f*. *See also* ankle; C spine; finger; hip; neck; shoulder; wrist
  plane and direction of movement, 7, 8*f*
flexion contracture, 13, 61, 179, 179*f*
flip sign, 257, 258*f*
fluid wave of knee
  checking for
    regional musculoskeletal examination of knee, 141
    right knee, 149, 149f
  small effusion, 53, 53*f*
    right knee, 55–56, 56*f*
  suprapatellar pouch and, 146
focal tender areas, 197, 197*f*
  of spine, historical context of, 238, 238*f*
foot, dorsum of, sensation assessment, 258, 259*f*
foot and ankle
  lateral, sensation assessment, 258, 259*f*
  sensation assessment, 258, 258*f*
foot eversion and dorsiflexion, 255–256, 256*f*
foot inversion and dorsiflexion, 255, 255*f*
forefoot, 66, 66*f*
fracture. *See* specific fracture
frozen shoulder. *See* adhesive capsulitis

G

gait
  abnormalities of, 218, 219*f*
  examination and, 85
  inspection of, 235
  observation of, 22, 22*f*, 30, 74, 75*f*, 234

general musculoskeletal
examination (GMSE), 1, 25–86
  ankle examination, 29, 62–64, 62f–64f
  categories of abnormality, 27
  clinical use of, 2, 2f
  clinical utility, 25
  components of, [illegible]
  conclusions on, 86
  essential concepts, 26
  introduction to, 25
  objectives, [illegible]
  overview of, 28–30
  practice checklist, 83–84
  range of motion, 29
  recording findings, 85
  skill building, 85
GH joint. *See* glenohumeral joint
glenohumeral arthritis, 119, 122, 127, 129
glenohumeral joint (GH joint), 90, 90f
  range of motion
    seated, 122–125
      abduction, 122, 122f–123f
      external rotation, 124–125, 124f, 125f
      internal rotation, 123, 123f, 124f
    supine, 126–127, 126f, 127f
glenoid fossa, 88, 88f
glenoid labrum, 90, 90f
gluteus medius tendonitis, 247, 247f
GMSE. *See* general musculoskeletal examination
great toe
  dorsiflexion, 255, 255f
  joints, 68
greater tuberosity, 92, 93f

H
hairy patches, 236, 237f
hand examination, 30–39, 30f–39f
  PIP joints, 31, 31f
Hawkins impingement sign, 102, 120–121, 120f–121f
head and neck
  alignment, 70
  examination, 18, 18f
heels, from behind, 18f
herpes zoster vesicles, 237, 237f
hip
  examination, 15, 16f, 46–50, 46f–51f, 51–62
    [illegible], 15, 16f, 50, 50f–51f
    low back pain, 244, 247–250
  flexion assessment, 14, 15, 15f, 234
  pain from, [illegible]
    examination maneuver, 250, [illegible]
  rotation, 15, 15f, [illegible]
hip range of motion
  external rotation, 248, 248f
  internal rotation, 248, 248f
Hoffman sign, 196, 215, 217f
humeral head, 100, 100f
hyperreflexia, 217

I
impingement, signs of, 102
impingement syndrome, 100–101, 101f
infections, 277
  spinal, 223
inferior articular processes, 191, 191f–192f
inflammatory spinal pain, 276–277
infrapatellar fat pads, 52, 52f, 138f
  anatomical position of, 137, 137f
  patellar tendon and, 144, 144f
  women, 144, 145f
infraspinatus muscle, 94, 94f
infraspinatus tendons, 111, 113
initial examination, 5
injury. *See also* whiplash injury
  ACL, 181
interosseus muscle strength, 211, 211f
intervertebral disks, 230, 230f
  anatomy of, 226, 227f
  load bearing by, 231, 231f

J
joint. *See also* painful joint; *specific joints*
  direction of motion, 7
  extension, 7, 8f
    plane and direction of movement, 7, 8f
  movement, 27
  neutral position for, 5, 7, 8f
joint (*Cont.*):
  plane, 7
  swelling, 28
  tenderness, 28
joint redness (erythema), 28

K
kiss the hand position, 12, 12f
knee. *See also* fluid wave of knee
  from behind, 10f
  alignment, during weight bearing, 17, 18
  [illegible], 146
  extension, 15, 16f, 179, 179f
  flexion, 15, 16f, 179, 179f
  inspection, 142–146, 142f
  problems, common, 180
  range of motion, 61, 62f
  reflexes, 217
  RMSE of, 131–182
    clinical history, 141
    clinical utility, 131
    essential concepts, 132–141
    introduction, 131
    objectives, 132
    overview, 141–142
    practice checklist, 180
knee effusion, 52, 141, 145, 145f
  large, 146, 146f, 153–154, 153f–154f
  moderate, 146, 146f, 151–152, 153f
  small, 146–150
knee joint, structural and functional anatomy, 132–141
knee joint line, 171, 171f

L
Lachman test, 141
  technique, 162–164, 162f–164f
laminae, 189, 190f, 228, 228f
lateral collateral ligament (LCL)
  anatomical position, 132, 133f
  assessing, 142
    integrity of, 167–169, 167f, 168f, 169f
lateral deltoid, light touch sensation, 212, 212f
lateral epicondyle, 43, 43f
lateral flexion assessment, 203, 203f
lateral masses, 184, 185f

lateral meniscus, 135, 135*f*
LCL. *See* lateral collateral ligament
lesser tuberosity, 92, 93*f*
ligaments, of spinal column, 230, 230*f*
ligamentum flavum, 230, 230*f*
light touch sensation
  fifth finger, 212, 213*f*
  lateral deltoid, 212, 212*f*
  skin, 234
  thumb and index finger, 212, 212*f*
lipomas, 236, 237*f*
lordosis. *See also* cervical lordosis; lumbar lordosis; resting cervical lordosis
  flattening of, 72, 72*f*
low back, RMSE, 225–278
  clinical utility, 225
  introduction, 225
  objectives, 225–226
low back pain, 195
  causes, 233–234
  evaluation of, OPQRSTU mnemonic, 233
  hip examination, 244, 247–260
  mechanical disease, 233
  nonradiating, 251, 251*f*
  patient history and, 234
  special testing, 251–271
  straight leg raise, 253
  systemic disease, 233
  visceral disease, 233
  Waddell behavioral signs, 260–263, 261*f*–263*f*
lower extremity (LE)
  examination, 9, 14–17, 15*f*, 29
  GMSE, 85
lower lumbosacral facet joints, 250
lumbar disk herniation, crossed straight leg raising sign, positive, 253, 253*f*, 254*f*
lumbar extension, 74, 74*f*
  assessment, 234
lumbar facet joints (apophyseal joints), 192*f*
  spinal segment stability of, 231, 231*f*
lumbar flexion, 20, 20*f*, 72
  assessment, 234
  normal, 73, 239, 239*f*
  observation, from behind, 240, 240*f*, 241*f*
lumbar kyphosis, 72–73, 73*f*
  range of motion and, 239, 240*f*
lumbar lateral bending, 21, 21*f*
lumbar lateral flexion
  assessment, 242, 242*f*
  pain, 242, 243*f*
lumbar lordosis, 18*f*, 72, 72*f*, 226, 226*f*
  range of motion and, 239, 239*f*
lumbar vertebral end plates, 231
lumbosacral extension, assessment, 241, 241*f*
lumbosacral radiculopathy, 275
  nerve root irritation and, 251
lumbosacral range of motion, examination, 239–242
lumbosacral spine extension, 20*f*
lumbosacral spine flexion, 20*f*

M

malignancy, 238, 238*f*, 277
  spinal pain and, 223
MCL. *See* medial collateral ligament
McMurray maneuver, 172–174, 172*f*–177*f*, 176–177
McMurray test, positive, 177, 177*f*
MCP joints. *See* metacarpophalangeal joints
mechanical disease, low back pain, 233
medial collateral ligament (MCL), 132, 133*f*, 142, 165–167, 165*f*
  assessing, 166–167, 166*f*–167*f*
medial meniscus, 135, 135*f*
medial scapular border, 200*f*
meniscal tear, 181
metacarpophalangeal joints (MCP joints), 66, 66*f*
  examining, 67, 67*f*
  position of, 10, 10*f*, 31–32, 32*f*, 36–37, 36*f*–37*f*
    abnormalities, 39
metatarsophalangeal joint synovitis, 66, 67–68
mid supraspinatus palpation, 199*f*
mid trapezius palpation, 199*f*
midfoot, 64
midfoot joints, 65*f*
moderate effusion patellar tap, 59, 60*f*
modified Lachman test, 162, 163*f*, 164, 164*f*
modified Schober test, 265–266, 265*f*, 266*f*, 268, 268*f*
muscle atrophy, 143, 143*f*
musculoskeletal examination
  chief complaint, clinical context, 6*f*, 27*f*
  clinical history and examination, 194
musculoskeletal system, symmetry, 5
myelopathy, special testing, 215, 216*f*
myofascial trigger points, 197, 197*f*

N

neck
  examination, palpation, 196–198, 200
  flexion, 70, 70*f*
    assessment, 195, 201, 201*f*
  pain, 195
    axial loading and, 242, 243*f*
    nonradiating, 205, 205*f*
  problems
    common, 221–222
    less common, 222
  RMSE of, 183–223
  rotation, 71, 71*f*
neck extension assessment, 70, 70*f*, 202, 202*f*, 203*f*
Neer impingement sign, 102, 117–119, 118*f*–119*f*, 131
nerve root irritation, 234, 257, 257*f*. *See also* cervical nerve root irritation
  practice checklist, 273
  special testing
    biceps, 206, 206*f*
    brachioradialis, 206, 207*f*
    triceps, 206, 207*f*
neural arch
  anatomy of, 228, 228*f*
  pedicles of, 189, 189*f*
neurofibromas, 236, 237*f*
neurovascular assessment, 81–82, 82*f*
nucleus pulposus, 226, 227*f*

O

occiput-to-wall test, 268f, 270, 271f
odontoid (dens), 186, 187f
odontoid process, 187, 187f
olecranon bursa, 13, 13f
- swelling, 42–43, 42f

OPQRST mnemonic, 102
- pain assessment, 141

OPQRSTU mnemonic
- low back pain, 233
- pain assessment, 194

osteoarthritis, 100
osteoporotic compression fractures, 276

P

pain. *See also* chronic neck pain; chronic pain syndrome; low back pain; referred pain
- AC joints, 109, 129
- active range of motion, 203, 204f
- assessment, 102
  - OPQRST mnemonic, 141
  - OPQRSTU mnemonic, 194
- from hip, 249, 249f
- hip range of motion, 248, 248f
- from lower lumbosacral facet joints, 250
- lumbar lateral flexion, 242, 243f
- passive abduction, 123f
- patellofemoral, 181
- proximal arm, special testing, 206, 206f
- range of motion, 49, 203
- spinal, infection and, 223
- threshold, fibromyalgia tender point assessment, 76

painful joint, range of motion, 6
pain-related behaviors, 235
palpation
- AC joints, 107, 107f, 109f
- finger joint, 68
- low back, 237–238, 237f
- mid supraspinatus, 199f
- mid trapezius, 199f
- neck, 196–198, 200
- PIP joints, 34–35
- plantar fascia, 63–64
- SC joints, 102
- spinous process, 238, 238f
- suboccipital muscle insertions, 198, 198f–200f

palpation (*Cont.*):
- trochanteric bursitis, 234
- upper trapezius, 199f

passive abduction, painful, 123f
patella, 132, 132f
patellar apprehension test, 157–158, 157f
patellar dislocation, 158
patellar reflex test, 254
patellar tap (ballotable patella), 59, 60f, 132, 133f
patellar tendon, infrapatellar fat pads, 144, 144f
patellofemoral joint, 132, 132f, 154–158, 154f–157f
- examination, 61

patellofemoral pain, 181
patellofemoral pain syndrome, 181
patient care, effective, 4
PCL. *See* posterior cruciate ligament
pedicles, 228, 228f
pelvic droop, 244, 245f, 246f
peripheral joints, direction of motion and, 5
pes anserine tendon, 178f
physical examination, 4. *See also* complete physical examination
- athletic preparticipation, 5
- low back pain, 234
- techniques, for ligaments, 134, 134f, 135f

pigmented spots, 236, 237f
PIP joints. *See* proximal interphalangeal joints
plantar fascia palpation, 63–64, 65f
plantar reflexes, 218, 218f
plantar surface of foot, 68
positive compression test, 267–268, 268f
posterior cruciate ligament (PCL), 133, 134f, 135f, 142, 170, 170f
posterior longitudinal ligament, 230, 230f
prepatellar bursa(e), 136, 136f, 144, 144f
prepatellar bursitis, 181
primary providers, new instruction for, 4
proximal arm pain, special testing, 206, 206f
proximal interphalangeal joints (PIP joints)
- abnormalities, 34
- finger extension assessment, 10, 10f
- hand function, 11, 11f
- palpation technique, 34–35, 34f, 35f
- of toes, 68

psoriatic arthritis, 100
psychological distress, 237, 238
- indications of, 260, 260f
- straight leg raise, 257
- symptoms, 257
- Waddell categories, 260
- widespread bony tenderness and, 237, 238, 239f

R

radial head, 44, 44f
range of motion, 28f. *See also* hip range of motion; shoulder
- active, 5, 6, 7f, 27, 28f
  - pain, 203, 204f
- GH joint
  - seated, 122–125
    - abduction, 122, 122f–123f
    - external rotation, 124–125, 124f, 125f
    - internal rotation, 123, 123f, 124f
  - supine, 126–127, 126f, 127f
- GMSE, 29
- knee, 61, 62f
- lumbar kyphosis, 239, 240f
- lumbar lordosis, 239, 239f
- lumbosacral, 239–242
- pain, 49
- painful joint, 6
- passive, 5, 6, 7f, 27, 28f
- shoulder, 46
- shoulder elevation, 102, 103f

rashes, 236, 237f
referred pain, 111, 112f
- cervical spine, 130
- visceral, 130, 219

referred visceral disease, spinal pain and, 223
regional musculoskeletal examination (RMSE), 1, 2, 62
- clinical use, 2f

regional musculoskeletal examination (RMSE) (*Cont.*):
 of knee, 131–182
  clinical history, 141
  clinical utility, 131
  essential concepts, 132–141
  introduction, 131
  objectives, 132
  overview, 131–182
  practice checklist form, 180
 of low back, 225–278
  clinical utility, 225
  component parts
   inspection, 235–236
   observation, 235
   palpation, 237–238, 237*f*
  overview of, 234–235
 of low back I, practice checklist basic examination, 272
 of low back II, practice checklist
  nerve root irritation, 273
  sacroiliitis/spondyloarthropathy, 274
  spondylitis measurement set, 274
  vascular disease, 274
  visceral disease, 274
 of neck, 183–223
  clinical utility, 183
  component parts, 196–219
  essential concepts, 184–195, 184*f*–195*f*
  introduction, 183
  objectives, 183
  observation and inspection, 196
  overview of, 195–196
  practice checklist form, 220–221
 of shoulder
  clinical history and, 102
  clinical utility, 87
  component parts, 102–130
   inspection, 102, 103*f*
  essential concepts, 88–102
  introduction to, 87
  objectives, 88
  overview, 102
  practice checklist form, 128
resting cervical lordosis, 195
rheumatoid arthritis, 180, 223
RMSE. *See* regional musculoskeletal examination
rotator cuff, 91–97, 91*f*
 degeneration, 113, 113*f*
 function of, 97, 97*f*
 tear, 111, 113, 113f, 118, 119*f*, 129
 tendonitis, 129
ruptured anterior cruciate ligament (ACL), 161*f*
ruptured posterior cruciate ligament (PCL), 170, 170*f*, 171*f*

S

S1 root weakness assessment, ankle plantar flexor strength, 256, 256*f*
sacroiliac joints (SI joints), 232, 232*f*, 233*f*, 264, 264*f*
 maneuver affecting, 267–268, 267*f*
sacroiliitis
 examination for, 264–270, 264*f*
 practice checklist, RMSE, 274
sacrum, 232, 232*f*
SC joints. *See* sternoclavicular joints
scapula, 88, 89
scapulothoracic joint, 88
scoliosis, 73, 73*f*, 240, 240*f*
 observation, from behind, 240, 241*f*
screening examination. *See also* specific examination
 categories of abnormality, 6
screening musculoskeletal examination (SMSE), 1, 5–24
 clinical use of, 2*f*
 clinical utility, 5
 component parts, 9–22
 essential concepts, 6–7
 introduction, 5
 objectives, 5
 overview, 9
 practice checklist form, 23
 recording findings, 24
 skill building, 23
sensation
 assessment
  dorsum of foot, 258, 259*f*
  foot and ankle, 258, 259*f*
  medial foot and ankle, 258, 258*f*
 fifth finger, 212, 213*f*
 to light touch
  fifth finger, 212, 213*f*
  lateral deltoid, 212, 212*f*
septic arthritis, 180
shoulder. *See also* regional musculoskeletal examination
 abductor of, 93, 94*f*
 anterior instability testing, 125, 125*f*
 elevation
  range of motion, 102, 103*f*
  symmetry and, 102, 103*f*
 examination, 14, 14*f*, 18–19, 19*f*, 45–46, 45*f*–46*f*, 102
 external rotation, 14, 14*f*
 external rotator of, 95, 95*f*, 96*f*
 flexion, 14, 14*f*
 flexion assessment, 46, 46*f*
 impingement, 129
 instability, 130
 internal rotation, 14, 14*f*
 internal rotator of, 96, 96*f*
 problems
  common, 128
  less common, 130
 range of motion, 46, 102, 103*f*
 special testing, 206, 206*f*
 structural and functional anatomy, 88
shoulder effusion, 102, 103
SI joints. *See* sacroiliac joints
simulation spinal testing, 242, 243*f*
skill building, SMSE, 1–2
SMSE. *See* screening musculoskeletal examination
spinal column
 balanced curves of, 226, 226*f*
 ligaments of, 230, 230*f*
spinal compression fractures, 238, 238*f*
spinal fractures, 276
spinal infections, 223, 238, 238*f*, 277

spinal pain. *See also* inflammatory spinal pain
infection, 223
malignancy and, 223
spine
examination, 9, 30, 70
thoracolumbar, 19, 19f, 72
focal tender areas, historical [illegible]
spinous processes, [illegible], 228, 228f, 230, 230f
palpation, 238, 238f
spondylitis, examination for, 264–270, 264f
spondylitis measurement set, RMSE, practice checklist, 274
spondyloarthropathies, 223, 268, 268f, 276–277
RMSE, practice checklist, 274
Spurling maneuver, 195, 214, 214f
squatting, 142, 143f
stacking joints, 228, 229f
standing posture and alignment inspection, 235
sternoclavicular arthritis, 130
sternoclavicular (SC) joint line, 106, 106f
sternoclavicular joints (SC joints), 45, 45f, 90, 106
palpation, 102
straight leg raise
lumbosacral radiculopathy and, 251–254, 251f–253f
negative test, 257f
pain onset and, 253
positive test, 252, 253, 253f, 257f
psychological distress, 257
seated, 257, 257f
supine, 234
subacromial bursa(e), 102, 110–111, 110f
subacromial bursitis, 129
subacromial-subdeltoid bursa, 91, 91f, 101f
subdeltoid bursa(e), 110–111, 110f
suboccipital muscle insertions, palpating, 198, 198f–200f
subscapularis muscle, 96, 96f
subtalar motion, 63, 64f
superior articular processes, 191f
suprapatellar pouch, 54–55, 54f–55f, 56, 57f, 139, 139f, 147–151, 147f, 148f, 150f, 152f
fluid wave of knee, 146, 146f
swelling of, 140, 140f
supraspinatus muscle, 93, 93f
supraspinatus tendonitis, 111, 112f, 129
supraspinatus tendons, 101f, 111, 111f, 112f, 113
supraspinatus test, 102, 111, 111f, 112f, 113
swelling
AC joints, 45
joints, 28
olecranon bursa, 42–43, 42f
SC joints, 106
of suprapatellar pouch, 140, 140f
synovial, 44
of wrist, 13
symmetry, 6, 27
musculoskeletal system and, 5
synovial sandwich bag, 140, 140f
synovial swelling, 44
systematic musculoskeletal examinations, 1, 2
systemic disease, low back pain, 233

T

tender point examination, 29f, 195, 200, 200f
tenderness, SC joints, 106
tendonitis, 115, 116f
teres minor muscle, 95, 95f
terrible triad, 181
thoracic kyphosis, 18f, 226, 226f
thumb and index finger, light touch sensation assessment, 212, 212f
thumb examination, 37
tibia, 132, 132f
tibial sag, 170, 171, 171f
tibiofemoral joint, 132, 132f
total hip replacements, 49
hip range of motion assessment and, 249, 249f
transverse ligament, 187, 187f
transverse process, 191f, 220, 220f
Trendelenburg sign, 234, 244, 245f
positive, 246f
triceps muscle strength, 210, 210f
trigger points, [illegible]
trochanter, 247, 247f
trochanteric bursitis, [illegible], 247, 247f
palpate for, [illegible]
trochanteric syndrome, 247
tuberosity on lateral humeral head, 92, 92f

U

uncovertebral joints of Luschka, 193, 193f, 194f
upper extremities (UE), GMSE, 30, 30f, 85
upper motor neuron
lesion, 217
signs, 196
upper trapezius palpation, 199f

V

varus stress, 168, 169
vascular disease
RMSE, practice checklist, 274
suspected, 271
vertebra prominens, 194
vertebrae, common features, 226, 227f
vertebral body, 188, 188f, 189f
vertically integrated learning, 3
visceral disease, 277
low back pain, 233
RMSE, practice checklist, 274
suspected, 271
visceral referred pain, 130
special testing, 219

W

Waddell behavioral signs, categories of response, 260–263, 261f–263f
Waddell categories, screening for, 242
walking movement. *See also* gait
heel and toe, 235, 236f
phases of, 74, 75f

walking movement (*Cont.*):
stance phase, 22*f*
swing phase, 22*f*
web-based instructor's manual, 3
web-based skill building workshops, 3
web-based tutorials, 3
whiplash injury, 221–222
wrist
flexion, 11*f*
inspection, 11, 11*f*, 12, 12*f*, 39–41, 40*f*–41*f*
wrist (*Cont.*):
neutral, 11*f*
swelling, 13

Y

Yerguson test, 116, 117*f*